for the people, for a change

BRINGING HEALTH TO THE FAMILIES OF HAITI
ARY BORDES AND ANDREA COUTURE

BEACON PRESS : *BOSTON*

Copyright © 1978 by Ary Bordes and Andrea Couture
Beacon Press books are published under the auspices
of the Unitarian Universalist Association
Published simultaneously in Canada by
Fitzhenry & Whiteside Limited, Toronto
All rights reserved
Printed in the United States of America

(hardcover) 9 8 7 6 5 4 3 2 1

Library of Congress Cataloging in Publication Data

Bordes, Ary.
  For the people, for a change.
    1. Maternal health services—Haiti. 2. Birth control—Haiti. 3. Child health services—Haiti. 4. Haiti—Social conditions. 5. Bordes, Ary. 6. Health-officers—Haiti—Biography. I. Couture, Andrea, joint author. II. Title.
RG963.H2B67   362.8'2   77-88372
ISBN 0-8070-2166-0

FOR THE PEOPLE, FOR A CHANGE

Our task . . . is to find the few principles that will calm the infinite anguish of free souls. We must mend what has been torn apart, make justice imaginable again in a world so obviously unjust, give happiness a meaning once more to peoples poisoned by the misery of the century. Naturally, it is a superhuman task. But superhuman is the term for tasks that take a long time to accomplish, that's all.—Albert Camus

To Gental, who is what "underdevelopment" is—
the waste of human resources.

CONTENTS

Preface   xi
Introduction   xiii

PART I
1 That's The Way It is   1
2 Why It Is   22
3 What There Is   31

PART II
4 Getting Acquainted   41
5 Planting the Seeds   67
6 The Khrushchev of Fond Parisien   90

PART III
7 Not Quite Welcome   113
8 Warming Up   133
9 Welcome Back   159

PART IV
10 A Taste of Honey   167
11 The Pungent Taste of Rural Medicine   192
12 United We Stand   217
13 The Local Connection   241

PART V
14 The Harvest   266

Appendix   286

Index   293

PREFACE

I remember walking along Boston's Charles River once at the end of a writing day. My city seems at its most lovely then, the sailboats out, peaceful flags of perspective after losing it for the usual quota of hours absorbed in something, surely not all that important, but that's how you get something done.

The greenbelt along the river's edge was full of joggers, running off the day's frustrations and triumphs, getting their perspective back, bringing the physical in line with the mental, maintaining some balance. They smiled at each other and everyone through the strain and sweat of the arm-swinging, muscle-paining agony of it all, an almost masochistic pushing and stretching, virtually beyond endurance.

I remember one particularly spent passerby, sparkling in perspiration, his beard wringing out with it, some flying in my face as he passed. I thought I had seen him before, which meant he had run around the two bridges spanning the river—three miles—at least once. He looked like the personification of the "last lap" as he puffed toward the point where the greenbelt and the commuter-cluttered driver merge, just as a big yellow school bus inched along in the traffic. Two kids screamed out their bus window—"Faggot!"

He looked up. Enraged! "Meatheads!" he hollered back between gasps of breath, never losing stride, although clearly off-balance in other respects. "You try running five miles . . . jerks!" And he ran off with the true loneliness of the long-distance runner: gutsy, hard at work, by himself, misunderstood, under stress, sensitive to criticism, ridiculed by the stupid and narrow-minded, totally involved in his travail, with a broader awareness of what was really sane and healthy and a vision of the fulfilling finale.

If I have ever met the proverbial long-distance runner it is a Haitian public health specialist named Dr. Ary Bordes. He doesn't jog but he has made a l-o-n-g run for about twenty-five years, uphill all the way.

PREFACE

I first met Ary Bordes in Haiti in January 1972 and again in August 1974, but it was not until November 1976, and during the following months of on-site research that I came to know more about him and his work. This is his story as I interpret it. And I must say first off, there are things in this book he does not like, that turn his pure white hair a little blond, even brown, sometimes black.

Ary Bordes is a thin-skinned nationalist, fiercely protective of his country, amused rather than enraged by its foibles, passionately concerned about its reputation. He has most refined sensibilities about Haiti—which he loves. This book contains my impressions: what I saw, heard, think. I wrote it and I take full responsibility for its contents.

I interviewed Ary Bordes over a period of months, as he relived for me and recollected his experiences in late-afternoon taping sessions in the office of his private Family Hygiene Center, number 10 Impasse Lavaud, Port-au-Prince. Darkness comes early in the tropics, and when we began our talks at the end of his killer workdays, it would often seem much later. The air conditioner hummed hypnotically, and gradually a definite mood would emerge, an accumulation of the day's events and personalities. Through all those hours of taping together I found him to be a kind man who can be delightful company; intelligent and well trained; fiercely disciplined and compulsively dedicated. He can be petty, selfish, chauvinistic, and occasionally worse. He is a person like the rest of us, a superior person, an idealist of the best kind. He works terribly hard; he fights every day for what he believes; most of all, he knows how to win.

This book describes to date his daily construction, piece by piece, of a mosaic of a healthy Haitian mother and child: a labor accomplished at a significant personal cost, despite a virtual windstorm of bad odds, just about every natural, human, financial, and organizational obstacle you can think of. But he did it. Ary Bordes has succeeded in creating a model of maternal-child health and family planning, but most of all, he has succeeded in institutionalizing it in his country. It is imperfect, but it is there and growing, an accomplishment which has brought him international recognition and prestige.

This is the story.

I want to thank him for the pleasure I have found in his company. I have learned from him. May his dreams continue to come true. Also I would like to acknowledge the contribution of the General Service Foundation, whose grant made this book possible. Most of all to my sister Gonda and E.S.M.—my love and thanks for sharing it all.

Andrea M. Couture
Boston, 1978

INTRODUCTION

If art is really that lonely, laborious effort to expand and deepen human awareness of the world and of life.... If it is participating in the unknown, venturing into the insecure, breaking through to revelations, knowing the joy of surprise, sometimes finding out the very worst.... If it is to escape from the history of human error and to fight for nobility instead.... If art is these things, or even some of them, then there is a painting that must be mentioned. It hangs in the Art Museum of Haiti in Port-au-Prince, untitled, but words often are superfluous when image makes a statement. Faustin's is a very strong statement.

At his best Faustin is a highly sophisticated surrealist, gripped by the drama of his country's anguish, expressed not in the dream imagery of unconscious depths, but in the folk imagery of his unique culture. Haiti is a surrealist fantasy come to reality, lush with the remnants of African animism, Catholic religious belief, and always, fully lived instinct. A member of the second generation of painters who burst forth from this country twenty-five years ago, naive and joyful, and brilliantly maturing and exploding ever since—Faustin knows his country. He is a painter with a conscience. He is a patriot.

His huge canvas full of brooding browns, melancholy lavenders, and unadulterated black depicts all the elements of Haitian life caught up in a giant spiderweb. Everything, everyone trapped, carrying on with terrible strain, without indignation or protest. Despite demonic, destructive forces, and breathless kinds of cruelty, horror, and torture, there is not even the faintest visible struggle to throw the bondage off and let in the victory of light. The entanglements are too overwhelming, the fatalism too oppressive. Simply, there is suffering; there is stoicism.

A giant tree trunk drips with blood from the wound of an ax, the appropriate focal point of the work, for deforestation begun centuries ago by the uncaring colonizers ranks high among the reasons for Haiti's condition today. In the background, a spider weaves a web, fraudulent and hypocritical, dangling a parchment proclaiming, "Liberty, Equality and Fraternity," the battle cry of the revolutionary Paris masses. The wonderment was, with all those screams for human rights they never could quite bring themselves around to vote for the abolition of slavery on this island, then their lucrative colony. "Loa," as the spirits are known in this much-enchanted country, roam about the canvas, many malevolent, others very old and broken, disheartened, defeated, despairing. Then there are the animals, stubborn horses and cows, frightened and reluctantly yanked along; the most pathetic dogs, fur over bone without the apparent strength even to howl in torment. There are cooking pots brewing over charcoal fires; workers like ancestral slaves, bare to the waist and sullen of expression. All are caught up and dragged, sustained and supported by the supreme act of will and unrelenting tenacity of a black and most fatigued female figure, strained by the oppression of this burden but bearing it. Much of the back-breaking work which keeps Haiti lumbering along, albeit far behind its other Latin American neighbors, is done by its indomitable women. Caught in his own spider web, a Haitian Catholic priest appears governed by a black Virgin wearing a tiny speck of redemption, a bright, aqua-colored halo. He looks uncertain and confined, an understandable state of mind, for he prays and preaches in a country only very partially Roman Catholic, its masses worshiping infinitely more than a three-person Trinity. He is of recent vintage, for the French hierarchy long feared opening its ranks to local membership, steeped in voodoo, accepting everything visible about Catholicism, but in fact the competition.

Mostly, there are the all-encompassing and inescapable spider webs, gossamer white like see-through chiffon but as enduring as a monolith. Faustin speaks of doom.

Haiti is trapped, and some believe as hopeless as Calcutta. Many specialists in international development put this diminutive country not in the third world, but the fifth. Obvious as well as subtle and devious forces year after year have woven quite a web regardless of the superman wielding power from the white presidential palace downtown. Statistically, Faustin's webs look like this compared with other countries of the Americas: lowest per capita income, $88; lowest life expectancy, 48 years; lowest per capita calorie consumption, 1,850 calories; lowest per capita protein consumption, 40 grams; lowest literacy rate, 11 percent; lowest ratio of medical doctors, 0.9 per 10,000 people; lowest ratio of hospital beds, 8 per 10,000 people; lowest percentage of students to school-age population, 24 percent; highest infant mortality,

INTRODUCTION

147 per 1,000 live births; highest rural population density, 350 per square mile; highest urban-rural ratio, 80 percent to 20 percent; and on it goes, lowest per capita output of electric power, lowest agricultural productivity, lowest . . . highest. . . .

This is Haiti.

[PART I]

1

THAT'S THE WAY IT IS

"They tell you, 'You are in the fifth world.' What can that do to you? You are not even in the third world—you are in the fifth world! It means what? Be ashamed of yourself and look at us as the great ones? I don't admit that issue of being in the fifth world. We are Haitians and we are in Haiti and we should not be ashamed of our conditions and ashamed of ourselves. If we hold to that attitude and are ashamed we won't go forward and we will always be asking for help. This is why I am against that question of being ashamed of ourselves.

"For instance, you take some Haitians and they are with a foreigner and there are some things—some parts of the city or something—they will not show a foreigner. To me, if a foreigner wants to see—let him see everything! Why be ashamed! America was worse than Saint-Domingue two hundred years ago. So why should we be ashamed when at one time this country was one of the richest countries in the world? We are in poverty because so many things have changed. We had hard times. We had a beginning as slaves. We have not been able yet to unite ourselves into five million people. Okay, it will come. This is why looking at history helps you to accept your conditions.

"If someone wants to go to a country and criticize—you can go anywhere and criticize. But when a country is big it will have no effect because you can go and describe a slum area in America and what affect can that have? Nothing, because in general the country is a rich country. Poverty exists everywhere even in the midst of richness. Richness exists everywhere. Here you have people living as well as Americans. Now the question is to bring equality so that everyone can enjoy that *sun, that climate, those beaches, the mountains . . . so that everyone can enjoy it. I think that is what we should strive for."—Ary Bordes*

Day begins very early in a Haitian village. It is not so much the specificity of the hour as the action. The villagers stir groggily even while night has left dark daubs of purple in the sky. Purple is a royal color and the sky also has a majesty about it, but brooding with overhanging mist, like King Saul on his throne chair, neurotic, bitter, obsessed, perhaps, by the sad destiny of this country and the suffering ahead this very day.

The mountain chains left and right of the village rest still and worn, streaked with cloud cover now, but always a silent presence. They seem to bear witness to what happens between them and form a corridor enclosing the appropriately named Cul-de-Sac Plain, a deep geological depression between the country's central and southern mountain ranges. In time purple yields to lavender and soon the mountains become the palest blue; while muted in tone, their outline is starkly clear. The sky is tinged with pink and orange until bright sunlight begins to gain energy, finally breaking through to dominate with a dazzling, sparkling new day.

Daybreak for the people in this village is much as Homer recounted in his poetry thousands of years ago, "when the young Dawn showed again her rosy fingers, they put forth. . . . Apollo who works from afar sent them a favouring stern wind. . . ." This is the Caribbean, not the Aegean, so perhaps it is not Apollo, but there is a stern, constant, prevailing wind that sweeps through this village, a warm wind, all-embracing and inescapable, very much like the mistral of southern France, which is reputed to drive people crazy. It may well be the work of one of the "loa," as the spirits are called here. They are everywhere, exerting great control, and most capricious; once aroused, they can avenge themselves and cause great tragedy.

In the wind all of nature seems to crackle and groan as if in noisy protest against the burden of this kind of life. The palm trees appear so lithe and flighty from a distance, but standing under them, their leaves—like splintered paddles—crunch against the wind; the abundant mango trees moan with their breakage. Banana leaves and sugar cane and cornstalks and rice grass all sound and ultimately sway in perfect unison, a well-rehearsed corps de ballet, supple and fluid and governed by the force of the wind; a real pleasure to watch off in the distance, surrounding the village swishing this way, then that. Their rhythm is affecting, an easy flow and movement, an unstressed arrangement interconnecting elements of time and space in a somehow musical and aesthetic cadence. Grace seems natural to this country—and contagious.

Foolishness and anxieties can be swept away, leaving only the bare bones of life, finally free from fat and fluff.

The stillness of night's heavy silence begins gradually to split with the buzzing of birds, their chirps and squawks. The roosters are most noticeably up first, heralding the approach of light, lifting the lavender haze from the mountains. Tropical night was so thickly dark and almost solemnly hushed, a feeling of rolling in black velour, or taste buds saturated by too many cognacs, syrupy and oppressive. No electricity provides relief. There was the communication of crickets breaking the quiet, so it was hardly deadly still; in fact, it was strangely alive. There was disturbance. The night had a faint but definite pulse, the sounds of voodoo drumming off somewhere and the echo of singing voices, an awareness fringing consciousness and creating a feeling of disquiet. In time these sounds in the night become very familiar, their frequency almost a comfort. The gods are being taken care of. The spirits are never far from thoughts or actions; devotion is constant, as is terror.

With daylight come the soft sounds of hens clucking. A donkey brays loudly, some distance away, but the cry is still distinct and harshly unattractive. Closer and sweeter, the baby goats, all soft and sweet, suckle with obvious delight, tugging at their mother's teats, almost violently, jerking and pulling for nourishment and position with all their tiny might. Stoically oblivious, their mother calmly munches on a few strands of straw. Now the babies begin their morning cry for the human breast, struggling for it, protesting when they are not immediately gratified, the selfishness of instinct, the will to live vividly heard—in the healthy ones. When the baby's demands take on the bleating whine of the baby goats, that is when there is danger and death hovers near. A child is being scolded, gently—but then it is still early. People cough. Almost imperceptibly, they begin to use the path outside, their bare feet treading earth ... gently. Isolated sounds. Actually, it is quite serene around "la cour," the central courtyard of a loose grouping of huts and outbuildings occupied by blood relations. The wind is so forceful and incessant it carries all noise away, controlling sense, quieting life. That is what is most striking.

Gental is off down the path to fetch water from the water hole, about twenty minutes away, likely longer for a four-year-old, particularly given the necessary balancing act on the trip back. He is a familiar sight with that water bucket on his head and unsmiling face beneath. The spillage flashes in the sunlight, painting some parts of him black while others remain brown, a cross between a glossy and a mat-finish photograph. The heavy metal bucket brimming with water trickling down his face weighs a lot and the strain will show in his tense expression and taut neck and back on his return.

Haitian children seem to be cherished in infancy and begin a life of hard labor, unappreciated and unrelieved work, at around Gental's stage. As surely as the work comes the continual berating for their nonexistent laziness, and frequent beatings for alleged disrespect and disobedience—more honestly, displaced hostility onto defenseless children. There is much anger here—with good reason; parents are severe lest their children be "mal élevé," badly brought up. "You can always strike your child . . . even if he is fifty years old," one mother said. "It is a parent's right." She refused to be restrained even by the threat of summoning the corporal.

Gental wears only a short white shirt, his genitals bouncing along as he swings the water bucket to be filled. The shirt is no longer big enough to button over his huge belly, for Gental is occupied territory—a paradise for worms. He is a survivor—second-degree malnutrition. Everything about him betrays his struggle for life: his spindly arms, his knobby knees, that belly, his height of a two-, maybe at most a two-and-a-half-year-old. The sugar cane he sucks on with his left hand offers some short-lived caloric energy, but none of the protein he so desperately needs to grow and have a healthy existence, now and in his future years. His head is greatly outsized for the stunted growth of his little brown body, always a chalky color with dust because of his nudity. In addition to his strange head, Gental's lower lip protrudes. People think of him as ugly; frequently they make fun of him. His extreme sensitivity, his profound melancholy at the age of four, are heartbreaking to observe. The slightest tone of ridicule sends his big head burrowing for shelter in those skinny crossed arms. Like any hurt child, he is very, very good—too good—eager to please lest he displease and experience more rejection. It is with great speed that Gental responds to the command to get water.

Gental is doomed. His family lives off to the right and are very, very poor, even by these standards of poverty. Consequently, he will never attend school because school costs in Haiti. His family cannot afford to buy him the green-checked school shirt, the dark green shorts, and the plastic sandals—the uniform he needs to attend the school, a forty-minute walk down the Haitian-American Sugar Company railroad tracks to the nearby market town. He will not get the uniform, the books, the rote education, even though he is demonstrably highly intelligent. Gental can thread a film projector, a totally foreign object, confidently making his way through a maze of gears and gadgetry—after watching the operation once. Gental can construct multi-story buildings with toy blocks—when he has never played with blocks before nor observed multi-story buildings. He has extraordinary spatial and manual abilities; he could be an engineer, an architect. He will be a farmer, as is his father,

THAT'S THE WAY IT IS

as was his grandfather. Thus is Haiti's destiny perpetuated in another generation, illiterate and confined to the ever-weakening topsoil.

Yes, Gental says, he will go into the "gardens," what Haitian peasants call their farmland. No, he says, he will never marry.

A generation older, Antoinisse has a slowness of gait and weariness of gesture this morning, as if he has not slept well. In fact, he has not eaten well, not yesterday, or the day before, perhaps for so long, maybe never, that he begins each day tired, lacking energy for all he must face, the cruel burden he must bear, his struggle against impossible odds. The day literally must be survived. So much adversity can strike... drought, sudden illness, a hurricane ripping through his exposed fields and defenseless thatch hut. What can he really do should any of this happen? What can he fight for or against? There is firewood and there is water—what else is probable, for even these are not certain. The rhythm of this kind of life grinds along its own route, lugubriously, like an ox-drawn cart. It has always been this way for Antoinisse, as it was before him, as he expects it will be for his children and his grandchildren. As he says, "Cé conça sa yé" (That's the way it is). There is nothing to be done save the living of it, so Antoinisse begins this new day, as he must... but it is done slowly, without enthusiasm.

He is prepared, however, and has emerged from his "caille," his house, wearing his work clothes. On his head rests a beaten-up straw hat with its much-tattered brim rolled back a little along the edges, frayed from repeated removals to wipe the sweat from his brow. It is very hot under a tropical Haitian sun in an unsheltered field. The wonderment is whether the hat is ever removed, it is so perpetual a feature of Antoinisse. At the moment he wears an undershirt of some kind because it is still cool this early in the morning; over it is a khaki shirt with a military-surplus look, rolled up to the elbows, exposing the sinewy muscular development of his forearms.

Antoinisse has been malnourished all his life, but he has lived, following the basic tenet of biology—survival of the fittest. He is stunted, only about five feet tall, but those forearms tell the tale of his toughness and how he has made it this far, into his early fifties. Typically, he does not know his exact age. His faded red trousers show the right pant leg in pretty good shape, but the left has a big tear at the knee and is short and tattered, exposing his painfully bowed legs, which add further insight into the story of his malnutrition. He is barefoot, and the callouses on his feet are thick as elephant hide and, like his handshake, testify to his harsh life.

He saunters off to urinate someplace, courteously not too close to a neighbor's dwelling. There are maybe thirty latrines in this village. Antoinisse is too poor to afford such a luxury. On his return he lets the animals out of an adjacent pen area, characteristically made of interwoven sticks and roofed over like boxes. They are confining, inhospitable places and the animals run off to feed with delight, the goats moaning their pleasure, the pigs seeming particularly full of urine and energy as they charge off, grunting loudly.

Tante, Antoinisse's "wife" for twenty years, has been up and about herself, grabbing some straw nearby, igniting it with a hot charcoal brought from next door by her thirteen-year-old, blowing gently until the smoke rises hesitantly; then a little flame emerges and she walks around back to get a fire going for the breakfast coffee. This is morning ritual, as is her reach for the broom leaning against the hut to sweep the courtyard free of leaves, twigs, excrement from the animals, and loose dirt. She brushes dirt from dirt, along the hard-earth courtyard above the limestone base upon which this village stands.

Tante is a Rubens woman, all rounds of fat flesh, unwrinkled knobs of cheeks punctured by deep dimples, big buttocks, huge breasts, and a large, protruding stomach, very wrinkled from the twelve babies that have grown there in her somewhere post-forty-five years of womanhood. They've been healthy years despite the burden of her life. When she was three her skin turned light and she almost died, she says, but ever since then all has been well. In between pregnancies she has worked as a market lady, walking country roads with those easy strides she makes, her loping gait betraying dignity of carriage and determination of step poverty cannot disguise. While she has never ridden in a car nor been on a boat, she has traveled widely with those large flat feet she washes constantly, even to take a walk through the village, for she is a very proud woman. Her marketing has taken her as far north as the seacoast town of Archaie and to Gonaïves to buy beans. She liked doing commerce and her husband did not mind her absence, she says, because she sent money back for food and clothing for the children.

Tante has style. In a single gesture she can squat, unself-consciously pull down her panties and pee, pulling her panties up as she rises—with a sweeping gesture as attractive as the pirouette of a ballerina. Her purple satin headscarf for special occasions like Thursday market days has the rippling softness of whipped cream on French pastry from her high-fashion knotting. Just as her walk sways, her voice tinkles with aristocratic modulation, her laugh comes with crackling eyes showing through the fingers shyly covering her fat face. Her eyes film with sadness when she pays a call on a sick neighbor. She butts into every family fight she can find, participating and negotiating, never minding her own business.

At Saturday-night voodoo dances she sings lustily, with outstretched arms waving in rhythm with the drumming. On the return trip in total darkness down the railroad track, she incessantly giggles because the other dancers were so bad compared with her ever-so-flowing movements, her entire body into it, pelvis oscillating in unison with the music, in effortless and enjoyed undulations. She is the star of the show. Her god is Guédé, a most passionate "loa," and when he mounts her, her sensuality bursts forth; she grinds away like a Mesopotamian fertility goddess. Once in her frenzy she grabbed some hot peppers and mashed them into her genitals and noticeably walked a little differently the following day.

Her tendency to giggle can turn into uncontrolled, rock-a-bye, fall-apart guffaws, particularly when she attends an evangelical church service. The village boasts one such house of worship. She goes, not for religion, but for entertainment: the comedy of testimony, the pleasure of singing, the gleefulness of chance happening, like a mocker passing gas through the open window, smelling up the place, creating havoc—convulsing Tante. A beleaguered minority, the evangelicals spat back out the window, retaliating for the outrage. Tante rules her children with an iron hand, and this gentle, lovely lady can turn into a sadist in an instant, eyes flashing, grabbing a stick, striking blow after blow, not quitting for a long time. When she asks for water, her children run.

Today she wears her trusty pink dress with a sweater so old its original red has arrived at the brownish purple stage, but it provides warmth. Her dress is starkly simple in design, as are the dresses of all peasant women, homemade with just the essentials: a bodice, short sleeves, no collar, a gathered skirt of mid-knee length. Nary one ornamental button, bow, stitch—the skeleton of a dress, almost childish-looking, like a kindergarten school plaid. On her head is the characteristic bandanna of Haitian women, as required as the Haitian man's straw hat. Today her scarf is of green and white checked material, likely a schoolboy's discarded shirt but tied with that definite flamboyance and pervading ease characteristic of her strength of personality. Tante's inner space is a sane and healthy place full of savvy and practicality. She could make it in New York, where, perhaps baffled by the subway system, she would walk.

The two boys return with their tasks accomplished, firewood from one, fresh water from the other. The eldest, Bradifey, is seventeen. He looks twelve. Frisnal is thirteen. He looks eight. This is what malnutrition really means—retarded growth and everything else. Bradifey brings his father a white enamel cup filled with water and Antoinisse scrapes his teeth clean with a finger, repeatedly gargling and spitting until the cup's contents are empty. That done, Bradifey is waiting, exchanging the empty cup for one with strong, locally grown coffee, just brewed in the cooking outbuilding in back. Antoinisse begins his breakfast seated once more and pulls out a corncob pipe from a pocket.

This long, silvery piece of nature has room enough for four people to socialize and is a gathering place evenings, like a park bench. There is an aura of vagrancy about this man this moment, his wizened, ravaged face, prematurely and cruelly aged, a stubble of gray mustache and beard, more a goatee, surrounding his gap-toothed mouth. He munches on some cassava bread, disk-shaped and sour of taste, made from bitter manioc flour. On his face is a vacant expression as he surveys the scene of his destiny. He is physically present, but so very weary, kin to a broken man in Central Park with the might and armor of skyscrapers in the background, but no longer an active participant. Absentmindedly, he fingers the torn edges of his trouser knee, closing the gap, which shows wide open again with the slightest body movement. He covers the tear once more and pulls out a corncop pipe from a pocket.

Like a solitary line of poetry there is a fragile beauty about this village which the starkness of poverty cannot intrude upon. A few doors down, Maria, Antoinisse's fourteen-year-old niece, has brought out the sleeping mats to air. While clearly not cushy comfortable, the mats, flung against the side of the hut, provide a visual lyricism, a softness of color and texture: pale cornsilk yellow, long, skinny shapes bound together by broad, weaving lines of tied knots; resting against the whitewashed look of the hut's wall, metallic in the early-morning sun and shadows.

Typical of the housing in the village, the hut is of wattle-daub construction, a woven infrastructure of tall sticks, human-height with a bit to spare, branching out of the four main corner points with two other supports halfway down each side to make the interior division into two rooms. The sticks are intertwined with twigs and branches and the whole arrangement is called "clissage." It is filled in with a mud and limestone mixture. The floor is of pounded earth; the roof gradually peaks and is rounded off with layer upon layer of straw. Protruding from the front is a little sun porch supported by two more beams retaining the shape of their ancestry. This "tonnelle" is also covered with straw, flat on top and sloping toward the front. It is the minimum of a house, walls to shelter from the wind and provide a roof over your head, not all that reliable in a rainstorm and subject to the visits of Haitian snakes. They drop in from time to time, very thin, and fortunately, not poisonous.

When the houses are new there is an immaturity about them, the freshness of a young sparrow, all soft creams, grays, and browns; then, with the weathering of nature comes a mellowing. The thatch turns from brown to gray, gets bushy-haired and tousled, requiring that a heavy branch be placed here and there to keep the roof in place. Just like an expressive, lined old face with sagging muscles, the plaster chips and cracks, breaking off in hunks here and there, revealing the pockmarks of the "clissage." In time, the house gets to look very trembling and vulnerable.

The single front doors of the houses and their side window shutters fit into their rough-hewed frames, pieces of puzzle, crooked, curving and grooving into the space, planks braced by crosspieces attached with metal hinges. All are essential and closed tightly at night to prevent the intrusion of malevolent spirits, in the process trapping every virus and bacteria exhaled and coughed by the family, maximizing the chances of infection. Just as inescapable are the facts of sex. Haitian children learn early and naturally about this part of life. Sexuality is never denied or embarrassing, but it is postponed until late adolescence.

The saying goes there is not a straight line in all of Haiti, and hostesses of the capital are always fixing askew tableclothes, mumbling complaints under their breath about the incapacity of their maid of twelve years to line cloth edge with table edge. Here too. The doors, the shutters, the corners of the houses, the roof lines, the thatch edges—everything—is crooked, right out of the nursery rhyme " . . . they all lived together in a little crooked house." The houses are grouped in crooked circles, sometimes just a few, or as many as a couple of dozen, depending on the size of the extended family. There are eight such houses in Antoinisse's "la cour." Each leads off to another in jigjag fashion, repeating the motifs of blue doors, straw . . . echoing each other in ever-diminishing line and color. Like a prism they subtly refract the hue of time. At noon the whitewashed limestone is ablaze with sunlight like a captured hearth, blinding, while in afternoon the huts assume a faint lavender, turning delicate gray with evening and coming up pink with the next dawn.

"If you see nothing outside, there is even less inside," one villager said. In the front room was a pile of rags in one corner and a branding-iron hanging from a nail embedded in the wall. Behind the inner mud wall relieved with a door space there was a single line of rope strung across with more rags, likely the family's clothes. In a corner on a straw mat was a baby bedded in rags, the tenth child fathered by this man, living with his third wife. The baby was tightly bonneted with two hats and heavily clothed not only to keep him warm, but to make him strong of body and personality in his years ahead. "My mother has pinned me up very well," grateful children say when they demonstrate energy and autonomy. The baby rested quietly in the windowless darkness and stale air on a bright, sunny day.

Houses are for sleeping and for sex. Haitian living takes place outdoors. There is little privacy; there is great community. To stroll among these extended families, through these courtyards and along these footpaths, is to experience lilting greetings of good day, warm arm waves of recognition, offers of hospitality, shy but interested company, friendship. The overweening impression is of considerable kindness and authentic empathy of people bonded by mutual suffering, relieved through togetherness, touch, and laughter. Women kiss noisily; men hug grandly; a hand reaches over to squeeze another with tender caring when the eyes betray the anguish of a sore soul. The faces are open and expressive. The eyes stare and look through, intimately seeing the spectrum of emotionality: true feelings of pleasure, anger, tiredness, sadness, joy, without sophisticated masking or complications of complexity. Often there is a strange repose and peacefulness of features. The physical beauty—outright sensuousness—is a constant source of disbelief.

People greet each other with great gentleness and politeness, doffing a hat, offering a hand. Smiles come in a flash of big white teeth, strongly rooted in jawbone, according to one dentist, because of the chewing of sugar cane from an early age. And the smiles come easily. Any occasion to laugh is seized, the littlest thing: a child carrying four pieces of firewood and dropping one; a woman spilling water as she engineers the pot to her head; a slip in the mud. It is all welcomed with ready laughter. At every turn comes the extension of a straight-backed chair, or perhaps some water. They have nothing else to give but themselves, to share time, talk, togetherness.

To the stock comment in any culture, "How are you?" comes the reply, "Oh, no worse off than yesterday, thank God." Haitian peasants understand envy as well. Their greatest fear is to arouse the ire of another, to provoke someone into putting a curse on them, making their lives suddenly worse than Job's. Aggression is expressed through the intervention of the spirits, hostility's intermediaries, and physical violence is extremely rare. Rather, tenderness is the gestalt. It is not unusual to hear people humming as they make their way along a path to the laundry stream or out to the fields, a pleasant sound in the wind along a route bordered in orchidlike white Lillian blossoms.

Movement is casual. There is no hurry. People cluster in front of a house in different body postures, sitting, standing, kneeling, squatting, like live mahogany sculpture in the shade, making netting, gossiping, shelling beans, playing checkers, repairing a chair, or silently enjoying the presence of kindredness. A crow cries from somewhere, disturbing the profundity of silence. The external wind blows and blows. Time melts away from one day to the next, without urgency, and particularly, free of change.

It is always the same. A father passes by, trailed by his young son carrying the garden hoe and wearing a pint-sized straw hat. It is time for brown-bean planting and the next generation is learning its occupation. Goats, pigs, chickens feed freely, finding something here and there, getting tangled in scrub brush or the cactus patches relieving the village's limestone flatness. Almost obsessive, water constantly comes and goes, its necessity to human existence eloquently evident. A ten-minute walk to the rear of the village finds the laundry, with vigor the order of the day; washing, an act of purification and absolution, accomplished with incessant soaping and violent sounds of scrubbing, wringing out, and smacking of material against rocks. Back in the village, one of the few schoolboys sits on the ground, leaning back against his house to learn his lesson, parroting in French, which he only vaguely understands since Creole is his language. In singsong and mechanistically he chants: "Geography is the study of the earth and its inhabitants. We make a distinction between physical and human geography. The first studies ... " A few feet away an illiterate eleven-year-old threshes rice in a pot of water, grain sinking to the bottom, chaff rising to be tenderly cleared from the water surface. In addition, he has kept an eye peeled on his three-year-old sister, in keeping with the custom of giving an older child responsibility for the care of a younger sibling. Boys play soccer, not with a ball, but with a sock stuffed with rags and sewn tightly, while girls play "pinche," like jacks, eight or ten little rocks thrown into the air, to be caught in the open hand. The muffled tomtom of millet being prepared for cooking, alternating thrusts of a "manche," a large log pestle in a "pillon," a hollowed-out end of a tree trunk, beat out a rhythm, a message picked up a few courtyards over, by another duo of brother and sister in perfect coordination. A villager repairs the "clissage" of the pigpen, struck down by an angry burro's kick, while another re-upholsters the "matla" of his chair. Stacks of sugar cane are loaded onto the railroad car standing by the village for the daily ride into the capital's refineries. A woman in her vigorous late thirties quarrels with her husband, reaching over to hurl firewood in his direction, motivated by relentless rage. Next come a few rocks. A discarded and dented bicycle wheel turns and turns, absorbing the four men intent on their gambling, a simple form of roulette. An old woman in the brightest blue cotton dress, the cheapest material in Haiti, hits and kicks her donkey, immobile in a huge mud puddle. Suddenly she's in the muck—and she laughs. A white heron sits among the lily pads of the river, maintaining a regal watch over his domain. A dog is kicked, incredibly skinny and even more pathetic. Women breastfeed babies. Children are rebuked. Courtyards swept. Millet threshed. Children scrubbed. Birds chatter.

That's the way it is in the sunlight and the wind. Day after day. That's the way it is with the hunger and the sickness. Day after day. A baby cradled by its mother has so little strength, the child's arm waves in the wind. A two-and-a-half-year-old rarely walks, because he does not have the stamina to support his body weight and venture a step. A five-year-old looks aged and pregnant, her belly so distended by malnutrition, her little dress sticks out like a cartoon of an umbrella; her hair like tufts of reddish wool also protruding from the roots. She walks with great fatigue and discomfort, suddenly losing bowel control with diarrhea, leaving a puddle behind which a pig quickly comes to lap up.

Any walk through this village easily reveals thirty to forty nude children with obvious and advanced malnutrition, their stomachs huge with it and with assorted intestinal parasites; heads outsized; shoulders negligible; limbs like pipes. There are runny noses from respiratory infections; swollen ears from poor hygiene. A two-year-old has the sad face and flesh tone of beaten old age, without the energy to reach for a toy. Kwashiorkor, a protein-deficiency disease, and marasmus, caused by lack of calories, and combinations of both are endemic, to the degree that health is the exception—not the rule. Very few children measure up to normal height and weight standards. An eighteen-year-old can stand four-foot-five inches; a five-year-old can weigh twenty-six pounds and look two; a three-year-old can weigh as much as a seven-month-old baby. There is diarrhea and vomiting routinely. Spitting and coughing from the burden of tuberculosis are matter of fact in many families. Illness and death are daily topics of conversation: "Edgar has been sick for two months." "That woman just lost her husband two weeks ago. She is left with six children."

Camil has been vomiting for six days, plus he has a cough and diarrhea, so now he is too weak to stand and his greeting is barely audible, more communicated with the movement of his lips than sound. His eyes are feverish, very yellow, and very, very sad. He fears for his life of thirty years and the impoverishment of his family, a wife and five children, the survivors of the ten he has fathered with this woman. The new infant is fat and healthy from the nourishment of her mother's breast, but the three-year-old has the telltale trace of orange in her hair from the herb teas, starchy gruels, and conspicuous absence of protein in her diet. The father looks as frightened as she this moment. He rests on a straw mat surrounded by cushioning rags, a sheet pulled up high to his chin, forming a tent-shape over his drawn-up knees. Helena sits with her husband, her eyes soulfully watching his progressive weakening with a direct ratio of alarm. She has notified the "houngan," the voodoo priest Joie, to come again tonight. Last night's treatment was not successful. Camil is worse.

On the third day of Camil's illness the village leaf doctor, Madame Londe, an expert herbalist, was summoned for her knowledge of stomach problems and inflammation. She charged one gourd for the treatment, twenty cents, to mix palm oil with rum, heat the brew over a fire, and massage it into Camil's stomach. No results. On the fifth day of his illness, the "houngan" was called, since the sickness appeared to be supernatural in origin, likely the work of a discontented spirit.

Camil's wife made the twenty-minute walk to Joie's "peristyle," the religious center for this village, easily accessible but just a little apart, appropriate to Joie's social status. The walk is often made by the fearful and the faithful, the sick and the vindictive. Like an after-hours place with all the hangers-on, amidst the goats and pigs wandering among the phallic symbols and forbidding voodoo crosses embedded in the hard ground of this compound, here could be found the potency of a widely respected inheritance of black and white magic, covering all categories of need. Here was Joie, an extremely big man, as if his "loa" had immunized him against the diseases of his milieu and the routine ravages of malnutrition. About six feet tall and big-boned, he tended to stand with his weight on his left hip, dominating casually, his left hand supporting the small of his back. His receding hairline edged away from a pushed-back forehead, flat like an Indian papoose. Beneath this strange physiognomy stared beady, laughing eyes, as if he knew all of life's little and big jokes; his mustache, relatively thick and trimmed; his wealth, showing in his black-rim glasses and wristwatch. He lived in this scattering of buildings, not all that different from any other peasant, but there was the "peristyle," a place of many moods and wonderments. He agreed to come.

That night he pleaded with the family spirits, promising to fulfill all wishes. The ceremony was simple: candles were lighted; mystical designs, "vèvès," symbols of the spirits, traced on the hut floor with cornmeal; the family led in the recitation of many Catholic prayers, hymns, litanies, and special chants. Then, a meal was prepared and buried under the threshold of the door for the spirits' appeasement and consumption. The climax came with Joie's loud pleading, his crying out in desperation, very dramatically imploring the spirits to "Please, loosen your hold on Camil! Set him free to work once more for his family! Whatever offense will be generously undone, any neglect of your will, speedily rectified, just so Camil gets well!!"

Today he is not better. The illness appears to be even more serious than a sulking family spirit and there is the beginning of real dread, even terror. An enemy may have sent a dead man to possess Camil. Tonight there must be an exorcism, which will cost many animals and be most painful for Camil to experience. He will be spoken to roughly, threatened, massaged with foul-smelling liquid called "beng," sprayed with rum, spit upon—all designed to displace the ghost residing in his body. Despite his weak condition, he will be forced to sit and stand, maybe even danced and jumped over and stomped upon, even prepared for death. His limbs will be bound with strips of white cloth; his jaw tied shut; a rope stretched above his body, with little pieces of red cloth attached. Food will be prepared in little gourds and passed over his body in an effort to entice the spirit out for a good meal. The same procedure will be followed with a live chicken. Next, the rope above will be untied for the ghost to exit from Camil and a neighbor hired to throw the food and the rope into a distant field or perhaps the cemetery. At that moment Joie will demand that Camil stand and identify himself, whose ghost he is, where he comes from, and which enemy sent him. Should Camil not know the answers, he will be threatened and scorned, a flame lighted under his eyes to terrorize him into revelations. There is much distress in Camil's house today. His eyes are round with fear and yellow with infectious hepatitis.

Life goes on. New life too. Three or four new lives enter the world of this village every month, their mothers aware of their pregnancy through the cessation of menstruation, more reliably confirmed from the massage test of midwives and card reading of Joie. Naturally, the husband is the first to know, quickly taking magical protective measures by buying certain potions to guard against the spirits that eat children. The potions mix herbs, insects, and animals with a high-class brew including a frog, so like a frog, anyone coming at night to drink the blood of the fetus will get a swollen belly and die. A horribly bitter potion is purchased to make the mother's blood bitter so any werewolf will gag and spit up the child's blood he has sucked; the mother gags too as she drinks the defense. In the third month, she begins to take a purgative called "lok," a mixture of castor oil, grated nutmeg, cinnamon, anise, sugar, garlic, bicarbonate of soda, sugar, and the juice of a sour orange. She will have three such treatments during pregnancy so her child will have clean blood and insides as well as health and beauty outside. Plus, there's a bonus: "lok" also prevents stomach pains and rashes in early infancy.

The child grows in one of the three sacks of the female stomach—the other two serve as receptacles for food and liquids—nourished by menstrual blood fed through a hole in the midpoint of the infant's head, evident at birth by the fontanels. Like house-building, each day God adds a little more to the child's development as the woman sleeps; it is very dangerous for her to awake suddenly during pregnancy. Her pregnant cravings are speedily accommodated as the child's will; sexual relations continue, considered helpful for the open uterine canal at birth.

"Woy! Woy! Give me room to get through. St. Ann good mother! Everybody answer the song for me!" screams Clairinoi in her labor, occasionally turning against her husband, her face bitter and enraged, her voice high-pitched and hoarse, cursing, "Look what you have done to me!" She tries to bite and punch him but he jumps out of reach, accepting her anger passively but with alacrity. "Oh, God, help her. Help her! Have mercy on her," holler very close and sympathetic family and friends, permitted to participate, sharing her travail, ministering to her comforts as much as possible, urging her to "push" with each contraction.

Very old and completely toothless, the midwife Sainçoila arrives in dirty old clothes, her shapeless dress falling off one exposed shoulder, revealing flesh with the consistency of original protoplasm. Her fingernails seem particularly dirty. Only after the delivery will she bathe and put on clean clothes. This is the way Sainçoila has been delivering babies for forty-five of her seventy-four years, a power, concentrated in her magic thumb, inherited from the spirits of her grandmother, also a widely respected midwife. A little sign outside her simple house advertises her many services. It reads: "Syrup for gaz, colic, bile, Madame Sainçoila, sage, syrup for grippe. Takes care of children and prepares lok." There is something classic about this old woman, a mother long ago, grandmother of fifteen, with sunken cheeks and flabby breasts, the long "wisdom" hairs on her face like a Chinese sage.

She immediately calls for castor oil and a bowl in which she floats seven small candles to insure divine intervention in the birth; sprinkling water and asking God to open the way, spreading out an old sack in front of Clairinoi's now open legs. Then she prays to the "marassa," the god of the twins, the source of all her supernatural powers, for Sainçoila has always known she was exceptional for this reason—a twin. She still gives food to her dead twin sister, now a goddess, very violent, temperamental and touchy, she often complains, requiring constant attention and thousands of precautions. It had always been like that, she says, with an accepting yet heavy sigh from her burden, quoting the proverb in a sad voice, "Twins don't get on." She shakes her head widely from side to side at all this difficulty, despite the fact that her parents had been so careful to divide their food equally, make their clothes identical, praise them both at the same time.

Sainçoila sits in a little chair, her body posture really a squat, legs wide apart, as her "patient" screeches in pain. She encourages her outbursts, considered therapeutic and helpful to birth. Bathed in sweat now, Clairinoi will deliver her fourth child as she has the others, in a sitting position in the front room of her house with all the doors and windows shut tight against cold and spirits. The midwife has dipped her hands in the bowl of now heated oil and starts to massage Clairinoi— roughly, eliciting protests, but it is necessary, although uncomfortable, to turn the child around from a standing position for entry into the world head first. The massage continues, as does Sainçoila's chanting:

"Oh, St. Margaret, deliver her for me. Mother St. Ann, Virgin Mary, all Saints in Heaven, deliver her for me. Bring her through. Here is how I will shake her womb." She violently massages. Clairinoi hollers out in agony, writhing and moaning to escape the motions of those hands unmercifully clutching her abdomen. From time to time Sainçoila leaves the hut and paces outside, passing the hours. Finally, shoulders emerge ... the mysticism of birth. A son.

He does not cry out. The onlookers grab plates for just such an eventuality, drumming with spoons, clapping their hands to wake the baby. He cries. Clairinoi is escorted to the rear room for a lukewarm bath, and only when she is resting on her straw mat is the baby's umbilical cord cut, so very carefully and without pulling, since it is the beginning of the baby's intestine. It is cut with a large door hinge, the length of the stump very minutely determined since it dictates the size of the child's genitals in adulthood. The stump is then covered with grated nutmeg and wrapped in a cloth soaked in castor oil. All of which welcomes the tetanus spores to germinate into a lethal bacillus, 100 percent fatal if untreated. The old midwife has squeezed a few drops of blood from the cord into the baby's mouth and poured down some "lok" to assist with his first bowel movement. Now she washes the blood from his body in lukewarm water, shaping his "broken" head and closing the fontanels, massaging the head with more grated nutmeg, finally doubly bonneting the baby and taking him to rest with his mother. Meanwhile, the father has dug a hole under the threshold of the door separating the two rooms, where the placenta is placed with hot charcoal and salt thrown on top, the first to insure speedy drying of the umbilical stump of the child, and the second to prevent odors and provide proper healing of the umbilicus. Clairinoi begins her five-day confinement in the house with her new son.

Antoinisse was born in his village, and except for a few trips to Port-au-Prince, forty cents by "tap tap," Haiti's public bus, this is life as he knows it. His father had two children with Antoinisse's mother, then left to cut sugar cane in the Dominican Republic, never to return. Later, his mother began living with another man so Antoinisse has a half-brother and a half-sister in a nearby "la cour." His mother died three years ago, he says, and the end was difficult because bad spirits had entered her body, causing her to walk around talking to herself like a crazy woman.

Antoinisse has had his problems with the spirits too, he confides; he does not know why since he has done his best to venerate his ancestors and fulfill all his obligations, as much as he could possibly afford. He speaks pleadingly, as if the "loa" might be listening and receive the message, ceasing the poverty and ill fortune which have so constantly beset him and his family. He never addresses his future directly lest the gods be provoked by his expectations. "If God wills it . . . if I am still here . . . " is the recurring parenthesis. His greatest fear is that someone will go to the "houngan" and put a curse on him, killing him with black magic, for which there is no defense. Or perhaps he could be put in jail if someone said he spoke ill of the government, something, he emphasized, he would never, never do.

Antoinisse began living with Tante when she was in her early twenties. Her precise age is unknown, but she knows she was born in the Dominican Republic, where her mother lived for thirty-five years, bearing eight children. Ultimately her mother returned to Haiti and has lived in the capital for twenty-two years now, in Portail St. Joseph, one of Port-au-Prince's five main slum areas, where she struggles to live, selling soap, toothpaste, pots and pans, and a few cooking utensils. There is no one to help her, and often she sleeps all night in the street to keep a prime spot in the market area.

When Tante was a very young woman she lived in another village with another man with whom she had three children. She left him, she says, because he was lazy and would not work; when the children were sick, he refused to spend money for the "houngan" to care for them. Only her first child, a daughter, lives. The second baby, a son, died at seven days, probably of tetanus of the newborn; the third child, another daughter, died at two-and-a-half months, of fever and diarrhea. Her first-born, Diana, has lived with Tante's mother since she was six because it is so hard to care for children in the poverty of village life.

Now twenty-one, it was very bad for Diana two years ago last July, Tante recalls. Her body went all stiff, her skin yellowed, and she was in great pain. Her bone joints seemed to calcify and in time she could not even dress and had to be taken to the hospital. She had been having problems with a man, Tante added, and a few months later became pregnant. Hysterical paralysis is a form of mental illness among Haitian peasants. Diana no longer lives with this man nor does he provide for his child, a daughter, who weighs eleven pounds at thirteen months and is on the road to marasmus.

Tante was alone for a year and a half before she became "placé" with Antoinisse. They would prefer to be married, he says, because God likes that better, but there never was enough money for the ceremony. Tante has been a very fertile woman and there are two other daughters living with a sister of Antoinisse's in the capital, doing chores in exchange for care, virtual indentured servants since they were sent to Port-au-Prince at the ages of five and three. They are now nineteen and seventeen. In the village there remain the two boys to help with the work, and a three-year-old daughter.

These have lived, but the others died and caused them both great sadness. All the children were sick as babies, with diarrhea and passing blood. They often speak of the dead children, they said; some had begun to talk and have their own personalities when they were taken from them. One son died at two and a half of fever and diarrhea despite every effort and cost to save him. They even tried taking him to Port-au-Prince to see a doctor at the hospital, but he died of dehydration on the thirty-five-mile trip and they turned back heartbroken and buried him. The next two children lived, but then a son died at four, all swollen at the end, his hair dry and red and falling out in patches—likely kwashiorkor. Then a daughter died at two of the same illness; the next child, another daughter, died very quickly, seven days after birth—tetanus.

Now the three-year-old is all swollen about the lower face and neck from advanced tuberculosis and Tante holds and smiles at this baby constantly, cheering her on, it seems, with a rush of maternal love, no antidote for the "microbes" eating away each day at her diminishing strength. If it were possible, Tante says, she would have preferred not to have had so many children because of all the worry and care they have taken, so often ending in death, six deaths out of twelve births. Perhaps soon the figure will be seven out of twelve. None of the children has gone to school because of the money.

For Antoinisse it was particularly bad about twenty years ago when the spirits sent him vomiting and weakness for five months. He was near death and Tante desperately paid four big pigs, twelve goats, their one mule, almost all they had, to the "houngan." Finally, the magic worked and Antoinisse became better, although never as well as before. The illness left him with very poor eyesight, particularly in his left eye, and also affected his hearing, totally in the left ear and partially in the right so Tante must do the negotiating for the irrigation and a lot of the talking for other purposes. When Antoinisse speaks, which is rarely, his voice is gruff and gravelly, voicing mostly complaints and demands. He is a frustrated and burdened man, lashing out at his children in an instant, particularly Bradifey, whom he sometimes ties to a tree and beats for an offense of the day before. Tante claims Antoinisse strikes her every day.

It all would be different, Antoinisse says, had he been able to use the inheritance of spirits from his "houngan" grandfather and train him for the "asson," the voodoo-priest rattle, comparable to the cardinal's hat of Catholicism. Antoinisse is a "houngan macoute," a paraprofessional of sorts, with definite supernatural insights and powers from beckoning spirits, but he lacked the funds to acquire the extended technical education into the names, characteristics, signs, tastes, and ceremonies of the "loa," their moods and vanities. Always, there has been no money.

THAT'S THE WAY IT IS

Occasionally when Antoinisse has drunk too much rum he ventures into the home of his family gods, still-lifes at every turn, old rattles, crumbling pottery from ancient offerings, indistinguishable pictures on the walls, and bursts into spontaneous and finely patterned banging on the old yellow and red drum of his grandfather. He seems vigorous then, happy and spirited. But that is a rare mood. He is not drunk now and sits on his log, unconscious of his pampering and pruning of his closely cropped hair, finally moving ever so slowly, placing a banana in his straw shoulderbag for lunch, grabbing his only farm implements, his hoe and machete, for today's work in the gardens.

It is confusing to walk to Antoinisse's garden. First, he follows along the railroad tracks for about ten minutes, passing the rich and obvious fertility of other farmers' holdings, hearing their good fortune—rippling water running through irrigation canals. The corn luxuriates in the sunlight, pulled toward the sky, leaves lusty with growth. A peek down the rows reveals more than one villager shining in the sun, shirtless, rippling muscles developed laboriously over a lifetime in this wind, with those scraping motions of a heavy hoe digging at resistant earth.

Then, Antoinisse hangs a left past sugar cane growing greenish brown on the right and twelve-foot corn plantings on the left. Shortly, another left, then a right, through the zigzag patchwork of other gardens, passing another pedestrian, a five-year-old, it seems, with the inevitable water bucket balancing on her head. Here is the very best land of this village, almost black, dark with organic life and abundantly humid. Antoinisse owns only one carreau, just over three acres, divided into three locations—none of them here. His father's many progeny took each an equal share, equally unable to support their generation's families.

Antoinisse silently greets another farmer returning from the fields, putting an arm affectionately around his shoulder—connection, gentle touch—and moves along. He takes another left, passing an irrigation-ditch bridge made of cornstalks, in disrepair, and reaches over to grab some nearby water-crescent leaves for a refreshing chew. Finally, he has arrived.

This is his very best plot because accessible is a wonderfully clear waterhole, its mud bottom visible through the blur, inhabited by little fishes and surrounded by maisonbelles leaves and the snakelike roots of distant trees that have crawled all this way for moisture. The roots look ominous, almost treacherously tangled, but Antoinisse disputes that impression. The spirits that dwell here are all white and long-haired, he says. Damballah particularly is a good-natured snake spirit who likes to hang around waterholes, make rain, and climb trees; Simbi is said to be very well mannered and intelligent.

On the surface, Antoinisse's field appears highly productive, a melange of foods, but upon closer consideration, protein-low. There is sugar cane, of course, rice, hard bananas, plantains, and the corn that Antoinisse is planting now. Also, there are watermelon, pumpkins, lima beans, papaya, and some coconuts from a few palm trees clustered on the plot and singing in the prevailing wind. He also grows a little cotton, fresh with yellow flowers and good for stuffing mattresses, some tomatoes, eggplant, mushrooms, and a touch of shallot. The corn he works with is for eating because there is not enough land for a large planting to sell at the market. The sugar cane unfortunately must be shared with another farmer because Antoinisse has only one grown son to help him with the work and must pay another man to assist with the harvesting. Would that he had more sons, he says, noting that daughters, however, care for their parents in old age. He understands crop rotation and once the cane is grown will plant rice and sweet potatoes three times before he grows more cane.

Antoinisse works with his hoe, much taller than he, and seemingly more heavy than necessary. The iron plate is attached to the pole by a spike stolen from a railroad tie. He leans over to work more closely, the voodoo beads around his neck dangling near his land, this earth that supports and breaks him at its whim, nature from which all life and death cycles get their impetus. The eternal wind plays around the trees, through the cane and down the corn rows, almost noisy with laughter. Mocking. There are no other sounds save a lonely crow's cry. The mountain chain contorts colors all day long. Like marine fatigues now, all green and brown spots, patches of savage growth with lovely lavender flowers on close inspection, nameless beauty, juxtaposed with eroded land with only a stubble of trees remaining across the mountain tops, spotty and unattractive. A place rich in cactus so poor in water, pulsing with energetic sunlight. As afternoon approaches for a visit, the mountains wear pastel blues, almost aquas, speckled with navy from the clouds overhead, later putting on pinks and purples.

Occasionally Antoinisse stops for a smoke of home-grown tobacco, leans on his hoe, confronting almost eye level the scarecrow that does double duty, guarding his seeds from birds and supplying magical insurance against evil. The cow skull stares back with the multi-colored streamers it wears, floating nonchalantly in the breeze. Antoinisse sits almost suddenly, squatting, head in hand, a habit and posture that can endure for hours. He is in suspended animation, almost meditation, arrested in self and time, looking at his own mirror. His is a most integrated work-leisure day. Work spills through the day, easily accomplished in less time, or perhaps, more accurately, more concentrated work time. He lives each day this way, for Antoinisse has never taken a vacation from this way of life.

What is he thinking? "There is no money," he says, a practical peasant pondering. It is usually so—the water, the weather, the money, the children. He worries about them all, all the time, for Antoinisse is an anxious person. One of his big concerns these days is $10, finding $10—about 20 percent of his annual income. That is what a neighbor has demanded for a share of irrigation water that one of his plots completely lacks. He is very vulnerable now. The land is getting very dry, the crops beginning to wither; without the money, the planting will die, losing the life essential to produce the food essential to the lives of his family. He must get some money! The $10 is far beyond his means but never far from his thoughts these days. Antoinisse believes the price is excessive and quotes an old Haitian proverb, "A dog has four feet but he cannot travel four roads at once." He hopes to negotiate the price, he adds, suddenly absorbed in thought once more.

Another hour's work and he responds to the mountain's sundial, returning home with what he has found to feed his family, corn and sweet potatoes. Yesterday he brought bananas, beans, and rice. On feast days there may be chicken, but most likely not. Sometimes there is lunch, a little midday snack of sugar cane or fruit, a baked sweet potato or piece of cassava bread. More often there is only a morning and an evening meal. The reason is simple. There is no food. As Antoinisse puts it, "You eat what you find in the gardens."

2

WHY IT IS

"Nothing annoys me more than those people who say nothing can be done with this country. I don't see how people can say that! You know some Haitians might say that and many foreigners say it . . . this is their way of looking at it. But if they would try to understand what happened, this historical background of all the problems we face. Then, I don't think they could think like that.

"We had the only slave revolt that was successful. They were slaves who didn't know how to read or write, organize, anything. All they wanted was to be free men and not be oppressed by a few and exploited. Instead of looking at us like that, what did the big powers do? They crushed us! Then they left us in isolation. Then they pushed us one against the other. The foreigners here were the ones paying for revolutionaries. In order to make money and benefit! They didn't help us organize ourselves! We stayed 115 years, fighting each other so we could not develop.

"Then, there was the question of prejudice. Haiti was the only black republic and presented everywhere as a group of Negroes unable to govern. People really enjoyed that. This was the image that all the big powers wanted to present of Haiti—a group of Negroes, inept, ignorant, not able to do anything. So they kept us that way. And then, well, we helped them because instead of getting together, we fought against each other. Also, since we had been free so long, we did not benefit from the organizational know-how of the more organized countries as did a lot of the small islands around us. But you also can see that Haiti is different because we have been able to maintain a certain cultural identity . . . . "—Ary Bordes

WHY IT IS

As the saying goes, Christopher Columbus landed on the shores of this island he called Hispaniola, a corruption of the Spanish "La Espanola," kissed the ground, thanked God for his safe arrival, and asked where the gold was. There was gold. Nice yellow flakes in the riverbed of the Yaque del Norte. Needless to say, the Spanish established a colony, La Navidad, on the northern coast.

It is here that the tragi-comedy of Haitian history began with that first wading ashore by Columbus and this land's initial experience with international forces which have harassed and crippled its development from the outside. While inside, virtually hereditary policies and practices generation after generation have caused this country's power elite to sin against the high ideals of the first black republic of the world and the second successful revolution of the Americas.

From the beginning the buzz word was exploitation. In a mere fifteen years, less than one Arawak generation, the variously estimated indigenous population of one-half to one million Indians was reduced to a mere 60,000 survivors; 140 years later there were less than 500.

Somebody had to do the work other than the Spanish, and the first African slaves began filtering into Haiti as early as 1503, finding a new and brutish life in the mines and on the plantations. In 1517 Charles V signed the authorization for 15,000 African slaves to be shipped to the colony called San Domingo, a fateful move, initiating an importation that would rise into the millions before rage and dignity overcame cupidity and sadism. In 1697, the Treaty of Ryswick, concluding the War of the Grand Alliance in Europe, ceded Hispaniola to France, creating the colony of Saint-Domingue, the French translation of San Domingo.

Now the success story began in earnest—as did the abuse. Today Haitian automobile plates boast the epithet "Pearl of the Antilles" because of those olden days when Haiti was the wealthiest colony in the new world, the biggest jewel in the French imperialist crown, the envy of all of Europe. Trade from this little island exceeded that of all thirteen North American colonies reporting to the British. Some years it took 700 ships and over 80,000 sailors to haul all the loot to France. "Wealthy as a Creole," the term for anyone born on the island, became the "in" line.

The white aristocracy numbered only 36,000 at the time of the French Revolution, overseeing more than 500,000 slaves, drained decade after decade from western Africa. Millions of them came, slaved and died doing it, with a complete turnover taking place every twenty years, wiped out by living conditions truly defying description.

Just as the Nazi camp guards deteriorated, so the slave system was destructive to the masters as well. Saint-Domingue became a location of degraded human life, monotony, tropical disease, loneliness, and depravity. Race became an obsession. The degree of whiteness and blackness numbered 128 possible combinations, the more white despising the more black with an open-ended degree of animosity and envy.

The system was bad but dazzling. Between 1783 and 1789 production doubled, slave importation almost tripling to 40,000 a year. Then came this strange cry from across the Atlantic: "Liberty, Equality, Fraternity!" Incredibly, the French revolutionaries withheld judgment on the question of the abolition of slavery itself. But the word had been passed.

Tropical thunder and lightning filled the night of August 14, 1791, in the depths of the Bois-Caiman of the Northern Plain, where the representatives of two hundred slave plantations joined their leader Boukman, a gigantic black and voodoo priest, Jean-François Biassou, and a little man named Toussaint, coachman of the Breda plantation, ugly, silent, steely-eyed, and forty-five years old, aged and gray by slave standards. Many Haitian historians consider this man the most extraordinary figure in their country's remarkable story. Not the least of his many achievements was his masterful outfoxing of the French, British, and Spanish forces, all desperately maneuvering to seize control of the colony and suck its riches. With France and Spain warring with each other in 1793, Toussaint joined the Spanish with 600 black troops, against the French. Soon his army numbered 4,000 angry blacks loyal to the death to this charismatic leader. In the summer of 1794, with the British suddenly deciding it was more in their self-interest to champion the cause of the whites and Mulattoes, Toussaint switched allegiance back to the French, joining them in routing the British in brilliantly executed military campaigns, leading to his appointment as Lieutenant Governor of the island. His skillful military tactics combined with deft political calculation soon made him undisputed leader of this island, once rich, now utterly exhausted and destroyed by 10 years of burning revolution.

Reconstruction began. Toussaint proved to be as outstanding an administrator as a general, founding schools, rigidly enforcing work on the renovated estates, negotiating contracts with England and the United States, drawing up a constitution sent to France for ratification, working hard to persuade the skeptical world of the competence and enlightenment of this first black republic, worthy of their respect.

Napoleon, however, was no fan and throughout 1801 he prepared for the launching of the largest expeditionary force in history—eighty-six warships packed with troops to destroy this "gilded African," as he called Toussaint, restoring slavery and French dominance. The

French landed on February 5, 1802. On May 6 Toussaint agreed to an armistice, but rather than being permitted to retire to a plantation as agreed, he was betrayed, taken prisoner, shipped back to France in the warship appropriately called *Le Heros*. Incarcerated in a wet prison cell in Fort-de-Joux in the Jura Mountains, he died April 7, 1803.

His deportation, however, along with the news of the restoration of slavery on the islands of Guadeloupe and Martinique, aroused his countrymen. Led by Jean-Jacques Dessalines, the revolution ruthlessly rekindled, assisted by an opportune outbreak of yellow fever. The weakened and sick French troops were pushed closer and closer to the sea until on December 4, 1803, the island was free at last, after one of the bloodiest fights for independence in recorded history. Dessalines was proclaimed Governor-General-for-Life in the city of Gonaives on January 1, 1804, beginning a tradition of absolutist rule perpetuated throughout Haitian history. He was a tyrant—"the laborers can be controlled only by fear of punishment and even death," he said, while adjusting his wig and plumage, his uniform despite the sticky, tropical humidity. The country pretty much divided into laborers and soldiers, the subservience of the many to the few, populating a land utterly devastated by war. Disillusioned but not out, finally they rose up against this ruler who modeled himself after Napoleon. In 1806 he met his final destiny—assassination. It was to be only the first.

Learning their lesson with military absolutism and recognizing the value of separation of powers, the Haitians created a republic. It was good on paper, but when Henri Christophe was elected president, he promptly mustered his army, moving toward Port-au-Prince—so much for separation of powers. He was not successful, however, and Haiti split for the next thirteen years into a Northern Kingdom, ruled by Christophe, and a Southern Republic, governed by Alexander Pétion. They were diametrically opposed regimes, with Christophe's methods fruitful, Pétion's not. Sadly, the failure became the model for the country's future.

Christophe had been born of free Negro parents on the island of St. Christophe, whence his name. A waiter in the Crown Hotel in Cap François, he could neither read nor write, but he had learned the ways of the world. A proven military commander, he governed with equal authority and ability, firmly basing his kingdom on the work ethic and discipline, education and culture, master building and elitism.

His accomplishments are legion—vigorous agricultural development, roadbuilding, commerce, universal education, solid currency, a seven-part code of laws based on the French model. Following some of the policies of Toussaint and Dessalines, the people were bound to the earth as before, but allowed to make a profit, one-fourth of their yield.

They awoke to a bugle call in the morning, worked regular hours, were lashed for laziness, had Saturday afternoons and Sundays off. Each morning he checked into the state of warehouses, customs, and his treasury, growing each year with $3.5 million in revenues, greater than at any time since 1791.

Nevertheless, rebellion broke. Semiparalyzed by a stroke and unable to mount his horse, Christophe took his own life with a gold bullet through his heart, October 18, 1820. He left behind a treasury with $6 million worth of silver coins he had minted; an ungrateful and landed nobility scornful of his final weakness and infirmity; triumphant cries echoing through the land, "The King is dead!"

Pétion by contrast died two years earlier as unflamboyantly as he had lived, virtuous, compliant, and melancholic to his premature end at the age of forty-eight. An easy-going sort, his regime in the South featured laissez-faire carried to an extreme and charted Haitian land tenure on a course dooming its people to subsistence agriculture.

With iron-fisted Christophe and compliant Pétion gone, Haiti united under Jean Pierre Boyer for the remarkable span of twenty-five years, the longest term of office of any Haitian head of state. What he is most remembered for is his effort to resurrect the economy of the country along the lines of the policies of Christophe through the Rural Code of 1826. He failed miserably. It was the last attempt to reverse the tide in agriculture and turn the land back to the prosperity of the colonial period. The peasants simply had been free too long and the thought of again being bound to the soil with a production quota hanging over their heads was too close to the hurt of the lash for comfort. They ignored the decree and followed the French inheritance tradition, as was the custom in everything. Primogeniture did not apply. Land was equally divided among the sons upon the father's death, generation after generation, to this very day.

Something else happened during Boyer's years in the executive seat, more subtle but as enduring in impact. As the land was parceled and parceled, likewise the society increasingly broke apart, an irreconcilable cleavage, an elite—light-skinned, French-speaking, classically educated, nonworking—controlling the destiny of the peasant masses—black, Creole-speaking, illiterate, and very much working. No middle class existed to act as a buffer to these class antagonisms. Skin color ruled as supremely as it had during colonial times of the infamous 128 varieties.

Diplomatically, Boyer was understandably preoccupied with his country's poor face in the international community. Haiti had only "de facto" recognition of its sovereignty after all these years, with even France refusing to concede "de jure" recognition. This indifference and worse toward the world's first black republic seemed intolerable. In 1825 Haiti agreed essentially to buy its recognition from France, paying 150 million francs in five equal annual installments, a price the country could hardly afford despite Boyer's salary cuts and other economies. King Charles X published an ordinance granting independence, which of course Haiti already had, in exchange for this compensation for colonial property losses.

Haiti had tried to be a good neighbor, hopeful of friendship and notice of its revolution, courting the affection of other countries and merit of its existence with various maneuvers. The first president, Dessalines, had offered brotherhood to the Venezuelan patriot Francisco de Miranda. Petion provided safety to Simón Bolívar after his two defeats by the Spanish and equipped him for his third and unsuccessful assault on Venezuela, ultimately triumphing to create the Gran Colombia. Revolutionary Christophe had been among the eight hundred Haitian "volunteers" fighting the British in the American Revolution, alongside Washington at the siege of Savannah in 1778. Somehow none of this seemed to matter. When the first independent countries of the Americas met at the Congress of Panama in 1826, convened by Bolívar to promote an inter-American alliance—Haiti was not among them.

Why? Heavy economic dependence on the slave system. "The United States could never welcome Mulatto consuls or black ambassadors from Haiti," spoke the representatives from Missouri on the Senate floor, "because peace in the eleven states of the Union would not be preserved if these Mulatto consuls and black ambassadors were permitted to reside in our cities, travel throughout the country and, so doing, instill in our black citizens a spirit of revolt in order to benefit some day from the privileges and honors bestowed upon the Haitian representatives." Added the senator from South Carolina: "Our policy toward Haiti is clear. We will never recognize its independence." Hardly an isolated position, the Colombian minister for external relations told his delegation flatly, "Colombia is reluctant to entertain with Haiti the generally accepted relations of courtesy between civilized nations." So it was for decades. Black Haiti was ostracized by its definitely white and allegedly revolutionary counterparts in the Hemisphere.

Clearly, Haitian internal turmoil caused some of this "hesitation" through these years, sometimes called the Haitian Dark Ages, with government after government reaffirming at the minimum certain unfortunate characteristics. Statistically from 1804 to the American occupation in 1915, Haiti had twenty-six chief executives, a veritable procession of generals, presidents, kings, and emperors, of whom nine died in office, four of old age and illness and five from suicide, firing squad, or ambush; seventeen escaped into exile in the nick of time;

only four completed their terms of office or died peacefully; many just gave up in disgust and despair. It wasn't a very good record.

Throughout these decades the revenues of the country's coffee tax found their way into the pockets of the Mulatto elite despite the tyranny of a succession of black presidents . . . always at the expense of the peasant masses. A painful pattern had developed through this succession of dictators. A military oligarchy controlled the executive. The executive in turn promptly attempted absolutism. Personality, not ideas or platform, dominated politics. The opposition wanted overthrow. Every chief executive wanted to be President-for-Life. Paternalism kept the peasant down, poor, uneducated—and manageable. This is the gene pool of the Haitian political inheritance, stirred for over a century, and still viable today.

In between there occurred something called the U.S. occupation, officially dated from 1915 to 1934 when U.S. Marines departed the island, but nonmilitary United States presence continued for years later and economic influence appears perpetual. Pretexts were not hard to come by for this long visit. Political and economic chaos prevailed. Six presidents had held office in four years: one blown up in a palace explosion, the following four ousted by revolution, and the last, President Vilburn Guillaume Sam, chopped to pieces by a mob infuriated by his general's massacre in a nearby prison of all political prisoners, 167 of them. That was just what the United States had been waiting for. The marines landed that day at Bizoton and quickly gained control of the major points of the capital.

As might be expected, economics also figured in this decision for military intervention. World War I had begun the previous year and Haiti owed money to both France and Germany, making Washington skittish about the possibility of a concession of a naval or coaling station to the Europeans in their own backyard. Also, rampant corruption and borrowing by Haitian presidents had permitted the United States gradually to gain mortgage control over the National Bank and the National Railway Company. By 1914 the Haitian gourde had fallen to a low of 10.5 cents with the national debt taking 80 per cent of the revenues and the government unable to guarantee the dollar bonds of the railway. The American investment was slowly moving out to sea. This simply would not do. The Marines came in with the next convenient tide.

In the beginning the Americans built roads and bridges, hospitals and clinics, telephone lines and electric systems, salting wounds in the process. Peasants were required to work on road-building projects, a little bit of forced labor revisited. The American High Commissioner had a penchant for vetoes when his suggestions were not speedily heeded. The

WHY IT IS

word "bi-cephalous"—a monster with two heads—became descriptive of the puppet governments. The enforced right of foreigners to own land also aroused deep suspicion. The Mulatto population substantially increased, courtesy of a sexually-active Marine contingent. American officials appeared just a little too interested in the amortization of Haiti's foreign debt more quickly than the timing of agreements demanded, siphoning funds needed for development. American capital found a way to grow a little something. By 1930 seven American-owned companies controlled over 50,000 Haitian acres, having actually purchased only 13,000 of them.

Needless to say, many Haitians wanted the U.S. out. For four years, 1918-1922, a guerrilla war raged, the so-called Cacos War, with Benoit Batraville and Charlemagne Péralte leading bands of armed peasants against the Marines. An estimated 6,000 Haitians died in these clashes, which pretty much ceased with the nailing of Péralte's dead body to a barn door to inhibit further thoughts of rebellion against the occupiers.

In October 1929, students at the Central School of Agriculture called a strike which spread rapidly to other schools in the capital and towns. In December, a group of peasants in the South had been machine-gunned in their entirety by a company of trigger-happy Marines, a slaughter called "Marchaterre" for the small village nearby. Other Haitians were killed in reprisal for sniper shootings at St. Marc. National feeling switched from passive and sullen acceptance of the American presence to outranged aggressive moves for ouster. Troops were withdrawn in 1930, with an American fiscal agent remaining to control customs until the Haitian debt had been paid.

In an election free of American interference as well, Senator Stenio Vincent, a constant opponent of the occupation, came to power for a six-year term of office in 1930 along with many anticollaborationist senators and deputies. But international events cracked the pilings of his base. Thousands of Haitian sugar cane cutters were slaughtered in the cane fields of the Dominican Republic, shot with carbines and hacked to pieces with machetes. The finger of guilt pointed decisively at the government of Dominican dictator Trujillo. He denied nothing. At the conference table the Dominican Republic expressed regret for the tragedy, promised to punish the perpetrators, and pledged an indemnity of $750,000 for the rehabilitation of the families of the victims—they paid only two-thirds. The crime just had not been adequately avenged and Vincent's hopes for a third term were tarnished. He decided to retire, albeit in a sulk, in favor of his Washington representative, Elie Lescot.

The Washington-Port-au-Prince link solidified like a bear trap during Lescot's term of office. Three of the six directors of the National Bank

were designated to be Americans and the Haitian economy geared up to assist the United States, at war with the Japanese and the Axis powers.
Lescot used World War II as a pretext for military rule. He went too far. Early in 1946 his imprisonment of two young journalists provoked a general strike in the capital. The military took over and Lescot got a ticket to Canada.

After months of turmoil and jockeying for power, Dumarsais Estimé was elected president August 16, 1946, and on November 22, a new constitution brought fundamental social and political change to Haiti—and blacks to the executive office. They found a standard-bearer in Estimé, also a black, soon to be followed in power by others, Paul Magloire, François Duvalier, Jean Claude Duvalier. These are the main characters of the Haitian contemporary drama, well covered by the news stories emanating from this country, never surprising given this history.

Estimé did take two giant steps forward for Haiti, in education and health care. However, his socialist tendencies included moves to create collective farms for the peasants and created more than a little consternation among the members of the ruling class. When he did the usual and tried to succeed himself, the military responded with an invitation to exile.

Lescot appeared briefly on the scene to set up a provisional government, called the Government Junta, the most popular member being Colonel Paul E. Magloire, who, sensing the tide, resigned to run for president, and won. From 1950 to 1957 Haiti made slow but steady progress, perhaps a little too fast for Haiti's finances, further milked by unprecedented graft.

The country was virtually bankrupt when Duvalier took over and began to build the fortress which stands this moment as impregnable as Henri Christophe's Citadel, a structure buttressed by U.S. financial and technical assistance, lest Haiti go left like Cuba, Jamaica, Guiana, turning favorite tourist resorts into socialist strongholds. The money comes in securely to the government of Jean Claude Duvalier and the U.S.-trained and equipped "antisubversive unit," the so-called Leopard Corps, today walks the streets as "tonton macoutes," also U.S.-trained, did during the days of his father's presidency. The period of coolness and passive-aggressive disapproval demonstrated in a pullback of foreign assistance during the Kennedy years later has yielded to strategic political considerations.

3

WHAT THERE IS

"I remember one day I had a talk with a young American who was here for a project. He was saying that Haitians were so backward and there were not many things that could be done about it. I asked him this question: 'Suppose you were able to move all the Haitians out and bring five million Americans to Haiti. What do you think Haiti would be in ten to fifteen years from now?' His answer was that most likely Haiti would be a developed country. 'Then,' I said, 'why are you pessimistic about Haiti's future and Haitians developing it?'

"We have our problems. We have not been able to get together as five million Haitians. We still have urban Haitians and the peasants. But this is something that is going to change. It will take time to change. Just give us the time to realize it! That's the way I look at it . . . because we are all human beings with the same capabilities. The only difference is that the Americans know how to read and write and have a higher level of education, so we simply have to bring Haitians to a certain level of education. Also, it takes time and a lot of work in civic responsibility—because political action will be based on civic responsibility. . . . We will arrive at a time that five million Haitians are educated and there will be no question of the country changing. That's first.

"Secondly, I think our way of life should not be a repetition of America, France, Canada, England. . . . We should find a way of life that is related to our position as a small, mountainous, beautiful island, not a rich country, but where people can live very happily. We do not have a harsh climate . . . we have the sea nearby . . . and all we really need to have happiness is getting together to improve some of the material *conditions with our own concept of happiness. We should be able to be happy with the donkey and the jet plane. In a country like this one, I don't think we should say the age of the donkey and the horse is gone and feel we are backward because we are using donkeys and horses. This is a country for donkeys and horses! We should be using them when we need them. The plane when we need it. The helicopter when we need it. And still have a style of life that joins the past and the present together. . . .*

"Foreigners want things to change rapidly because they have been used to a very advanced country and they feel things are going slowly here. For a person who is living here, there are many things that are static but there is progress being done. . . . But, I think, what we really need is progress in attitude, in the minds of Haitians, their understanding and their participation in the development of the country—all of them—and their belief in the fact that there are no differences between an urban Haitian and a peasant. That's the fact that needs to be accepted. It will take time.

"Also you must understand that there are many forces—national and international—delaying the development of less advanced countries. I do believe that the richness of the great countries is based somewhat on the poverty of the third world. If the rich countries are always going to be rich, then the poor will stay poor for a long time. The problem of the third world is that for the rich to be rich, they have to get what the poor need. We must do our share to try to get together as five million Haitians and not have the few with everything and the remainder not having enough—that's what we have to do ourselves. Also, there must be greater understanding in the society of nations that the rich cannot keep getting all the basic things from the small countries while giving them an idea of life in rich countries and keeping them poor. I think these are the two things that could be done.

"I have lived here for more than half a century and I can see that Haiti is coming out of a time of turbulence and now we are becoming conscious of the need for organization. This is the beginning of change. Now Haitians know the country needs to be organized. I do believe also that more and more the masses of Haitians are becoming conscious that we cannot stay like that over and over again. There are many people who are socially minded and feel that this cannot continue, either. And that's why we feel we should not be pessimistic about it. But it is going to take time and a lot of effort, a lot of idealism and a lot of suffering. But I think we will arrive. If some human beings think they can change the country why cannot other human beings do it when all human beings are equal. Either they believe in human equality or

WHAT THERE IS

they still believe that all human beings are unequal—which would be something horrible!"—Ary Bordes

On the map the Republic of Haiti's boundaries look like the outline of a mouth opened in a scream with two jutting peninsulas, north and south, open lips enclosing the Gulf of La Gonave with Port-au-Prince smack in the center. Within its territory lives a deeply wounded society, staggered by differences.

Haitians are divided by a profound and immense social cleavage: four million rural peasants and one million urban dwellers dominated by a refined elite constituting only about five percent of the total. The division shapes Haitian society into a pyramid with only the top of the peak scented of Chanel No. 5; a tiny and beleaguered middle class just, but still far, below, about two or four percent, blending domestic perfume and perspiration; and the rest, reeking of unadulterated sweat from unrelieved work. There is Paris and its aspirants and there is Africa.

Perhaps the polarity can best be summed up in two words—voodoo and Creole—what 90 percent of Haitians believe and speak, a unique religious and linguistic situation greatly contributing to underdevelopment.

A Port-au-Prince taxi driver will devoutly make a grand-style sign-of-the-cross as he passes Sacred Heart Church, the morning after observing an eight-hour voodoo practice. The same morning scrawled in white paint on the church wall is the rebellious graffitti: "Vive le Voodoo Ancien!" Roman Catholicism has been Haiti's official state religion since the beginning but it is taken by the more sophisticated elite with several grains of salt, used more as a link with the philosophy of the outside world and bulwark against the voodoo-practicing masses than for salvation. The middle class, however, are devout, needing not a bulwark but a fortified rampart to protect them from any similarity to peasant religious practices. For his part, the peasant feels no conflict at all in his multifarious pantheon of pagan African deities and Christian saints and angels and doesn't really need the Church since he is so Catholic already, he thinks. He baptizes his babies and has as Christian a burial as he can get, marries when he can afford to, and attends Sunday Mass for social and display purposes. But deep in his hurting soul and at every minor and momentous event in his life from birth till death, voodoo lives—as the graffiti proclaims.

From the Dahomean term for "god," voodoo basically amalgamates African animism and ancestor worship with Catholic ceremony and spirituality. It is a religion of considerable complexity, all-pervasive and centering, essential to peasant existence, so full of deprivation and suffering. Voodoo explains peasant reality regardless of how desperate, gives meaning to experience, provides an outlet for pent-up angers and frustrations, retribution against enemies, medical care for illness, dignity within a humiliating life, social control and the comfort of the group, divine intervention on request, and recreation in music and dance. It is intimate and personal, more effective perhaps than most religions believed in this world, albeit unacceptable to the elite and their devotees.

The same dichotomy holds true of language. French is the language of every newspaper that publishes, all formal public occasions, formal private occasions, the medium of culture, arts, and refinement. It is the official national language of Haiti, so stipulated in every Haitian constitution—and there have been many. Yet, only 7 to 10 percent of the population speak and write French fluently; the rest communicate in Creole. Again, isolation, illiteracy, and impotence are reinforced for the vast numbers of Haitians whose language symbolizes and underscores inferic• position, ignorance, and impoverishment.

Haiti's language problems compound the problems of Haitian education, which needs everything—buildings, teachers, books, water, toilets, budget, recreational facilities, supplies. Most of all, it needs flexibility. The regimentation of school uniforms is symptomatic of the extremity of authoritarianism lavished on students, forced to learn by rote. Lessons are memorized verbatim. Little wonder that less than 32 percent of the children in the five- to fourteen-year-old category are in school despite the fact that primary education for the first six grades is compulsory by law. The rate of attrition is phenomenal; only 2 percent of those who walk in the door make it to the primary school certificate. The government says about 400,000 children are in Haiti's schools at the primary level, with the urban-rural breakdown 275,000 to 125,000, despite the reverse population concentration. About 54,000 students are in secondary school nationally; 1,500 attend the university. Illiteracy throughout the population is variously estimated from 75 to 85 percent, with almost half the capital's people able to read and write some, while only one in ten can in the rural area—among the world's worst ratios. Haitian education gets about eight percent of the meager national budget, meager because of the land.

When Columbus found Haiti by accident in his search for Asia, he was delighted, noting in his diary details of "mountains of very great size and beauty, vast plains, groves and very fruitful fields." It is not like that anymore. The mountains do remain; in fact, the name Haiti comes from an old Indian word meaning mountainous land. Three great mountain ranges crisscross the country, piling off into the distant mist, floating islands of magic and mystery, and millions of people have fashioned a strange life on their hillsides. Less than 20 percent

WHAT THERE IS

of this country lies below 600 feet from sea level; about 40 percent virtually floats at elevations over 1,500 feet. Because of this only one-third of Haiti's 10,714 square miles can be cultivated, and cruel jokes are told about peasants falling to their deaths while tilling some precipitous cornfield. He has little choice for there are less than two-and-a-half acres—one hectare—of arable land for every 5.2 Haitians, compared with the one hectare per 0.5 average for the rest of Latin America. Haiti's rugged terrain negatively impacts on vital internal communication and transportation as well as basic national cohesion.

The land is worse off than any battered child, the victim of massive deforestation centuries ago and erosion ever since. One agronomist claims that what was grown on one acre a few years ago, now takes ten to produce. In 1977 Haiti imported tens of thousands of tons of rice, maize, and even sugar. There was famine in the North.

As far as other natural resources go, Haiti has over 100 rivers and streams making their way to the surrounding seas, slow and meandering, often dry; only one, the Artibonite River, is navigable. There are two inland lakes. That's it. Scarcity of water dictates to this country more firmly than any tyrant has or likely ever will. While oil exploration continues to cause excitement, the black gold has yet to be found. What has been discovered and mined since 1957 is something of a comedown, bauxite. Haiti is not believed at this time to have much mineral wealth.

Haiti's greatest resource is its people. The best is also the worst, for the people are this country's Achilles heel, its tragic flaw. Haiti is the third most densely populated area in the world after Java and the Nile River basin. People are everywhere, scraping and hustling to make it, to live through the day. The rural population density averages 350 per square mile—far beyond what is considered viable—compared with less than 36 per square mile for the rest of Latin America.

While Haiti's 2.4 percent annual population growth is not considered high by Latin American standards, a lot of that moderate picture is due to high infant mortality, at least double the Latin American average. Consequently the fertility ratio—the number of children under five years for each 1,000 women of childbearing age—is about the Latin American average, at 139 births. But with 147 more babies living rather than dying per those 1,000 women, the situation would change radically.

The facts are that Haiti's population doubled in the period from 1920 to 1960, from 2.12 million to 4.13 million; the census figures culled in 1950 and 1971 indicated a population increase of 1,146,000, or 37 percent over the 1950 figures. At the current rate of increase Haiti will have at least eight, possibly twelve, million people by the year 2000. Another factor to throw into the mix is the youthfulness of the Haitian population. The median age is only nineteen years; 42

percent of the people are under fourteen. There are a lot of potential mothers coming to maturity. Also, Haiti has the highest rural-urban ratio, with 80 percent of its people on the land; a generation ago it was 90 percent. Most urban dwellers crowd among the 500,000 inhabitants of the country's only real city, the capital of Port-au-Prince, with other bits of urbanity scattered in ten small provincial towns with populations under 50,000.

The masses of Haiti's people, in urban slums or in the countryside, suffer from malnutrition, the country's biggest health hazard. The situation becomes particularly acute during the summer months when the crops are not producing, so there may be a single starchy meal and incessant chewing of sugar cane for energy. On the average of his one or two meals a day the Haitian consumes 1,633 calories and 47 grams of protein, well under the daily intake of 2,654 calories and 68 grams of protein for the rest of Latin America. The story is really told in the faces and the bodies of Haiti—stunted growth, underweight, poor muscular development, premature aging, premature death.

The pattern that kills Haitians starts early, according to one study, with 11 percent of one-year-olds and those younger suffering from significant malnutrition, rising to 24 percent from one to six years of age, leveling off to 10 percent from six to twelve years. Given the hunger it is ridiculous to quote data on vitamin, mineral, and other deficiencies. The problem is not enough food, and what is eaten is not nutritious enough. Over 70 percent of all food consumed by Haitians is fruit and vegetable types; food crops most in demand are high in starch—corn, millet, manioc, rice. Meat is rarely eaten with any regularity in the countryside, and if some is consumed, it will likely be goat or pork. The nutritional status of the urban poor is somewhat better than his country cousin, 2,450 calories a day, with average protein figures not available; but meat is readily found in the city. The elite, of course, eat superbly.

Another major health hazard is the housing, both urban and rural. Only about 20 percent of the houses of Haiti are considered even reasonably satisfactory, and Port-au-Prince slums rival the worst in the world. A survey made in 1971 indicated that only 22 percent of the houses were constructed of wood and brick; the rest were inadequate. The figures report that well over half of the housing has only two rooms, 15 percent with one room.

There are only fourteen water-supply services in the entire country and none can really claim to provide safe, potable water. Only 7,500 of the capital's houses have water connections, with less than 4,000 others reportedly connected in the rest of the country. About 57,500 urban dwellers are within access of a public fountain but another

WHAT THERE IS

677,500 people depend on rivers as their water source, while millions of others lug the precious commodity in calabash gourds from a water hole.

There is virtually no sewage system in Port-au-Prince, with only 8,000 urban houses connected. The wealthy have septic tanks and cesspools; the poor have latrines, about 134,000 of them, or the minimal privacy and nonexistent sanitation of a wall or a corner for 687,000 other Haitians surveyed. In a tropical downpour the streets of Port-au-Prince overflow into everything, and the foul odors of this city are as characteristic as the braying of packs of watchdogs all night long and the rousing of roosters with the dawn. Only about 13 percent of the capital's housing has electricity.

The poor nutritional state of Haiti, combined with poor sanitation, affects health to the extent that the most generally encountered diseases and difficulties of a tropical climate are not Haiti's biggest problems. No less than 78 percent of all preschool deaths are said to be related to malnutrition and diarrhea. Malnutrition and tuberculosis compete for first place for Haiti's high death toll. While more and better-qualified medical personnel and better-equipped facilities are desperately needed, what would improve Haitian health more is simple—more food, potable water, and latrines.

And there is another unique problem. Louis Pasteur is not appreciated, but pouty ancestors and the spirits of the underworld are. Sickness and disease are considered supernatural in origin, spiritual rather than physical, and the voodoo priest is visited first for his diagnosis, amulets, prayers, and exorcisms. Medicine is swamped by superstition, ignorance, and fatalism. Often, there would be no alternative anyway, given the scarcity and distance of modern medical care. The best bet may well be the local leaf doctor, a skilled herbalist, with his remedies of camomile flower to reduce tumors, soursop for sedation, and wild plum leaf for chills.

Making it through the life cycle in Haiti is a feat, an enormous test of endurance which begins at birth. The survival-of-the-fittest axiom applies from the first cry of life. From 10 to 15 percent of all babies born die within the first eight weeks because of umbilical tetanus from poor hygiene practices surrounding birth. Tetanus of the newborn is the single most important cause of the high infant mortality, a situation which has continued in this country for two hundred years. At six months, 20 percent of Haitian mothers have weaned their babies on starchy gruels, bananas soaked in sugar cane water, and other foods conspicuously absent in protein. At this tender age the Haitian child already has begun to fall behind infants in more prosperous environments and has begun another round in this fight for life that persists every day that breath is taken. Undernourished and protein-starved, diarrhea further will loosen this precarious hold on life. About one-fourth of all children born will die between the ages of one and four years. The survivors are so weakened constitutionally that they have little resistance to disease in general. Chances are nearly overwhelming of becoming host to intestinal parasites. In one study done in 1975 of 2,000 people, 75 percent had parasites, augmenting rapidly by age. Pinworms and roundworms are endemic.

Then there is the burden of tuberculosis, the major killer of Haitians of all ages, with research indicating Haiti among the most infected countries in the world. In one large survey conducted in 1970 by the Haitian health department, three percent of those researched had active tuberculosis and 20 percent of those under fifteen were infected. You can hear it, infant coughing, old-age coughing, painful, prolonged coughing, a racking of the throat and lungs, a low barking sound that goes on and on. The figures on tuberculosis mortality vary according to source, from the official 3.3 percent provided by the Haitian Bureau of Tuberculosis Control, to 8.5 percent, claimed by the World Health Organization.

Valiant efforts have been made to eradicate malaria but the disease still debilitates people living in some areas, about 52 of the country's 560 rural sections. While it is no longer a major cause of death, about three-fourths of all Haitians living in malarial areas are said to have suffered from the disease at one time or another, or maybe many times. Intestinal infections are a major medical and public-health problem. Typhoid and paratyphoid are serious and endemic in a number of urban areas, unsolvable until urban sanitation is developed. Epidemics occur frequently during the dry months. Dysentery constitutes another major difficulty.

As usual, health organizations and services are centralized in the capital despite the effort to regionalize into eleven health districts nationally. Port-au-Prince's eleven hospitals are half of those available in the entire country; two-thirds of all doctors and nurses work in the capital. The ratio of physicians really tells the tale: six for every 10,000 people in Port-au-Prince and 0.6 for the rest of Haiti—and these are often based in provincial towns, not the mountains and valleys where Haitians are packed in each acre.

Haiti started out with very few health institutions and virtually no doctors. In 1808 a school of health was created for health officers and in the 1860s there were five hospitals in the country. At the beginning of the American occupation in 1915, the figure had doubled to all of ten. The brain drain has been formidable. From 1928 to 1960, 960 doctors were graduated from Haiti's medical school and over 70 percent of them left the country for greener pastures abroad. In 1972 the dean of the medical school went on record as saying there were 600 Haitian doctors practicing in the United States, 300 in Canada, 200 in France, and many others in Great Britain, other countries, and international health and development organizations. The situation was so debilitating that in 1969 a law was passed prohibiting trained medical personnel from emigrating. During the 1960s it was difficult to enter medical school without strong political backing, another factor in the shortage of physicians.

Most recent data indicates Haiti has about 550 doctors, counting the most recent medical-school classes in their entirety, before they get to the airport; 350 dentists; 500 nurses; and 2,000 paramedical personnel—to serve its five million people. Most physicians, probably 98 percent, do work part-time in the Haitian health department, often halfheartedly because of the low salary level and lack of any incentive system to reward performance. A professor at the medical school gets on the average only about $60 to $80 a month, which gives a good indication why Haitian medical staff depend largely on private practice for sustenance. About $1 per capita of the national budget is allocated for health.

While Haitian health continues to suffer, a lot has been accomplished, perhaps more in this single area of development than any other. But with malnutrition and sanitation such basic barriers to a more wholesome and secure life, the Haitian economy must improve first for any real breakthroughs to occur.

Haiti was the only country in the world that experienced almost no growth in the 1950s and 1960s, according to the United Nations. Data is really so insufficient to come to any hard facts, but the underemployment rate is thought to be about 60 percent of the labor force in the countryside and 40 percent in the capital. Others claim the truth is closer to 80 percent. There has been definite movement since Jean Claude Duvalier took office in 1971. The balance-of-payments situation is much improved, there is more tourism, better business confidence, new banks coming in all the time, foreign reserves rising to record levels, and construction also up. But with the perpetually expanding population, Haiti continues to have the lowest per capita income in the hemisphere.

To speak of the Haitian economy is to refer to the land and hoeing farmers, trudging market women, and cacophonous market scenes like an import from Senegal. Haiti is an agricultural country supreme; its obsession with the land is unique in the Caribbean. About half of the gross national product comes from this sector, with manufacturing and commerce respectively adding another 10 percent, and government, mining, utilities, and other sources rounding out the total.

Most characteristic of Haitian agriculture is the small plot size and subsistence level of production. Estimates are about 600,000 family farms nationally. About half of the plots are thought to be less than three acres and 70 percent, less than six acres—often split into two or more parcels. Another problem is the lack of cash reserve for credit and for emergencies like hurricanes and droughts, so the peasant is stuck with what little he has. His trait of suspicion, given the fear of inviting envy or thievery if he pulls a little ahead, has implications in his work habits, holding him steadfast in traditional ways. Few educational facilities are available to change his mind.

Growth of the domestic market is retarded severely by the narrow consumer buying power. Demand for goods and services can hardly be very strong when the vast majority of Haitians are farmers outside of the cash economy. Consumption patterns indicate most peasant families spend about half of their income on food.

The communications barrier has retarded the economy and everything else. Not too long ago telephone communication was pretty much limited to overseas calls from the West Indies Telephone Company office. Now telephones can be found ubiquitously in government offices, businesses, and private homes. They don't always work, but they more often do. Then there are the Haitian roads—or better yet, their lack. When the Americans came to Haiti there were 210 miles of passable road in dry weather in the entire country. By 1929 there were 1,000 miles of roads and by 1948, 1,700 miles. The mountains have created tremendous obstacles to opening up the countryside, breaking down the isolation and making Haiti accessible. French engineering and financial assistance this moment are changing that, and Haiti's new road system is one of its most exciting developments, with enormous potential to link all Haitians together into one national entity. Getting the goods, the services, and the resources into the countryside—when such a desire has existed—has always been a task on par with Sisyphus pushing his rock up the mountainside. The task has been left to bare feet and public buses—like Haitian markets, permeated with folk charm but hardly efficient.

These are some of the facts behind the suffering.

[PART II]

4

GETTING ACQUAINTED

"I was always interested in helping ... that is part of my inner self."

"When you live in a country like Haiti and have an opportunity to compare the conditions of work and of life, at the beginning of your work you can have periods of discouragement. There is what you would like to do and what you cannot do. The fact that organization might be better and more could be done. But you have to understand also that if everything were all right, we would be a developed country—that is the harshness of the reality. Your hopes and the reality. Sometimes you can have moments of discouragement; it takes a lot of strength not to be discouraged.

"I think I have reached the point now where I don't think I can be discouraged. I have passed the threshold of discouragement. I don't think I can be discouraged anymore. I know the country well and I know how to avoid failure much better and I know also how to limit the level of success. I know what to expect. I am more careful and I move more slowly.

"For instance, I don't aim too high. I aim closer to reality. I move just like a staircase, step by step, instead of trying to go very high. Because I have learned to cope ... I have learned the mechanism of underdevelopment. And once you learn the mechanism, you know you should not be discouraged by what you see around you. As a matter of fact, you learn how to change things and know the value of time. You learn that progress is going to be slow and expect some failure and not be discouraged by it."—Ary Bordes

In the early 1960s Haiti's lowest per capita income, high birth rate, and lack of international assistance increasingly attracted the attention of up-till-then cool North and Latin American neighbors. Haiti became a topic of conversation among international organizations convening here and there to provoke development and catalyze social improvements. "It was obvious that of all the needy countries in Latin America, Haiti was number one," recalls Miss Alice Sheridan, a frequent conferencegoer at the time in her capacity as director of medical programs for the Boston-based Unitarian Universalist Service Committee, a small social-service foundation.

"Those Latins fight like . . . ," she makes a spitting sound—very strange coming from a retired career "lady" in severe French twist, pearls, and tweed-suited correctness, "but when they agreed," she continues, "they AGREED! And they could supply the specialists in different disciplines, affected as they were by the same terrain. And to get them to agree was really something. It's quite an experience, believe me."

She had had many through her long and multifarious career, including a stint as editor of *Cosmopolitan* magazine and a job in public relations in the Hollywood heyday of child stars. She had been involved in administration at the Service Committee since 1959, what seemed sterile but made the wheels go round, kept her moving, and dealing with doctors—who only talked with each other, she discovered.

In 1963 the Organization of American States agreed on the acuteness of the Haitian nutrition issue and passed a resolution to that affect. The fact was noted well by the Interamerican Institute for Children, an organization committed to health development—particularly, child health. The institute had organized a series of conferences in different Latin American countries, always upon the request of the respective national government. Their job was to assemble international technicians and specialists to join with nationals and take a severe look at the medical, social, geo-economic, and cultural realities of a country. Then it would be the job of the host government to translate the joint recommendations into specific follow-up programs, hopefully backed by international assistance generated by the publicity and commitment aroused by the conference.

In 1964 Dr. Maria Luisa Saldun de Rodriguez, an Uruguayan pediatrician and director of the institute, began having discussions with the Haitian government and a large planning committee of eighteen Haitians involved in health. From these sessions emerged the National Seminar on Nutrition in Haiti, to be held in Port-au-Prince from May 30 to July 4, 1965. To be convened with the cooperation of the Unitarian Universalist Service Committee, the collaboration of the United Nations'

Food and Agricultural Organization and World Health Organization, the Williams-Waterman Fund of New York, and with financial assistance from the U.N. Children's Emergency Fund, it would be the first time Haitian medical professionals, social workers, agronomists, engineers, and nutritionists met in seminar.

The conference began with a formal reception in the presidential palace, where 700 screened guests waited an hour for the appearance of President François Duvalier, signaled by the playing of the presidential hymn. What followed was a two-hour ceremony packed with suspense. All stood as the frail-looking president, flanked by military aides and surrounded by his personal bodyguard, marched slowly down the long aisle to the dais, where he sat facing the participants but near an exit, just in case. The name of each guest was called out for a personal handshake with the president, making a rare public appearance. "It was all carried off with great aplomb," Miss Sheridan recalls. "President Duvalier had been ill so it was a great honor to have his presence, and he reminded us all that he was a physician and bringing health to the island was one of his greatest wishes."

In his address, also a rarity, he recounted his own efforts and praised the work of those who had eradicated yaws and reduced malaria, wishing success to those now searching for an answer to Haiti's malnutrition and related diseases. His text was distributed and later published in full in the local press.

"It all went very smoothly," she continues, vividly impressed by " 'tonton macoutes' all across the way in baggy trousers with machine guns under their arms . . . a command performance, but the tension was so strong. I remember pocketbooks being examined, but not mine—didn't look like a moll"—she laughs—"and this U.S. government official turning to me and saying, 'Alice, look at you and me, we're right in the line of that gun.' And you know . . . we were! That's the way they were operating. People were afraid and didn't go out at night except in groups of officials."

At noon the president left the assembly, escorted down the long hall by the military to the tune of the band. A disturbance outside the palace was quickly squelched with seemingly little force as guards inched an hysterical woman slowly down the stairs and drove her off in a commandeered car.

Miss Sheridan was accompanied to the conference by the chairman of the Service Committee's medical advisory committee, also representing the Foundation for International Child Health of New York, Dr. Samuel Z. Levine. Well into his seventies, he had begun to repeat himself, but that was ignored because he was full of the wisdom and humility of old age, at the finale of a most distinguished career. Short and stooped, fatherly and empathetic, Dr. Levine was a world-recognized pediatrician, a professor emeritus on the faculty of Cornell University, whom President John F. Kennedy had called in desperation to save his prematurely born infant when all else seemed hopeless. When he entered a room people rushed to greet a great man.

"We were the tall and short of it," Miss Sheridan comments laughingly of their height discrepancy and constant togetherness during the week's events. They had come to explore the possibility of setting up some type of health program in Haiti and paid close attention to the many papers presented at the conference and the Haitians they met.

Among other field trips they made a rugged hour-and-a-half drive in a rented Volkswagen over muddy deeply rutted, almost impassable roads, to inspect a nutrition center for malnourished children under one year in a village called Fond Parisien. "We went over these awful roads! I almost had a broken back!" she says, quite literally. She was jounced out of "the jalopy," fortunately landing on something soft, but nervous because of her history of disc problems.

While the roads are something embedded in her consciousness forever, so was the shocking malnutrition and sanitation along the route. "You could see the women washing in these filthy streams of water . . . going off to market with so little money, selling food to get other food . . . people hanging off the tops of buses. . . . It was terribly depressing in this day and age." They finally arrived.

At the center selected sick infants were being cared for by a locally trained high-school graduate assisted by rotating mothers from the village, all directed by Haitian medical specialists. There were a dozen or so babies about and food was being prepared and the mothers educated. It was a small project. The babies' progress was carefully recorded and after four months' supervision they were returned to their families, mostly cured or visibly improved, to be replaced by another group. The work by the Haitian bureau of nutrition was being funded by the Williams-Waterman Foundation, one of the conference sponsors. It was something.

But the highlight of the week definitely came on Tuesday, with the presentation of a paper on "Infant Malnutrition: Cultural Factors," by a Haitian pediatrician named Dr. Ary Bordes. "We were carried away by it, really. He was so low key and modest while the others . . . a few of them were real orators with all their charts and bombast, giving the impression that they could cure everything if they had the wherewithal. But he was, well, in the first place, he was more realistic. We didn't think this was just a dreamer coming through, but a man quietly saying, 'Now if I could'. . . ."

It was a well-researched paper, giving strong credit to folk beliefs and

GETTING ACQUAINTED

demonstrating an impressive knowledge of Haitian medical and social anthropology, plus a sympathetic portrayal of the meager financial resources available to the masses of Haitians and their long cultural isolation. It was scientific and disciplined, but the compassion for his people's suffering came through with a restrained intensity: "A country is built by the work of its citizens," Ary Bordes concluded. "And it can never really progress without eliminating from its territory the specter of hunger. The infinite sadness of our malnourished children in our hospital wards weighs heavily upon this entire country. It is in the eyes of its children that the spirit of a people is reflected. Until we have brought a smile to the faces of the children of our cities and countryside, our work will not have been achieved." He modestly left the podium.

"Dr. Levine nudged me and said, 'This man is really something. Maybe we should meet him and see if he sees any further.' That was the quality. Very sincere. It was low-key but hopeful, not for tomorrow, but for the future. He seemed to be looking over the Antilles at the future with silver laps of the waves and he expected them to come in. Plus, he had knowledge of what he was talking about and it was *practical* knowledge! But above all what impressed us—he seemed truly dedicated. That if he got a hand he would go forth and give this same spirit to the other people who wanted to, but did not have what he had to give." They resolved to pursue this man and his thinking further. Prematurely snow-white-haired, diminutive of build, wearing black-rimmed glasses, quiet of manner, almost gently sad, handsome except for protruding teeth, he seemed different.

He is. For one thing, Ary Bordes is a small-town boy, no Port-au-Prince-spoiled elitist. And you can take the boy out of Jacmel but maybe you never can really take Jacmel out of the boy, which is the way it sounds even today: "When I came back to Jacmel after visiting all the cities, I thought—is there a more pleasant city?! It is more pleasant than Saint Marc and Petit Goave, Gonaïves, than Jérémie, than Port-de-Paix. The only city outside of Port-au-Prince you might discuss and say you like better is maybe Cap Haitien . . . well, it is normal that I think like that."

Three days' horseback ride from Port-au-Prince through Haiti's formidable mountain barriers, Jacmel was a provincial, protective place to grow up, with a quiet and sleepy ambiance touched with the softness of life. There were few cars along its unpaved streets, even fewer radios, no water on Wednesdays, the hometown newspaper was called *The Bee*, and Mr. Poux once was the richest man in town, living in a big balustraded house with a conical-shaped tower on top, like a dunce cap. He made it in coffee.

This town of about 8,000 in Ary Bordes's boyhood once boomed with coffee trading to the vibrations of over 100,000 bags a year, half of the country's export in the flourishing 1890s. The town's elite sealed their social eminence with those coffee beans, their wealth peaking with the feats of Eiffel. Jacmel is an architectural jewel, one of the world's finest examples of the glory of forged and cast iron. Like a Mediterranean hilltown, it steps gradually back and up from the Caribbean shoreline of its port; its two-storied houses and commercial buildings pastel-painted and overwrought with ironwork; its provincial pedestrians slowly making their way along crooked, wandering streets up the hillsides.

Ary Bordes's Jacmelian roots date back to the 1840s, well fertilized with French influence and more than a garnish of human idealism. His great-grandfather had been in charge of the guard in Guadeloupe in 1793, where he lived with his three hundred slaves and strong political opinions. He was a liberal and considered a traitor for his views on human rights, ultimately forcing him to leave, but not before he had freed his workers. He settled on the Dominican Republic side of the united Haiti, then moved to Jacmel with the separation of the island again into two nations. Bordes's grandmother had a very big store in Jacmel, one of the biggest, which she maintained until late in life, when she moved to Paris, where she died. Her property on the town's main market square across from the white Spanish-style cathedral of St. Philippe and St. Jacques has been a store for the past thirty years, run by Bordes's uncle upon his return from twenty years of living in Paris. It is filled with little boxes of buttons, toys, and haberdashery items. His aunt had a fabric store; his mother's store featured glasses, enamel cookware, lamps, and other household goods. His father was a judge. Ary Bordes is a solid member of Haiti's merchant and administrative Mulatto class, the upper class of provincial town life, comfortable but aware that others were much richer, those coffee-merchant families sending their children to France for schooling.

Born February 26, 1924, his was a secure beginning with an entrenched pattern of life pursued precisely day after day, familial and supportive. The youngest child who reached outside for companionship, he had an older, often ill and troubled brother, and an older sister, all arriving quickly after twelve years of his parents' marriage. His father had been a lawyer and school inspector before being appointed president of the Jacmel court, a short walking distance from their home. Like clockwork every noon Bordes could watch his father coming down the street with maybe two or three other judges. Their court day concluded, they arrived at the Bordes home for one—and only one—cocktail, not indulged in, however, by his father, who solely provided hospitality, except when he indulged in a before-Sunday-dinner drink, a habit his son perpetuates to this day. About four or five in the afternoon the family would dress to socialize with relatives and friends, rotating tea and talk at different homes, just sitting, conversing, and enjoying company. Every evening his father returned home—Bordes knew it must be 7 P.M.

Strongly disciplined, Ary Bordes's father was an exceptionally quiet man, not active socially or very expressive. He neither smoked nor drank nor believed much in religion, as did his wife. Involved in a distinguished career, he took his work very seriously and did his best, always. He was a man of great integrity, an exceptional characteristic in a society which traditionally has had low salaries for public officials, virtually forcing and almost anticipating more "creative" sources of livelihood. His son took note: "What struck me most in the life of my father was his honesty. He would never have done anything dishonest or against his conscience and he stressed honesty," inculcating the trait in his son, a man of total, virtually fierce, integrity.

Ary Bordes is impeccably honest and never does many of the standard Haitian things, the "moon" syndrome, in Creole terms—patronage. He does not use the staff car for personal reasons; put a member of the family on the payroll; take a rake-off; absent himself from the job. And while low salaries and few opportunities make these human weaknesses very understandable, he will fight almost to the death against such behavior if within his managerial control.

His father cultivated idealism in his children and paid close attention to their intellectual development, and Ary Bordes often speaks of a letter he received from his father during his days as a resident doctor in the United States. It was so typical. "He wrote me to always keep my illusions and that would keep me going. Keep up your goal and try to realize it. That's the way to accomplish meaningful things in life," he told him—another lesson very evidently learned by a person who exudes optimism, refuses to be daunted by a defeat or dissuaded from an objective, no matter how long it takes.

The letter sounded a recurring theme of his childhood, as does every bookstore, which Ary Bordes cannot escape without a purchase. A book was ordered from France every month and eagerly awaited. Every July before vacation, eight or nine books would come, little volumes on Greek history, the Haitian revolution, the lives of insects and animals, to occupy productively some of the month's leisure time, teaching him to love to learn and have a lot of "shoulds."

Always growing, developing, overcoming, Ary Bordes is the archetypal eagle scout. "I am trying to develop that, " is one of his recurring phrases. While he reads no poetry or fiction, just public health—everything he can get his hands on—he is concerned about his one-sidedness.

One of his "shoulds" is to have another interest. He even tried to develop an appreciation for classical music in the fifties, a failure despite hours of listening and reading. Years later, in the late sixties and early seventies, he would succeed in developing a diversion from his work. Haitian art would be cultivated and collected passionately, more than an interest in the aesthetic, an expression of his powerful nationalism—another legacy of a father who would retire from the court only after a long career, well into his seventies, and who struggles today with the blindness of his nineties.

The governance of the household rested with Ary Bordes's mother, a fact of life he recalls vividly—"My mother was a very strong person, a VERY STRONG person," disciplined and authoritarian. "You had to be on time for food . . . if it were Saturday and you forgot about the time, well, she would say, 'Then you don't eat!' You had to come home and eat at SEVEN." To this day when 7 P.M. nears Ary Bordes gets edgy and heads home for dinner. Any venturing from the straight and narrow creates a discomfort that nothing is really worth. She died in 1970 but lives on in her son's sense of duty and awareness of the virtues of an ordered existence, which he is grateful for, along with his habit of reflection and silence—since there was little point in arguing with her. He is a vision of repressed rage forty-plus years later when he thinks of that time when he was thirteen and his mother refused to permit his bringing a bicycle, purchased with his own savings, on a family vacation because he needed it in good shape for school traveling. "I was SO MAD!" But he couldn't do anything save obey.

So Ary Bordes learned to listen and not to talk, developing a certain introversion and passive aggression, a tendency to be quiet, careful, patient, and very realistic. He thinks rather than bursts, making up his mind silently and deliberately about what he is going to do when the proper time comes and how hard he will push. He is very controlling and can be ruthless in his utter goal-directedness, like a bowling ball splintering the pins in the direct line of his path. Inhabiting a most highly pyramided authority structure, like most Haitians, he loves power and can abuse it, although through the years he has been tempered by experience. There is a gentleness and sweetness in this man, much shyness and sincerity, surfacing on the rare occasions he feels safe. He suffers when he sees things going the wrong way, although he has a remarkable capacity to let things flow. He is a fighter who has learned the pragmatics of trying things on for size and when to quit.

Also, Ary Bordes is a loner, not uncommon for someone who finds his fulfillment in his work. Rarely does he discuss a problem with anyone. He appears to have few close friends and is not often seen in large companies; he has few close collaborators, for the competition is fierce in Haiti, not the cooperation. From a few difficult experiences he has learned to go it alone with his vision and determination well contained within his inner self with very private complications. He is a driven man, compelled to do good for people, and while he does have a personal life, his work is by far the larger part of his life.

"I have learned to live with myself," he would say one day. "Although I don't like loneliness, I cannot say I suffer from loneliness," he would add, "because I think if I am lonely I feel lonely first and after a while I feel I am losing my time. Then I have to do something. Then I am not lonely anymore.... Then it is just normal life and I don't feel any pain anymore.... I value work a lot," he continued. "First I feel that it is worthwhile and makes you feel that you are more useful. And it helps overcome worries and takes the place of worry, because if your mind is occupied on the work, then you don't have time to worry. So I use work as a way of life.... As a matter of fact, I am very happy in my kind of work. I enjoy it, and as a matter of fact again, it is difficult for me just to get out of it because professionally I am a very happy person."

Ary Bordes does not like to reveal vulnerability—ever. If you listen to him ... he never gets discouraged ... never loses control ... never. ... The same for his country ... no racism ... firm backing from the health department ... any Haitian can be anything he wants to be.... He denies. But very obviously, he is an exceedingly fulfilled professional who likes being an internationally distinguished public-health specialist in demand to give papers ... receiving unsought funds. He has worked and he has succeeded, as was expected.

His family lived modestly but comfortably enough in a two-story wooden house graced with a double colonnade supporting an encircling balcony in the Bel Air section of town, on top of a hill, surrounded by relatives and friendly neighbors. In the beginning there was no electricity and never a car, typical of the lack of extravagance. Other values were stressed. Years later, when confronted with American materialism and many job offers abroad for more money and prestige as his reputation grew, he would remember what he had been taught. While impressed, deep within him came an emergency brake, a recognition of the importance of limiting material desires to a certain comfort level. There were other forms of happiness to be pursued. "The only worry I have about money is to see if I can't find the money for the work, to organize things and contribute to things ... ," he would comment, never seriously considering lucrative alternatives despite the stature of the position, the breadth of field. Ary Bordes is not ambitious in the usual sense of the word. He is ambitious for his country and his people. He is dedicated to his work in Haiti—period.

Mostly his boyhood was a happy time developing a centered personality, relaxed and friendly, someone who would like to laugh, and party later on. There was a pet rooster and a pet goat, a fascination with writing numbers ad infinitum and a curiosity about the goings on in the town slaughterhouse, kite flying contests, games of tops and marbles and groups of 20 and 30 children riding horseback along the beach Sundays. There were haircuts at Simonis', tiny candy balls to put on cakes from the corner pharmacy off the main square, also home for a large bottle of blood suckers used as a prescription. A trumpet call attracted his attention and he heard the towncrier reprimand bad Carnival behavior; he held the bridal train at the baker's daughter's wedding. The movie theater was silent with a very fat lady at the entrance who played the piano for such features as "Buffalo Bill"; there were concerts in the town square shaded by mellow old mahogany trees and parties with Haitian jazz and dancing at Chez Marcel's on the corner. Mostly there were walks. "I have spent evenings of my life walking, *walking* back and forth and around," he recalls. Groups of boys and girls, eyes open, virtually pacing along the town's main pier, beginning to sea tip and back again, infinitely, until the wood appeared to wear thin. At which point it was time to venture up the hillside to the main square and rotation around and around the mahogany trees.

It was a childhood of innocence, a generation behind its time frame, with those blood suckers swimming, silent films, transportation by horseback, and walks.

Plus, it was characterized by an absence of class distinction. As a child Ary Bordes played frequently with peasant children, disliking social barriers. The children would come by, call him out to play, and he would spend the day shooting marbles made of pebbles, chasing birds with slingshots, and visiting their families. He was attracted to the people and was liked in return, and particularly looked forward to vacation periods and more adventures with peasant friends outside of the town.

It was a liking that would persist. Ary Bordes is almost strangely democratic toward the masses of his countrymen, compassionate and respectful, considering the attitude of most members of his class. He has gone just about as far as a professionally educated upper-class Haitian can go in understanding what the Haitian peasant feels, believes, and needs, and he secretly fumes at elitism. He likes the people; he enjoys their company.

In addition, Ary Bordes's early years were spent under the American occupation, with the graffiti on the bases of the town monuments proclaiming the familiar, "Yankee, go home!" He remembers that angrily, and coupled with his experience with racism while doing his residency in the United States and graduate work in public health, he exhibits a range of ambivalence on through deep distrust toward foreigners. Very surely this includes the Americans who occupied his country during those formative years, knew more than he did when he attended their schools, and worse, upon whom he was to be so financially dependent through the years in order to fulfill his dreams. There is a big third-world defensiveness in this man, a single-celled layer of thin-skinned nationalism. He is always looking for the imperialist arrogance he knew as a child, and since he is looking for it, he finds it whether it is there or not. "He sets a tone of suspicion," went one opinion of his influence in the health department. There is something of the big frog in a small puddle about Ary Bordes. He can be intimidated by too much Harvard. He is a small-town boy who has made it big in the very big world of international jet-setting specialists, but remains provincial in some ways, which are really nationalism to the extreme. He wants Haitians running everything; Haitians controlling their own destiny. Even if they don't do it as well, he wants them in the slots. No more occupiers for Haiti. "Yankee go home" revisited.

Chez Les Rocs, an old wooden schoolhouse, gave him his first taste of education, a civilian school, pleasant but without memorable experiences, as was the College Bloncourt, a private school run by a Frenchwoman, which he attended from age six to eleven. It was in 1930 that he made his first trip away from Jacmel. He was six years old, and the city of Port-au-Prince seemed full of magic, with President Stenio Vincent's recent election and the capital's trees filled with lights. "That was too marvelous for me . . . such a big city, too!" Five years later at the age of eleven he was sent to Port-au-Prince for secondary education at the Small Seminary College of St. Martial, just like a British public-school boy prematurely separated from his family, only to be reunited two years later when his mother closed the store with his father's appointment to a supreme-court judgeship in the capital. It was 1937.

Although when he was sixteen and seventeen he really wanted to be a sailor, there were no maritime schools in Haiti at the time and Ary Bordes would choose medicine instead. In July 1947 he received his medical degree from the School of Medicine of Haiti, where he would be remembered for his student activism. Some say radicalism. He calls it idealism. The issues seem benign enough—improved administration of the school, better teachers, better courses, housing for the students, a cafeteria. It was Bordes's group that pushed for all students to wear white medical shirts rather than suits, cutting down on clothing expenses. They got that. A spirited member of the Association of Medical Students, he wrote articles in their journal and was a member of the delegation that got a hearing with President Dumarsais Estimé, airing grievances and urging reform. "We wanted change! To have a better school!" It was as simple as that—and naive. Various political interests often have used the medical students for agitation purposes, in keeping with their own disrupting tactics, something Ary Bordes was unaware of. Others were politically more sophisticated and in turn suspected his motives as politically motivated and self-interested maneuvering. Only in retrospect would he realize the political implications. At the time his mind was on medicine, not politics—a position that has not changed.

To this day Ary Bordes is known to be uninterested in political power per se. It has never been part of his dream. While consummately political, his political astuteness actualizes that old idealism for medicine, public-health medicine now. It is the work that comes first, always, and politics gets attention, use, and/or neutralization in order to help get the job accomplished. His position is clear and known, and the powers that ebb and flow let him do his work. Although politically Ary Bordes matured very late, he has learned well, and often has a defined strategy in mind. Not a natural, he has worked at it, as much as he could, reading books on politics, successful negotiation, body English, unconscious motivation, struggling to expand his awareness of the human factor's presence and dynamics in any endeavor. He has read a great deal about many things and has had ample opportunity to observe, calculate, and perfect the art of the possible in his highly political milieu. Politics undeniably impacts on his work and he values his work enormously. He does what he has to do. He didn't always, but he almost always does now.

Once an M.D. and in keeping with the state requirement, Ary Bordes was sent by the government to serve his medical residency, contributing to his country, which had educated him free of charge. He was stationed in Grand Rivière du Nord, outside of Cap Haitien, a town of about 9,000, situated along a riverbank, so not lacking the water resources that generally doom rural Haitians, and famous as the birthplace of the great Haitian writer and ethnologist Jean Price-Mars. It was one of the first locations where Americans established a clinic during the early years of the occupation, around 1922, and when he arrived the dispensary was still there—unfortunately, occupied by the internal revenue service. So his clinic was located in his home, which he shared with the local lieutenant, now a general. It was a comfortable house, yellow with gray doors, with its own well and a little garden in the backyard, where he grew vegetables. He was friendly with the neighbors across the street and liked to party at the Le Reveil Club across from the usual dominating white cathedral, rather posh priests' rectory next door, the military headquarters, and local masonic lodge, all encircling a bare main square.

It was an obscure town with few diversions, no running water, its market and slaughterhouse, severe sanitation hazards.

But it was his twenty-third and twenty-fourth years and he says he enjoyed his eight-month stay. He mixed his own drugs from chemicals he obtained on infrequent trips to Port-au-Prince, saw patients in his clinic or made housecalls, and was paid with some eggs, bananas, or plantains, and occasionally, a chicken. "The people in these little towns, you can really enjoy their company," he recalls warmly. "After a while everybody knows you and likes you. They get used to you and it becomes very interesting. . . . There's much to learn from the peasant society about health and disease in order to understand them. You won't find their ideas in books. You have to learn everything yourself."

It was a joyful and simple career beginning. He won the people's confidence quickly, thanks in part to the beginning use in Haiti of penicillin. One of his first patients had a bad face infection, so every three hours Bordes would give him an injection, sleeping on a cot in the sick man's house. The man was saved, as was an old woman with heart failure. He stayed around the clock in her house too, valiantly working to keep her alive, little by little succeeding. With these two cases, the word spread and his reputation began to be established. To this day he is recognized in Grand Rivière du Nord with excitement and pulled around to see the new running-water facilities, market, community development projects, and medical centers, rewarded with a chicken for his devotion years ago, in turn encouraging the artists' cooperative by buying wooden serving trays.

It was in this little town with his many cases of sick children that Ary Bordes began to understand the magnitude of Haiti's maternal- and child-health challenge. He decided he needed more pediatric training and after a month of work in Port-au-Prince left for specialization in the United States. The opportunity came when a Haitian friend from medical school, working in Chicago, sent him a newspaper clipping advertising for resident physicians at Kansas City General Hospital.

It was to be a learning experience par excellence: medicine, racism, materialism, marriage, intertwined with financial struggles, burdensome workloads, and a dependency on people and institutions that rankled like a vacation minus a bicycle.

Some other friends wanted to go too, so three Haitians shared a dormitory room, noisy with Haitian music and laughter, fraught with discussion and discipline. There would be a lot of conversation about whether to return to Haiti and Bordes's perspective would be different. The other two doctors would choose to stay on and, he often notes, die prematurely. Mostly the talk was of medicine. They had a lot of work to do. "We would go on ward rounds with the staff, and every day, mostly in the first year, there would be a few things we saw we didn't know. But the people around didn't know we didn't know. So during the day we would find out all we didn't know and then at night we would learn, and the next day we would know...."

While English presented its problems, he integrated himself well into the hospital and enjoyed Kansas City, but making that daily trek to the mailbox for Haitian news, every day expecting something, inaugurating a habit that still persists. He says he liked the city and the people, but he also experienced their limitations—racial prejudice—for the first time in his life, something he laughs about, but the clear impression is not so much then.

Ary Bordes is a brown-skinned Mulatto, the neon sign of elitism of his own society, albeit small-town; descendant of a family with close ties to Paris. While the money never flowed, it was not valued that highly. Pride and dignity were; class distinctions and prejudice were not. Clearly, he did not like prejudice applied to him. When Bordes left Haiti he only knew he was coming to a hospital in the United States. It turned out to be a Negro hospital, a state-supported facility with segregated wards. He was housed in a Negro neighborhood. He was given $50 a month, his food, and medical uniforms. There was not much spare change.

Ary Bordes never tried the white movie theater downtown. He did use the train with the segregated white and black compartments to be found south of the Mason-Dixon line in the late 40s. The conductor stood near the car, directing white people one way and blacks the other. Bordes was sent the other way. When the white compartment was full and there were still places in the black compartment, the conductor asked all the black passengers to move into one part, leaving the other area free. Then he put up a white sheet to separate the sections. Bordes recalls the experience, one of several in the same genre, and it is understandable that in his dealings with Americans and foreigners generally, his antenna are out for any hint of racism. He expects it. He laughs at the ridiculousness of it all, but his pride was stung years ago and it is only natural to resent such an affront.

His second year of pediatric specialization was at the Homer G. Phillips Hospital in St. Louis and involved a lot of hard work. It was a big ward and understaffed: "I got the impression all the black children in St. Louis were sick." He didn't like the city very well, either, and the following year transferred to Meharry Medical College in Nashville, where staff conditions were much better. He was the chief resident and the ward was smaller. But he found Nashville less than interesting.

Progressive through these three years of residency was his attraction to public health medicine. There was no particular inspiring figure or experience—"It was a slow evolution toward the fact that I wanted to come back here and follow a career that could reconcile personal and community interests. We all act by interest whether we admit it or not. And there are some low-type interests and some high-type interests. The main thing is to have a high-type interest that can also permit you to satisfy your own personal interests."

Ary Bordes decided that public health was a good way to try. He wrote to all the schools of public health medicine in the country, looking for a fellowship to obtain a master's degree. Most said they could not help, but Johns Hopkins School of Hygiene replied with a question. All he had to say was that he was going back to Haiti—"That was it. Everything was okay." But it would be tough going, his two years at Johns Hopkins his most difficult years in the States.

He was the only Negro in his class. His housing arrangements, provided by the university, were in a black neighborhood once again. He could not help noticing that blacks occupied the most menial positions at the university, floor sweeps or women serving in the dining hall. The hospital wards were segregated. He had a room and food, that was it. He made his own arrangements to survive by getting a job in the emergency room of a local Negro hospital—"It was hard!" He was in class all day and on call from 7 P.M. through the night, doing his readings and homework between emergencies. Monday, Tuesday, and Wednesday nights weren't too bad, but later in the week the action really hit with a fury, all night long—drunks, fights, cuts to be stitched, dressings to be applied. With so little sleep on Thursday night, during Friday-morning trips to school he could barely stand the light, usually sleeping during early classes in the afternoons to make it through Friday night, revving up for even more excitement over the weekends. Ary Bordes knows what it is like to struggle each day for a goal and get it despite fatigue, lack of money, hassles.

But he made it and received his master's in public health with majors in maternal-child health and school health in 1952. Later to be joined by his American wife and daughter, he returned to Haiti. "This is my place. I feel comfortable here."

It was as he had always planned. He was trained in social medicine and committed to improving the conditions of the masses of his people. He spoke of his strategy just before his return: "If I make the decision to come back, I must make the decision not to complain because otherwise I'll be complaining all day long." The previous year he had returned to Haiti on vacation at the time of an electrical blackout. He was reading—then, there was no light; he was taking a bath—no water; he was going along the street—holes. "There are so many things to complain about if you want to complain. So I made the decision to come back to Haiti and not complain. To accept the country and not be ashamed of the country. Because I think people should never be ashamed of their country! When you are ashamed, you are dependent! To be independent you must accept the conditions and try to change them. That's where I developed the philosophy of not complaining. I see the bad parts of life in Haiti, but I accept them and I don't complain about them."

But there were to be great frustrations ahead for many years, accompanied by a maturity and ever-strengthening inner self from confrontations with adversity—enough to challenge, but not so much to break.

From 1952 to 1961 Ary Bordes was director of School Health Services in Haiti, for which he received his government's "chevalier" order as a pioneer in this phase of health work—but he did not get much done. It was a great disappointment, beginning as he did with considerable enthusiasm, particularly in the first few years, trying to organize a national health program, fresh from a country where it was a priority item, discovering in his own that it was not; further, encountering the many constraints of an underdeveloped country.

He began typically—scientifically—with a survey of all schools in the capital to see what the health conditions were with the intention of providing a health record card for each schoolchild. But Haiti wasn't ready for that yet, he discovered. So he concentrated on improving the sanitation standards of the schools; immunizing the children against tuberculosis, diphtheria, typhoid, and tetanus; getting sick children— and sick teachers—treated; teaching the instructors to recognize illness and refer the ill for treatment; providing first aid; teaching the children about health.

All well and good, but he had NO budget. Each idea required a prolonged and generally unsuccessful negotiation with another facet of the underendowed bureaucracy, wrestling with even more critical problems than school health. "It took a little time for me to make this discovery," he says, almost sheepishly. "They just couldn't provide me with the means."

He met time after time with various ministries and departments, organizing sessions to get a widespread program of school health into the rural area: "We made a program but nothing came out of that." He came up with draft after draft of health courses: "I went to see the minister and gave him a program to change the school curriculum which didn't work too well." He received Bordes. They talked it over. No action was taken. He kept thinking. He kept working. He kept urging— "We insist one more time," he wrote the ministry, "on the need to create a section for maternal-child health." He saw the urgency immediately and his pressure goes back to a letter dated September 8, 1953, after one year in office, and sounds like a blowhorn in his correspondence and records throughout the 1950s. It reached the blocked ears of a health department dominated by clinicians whose training, ego, and every other orientation were toward curative, not public health, medicine.

Recalls a colleague and close friend at the time, Dr. Henec Titus: "I don't think we accomplished a lot. . . . We could just examine the child and not do anything else to cure or suggest anything important." He sounds discouraged just remembering it all.

The energy and zest for change with which Ary Bordes returned to Haiti hit a hurricane of limitations, literally. In 1955 Hurricane Hazel's wrath devastated the entire southern part of the country, destroying coffee plantations vital to the economic well-being of the area, creating a hunger and health crisis that would persist during years of reconstruction. Plus, in 1957 there was the beginning of severe political tension with the rise of François Duvalier and frequent ministerial shuffles. Haiti was a disaster area and school health, however worthwhile, would simply have to wait. Which meant, of course, so would the director, stunned by the discovery.

"This was my first professional shock, finding out about the limitations of what you can do," he recalls. "Also, understanding the administrative patterns, and learning how to deal with administrators and understanding the reality of the country. I think I had a very hard period where I was just in an office, not able to do many things. It's a period of my life that I consider rather nonproductive. . . . I had nothing much to work with."

There was personal trauma in Ary Bordes's life. The strains of a cross-cultural marriage ending, his son and daughter returned to the United States, arousing a profound sense of loss and defeat in his private life as well. It was a very difficult period to live through, a time of self-analysis and introspection, creating a wound which some say changed him irrevocably. The often-laughing and relaxed, party-going Haitian male, moved into himself, well-defended and not trusting, rarely to surface, except maybe among the peasantry, where there was little risk of hurt. Always there was the comfort and fulfillment of work, his relief.

He did his best to be useful, volunteering his services. In the 1950s he worked with the Episcopalian Sister John and her School for the Handicapped, with its many paralyzed children from a polio epidemic. Every Tuesday morning he could be found at a pharmaceutical house which provided low-cost drugs to the public. Bordes provided free consultation at the company dispensary and prescribed—"It was an idea that needed encouraging," he comments simply. He volunteered time in the schools as a health physician to see if he could build up a school health service as a self-sustaining, private organization. Each child paid $1 a year and received medical care—physical examinations, vaccination—but it did not really work. In another attempt at preventive medicine, while forced to do private practice for financial reasons, he developed an insurance system which is still widely used by Haitian pediatricians today. Parents paid $5 a month and the child was examined each month, never having a chance to get very sick. It also spared him the embarrassment of fee collection, another aspect of private practice adding to his distaste. Ary Bordes never signed a bill for over $200, regardless of treatment, in his seventeen years of practice. He believes medicine is a service, but the hard fact of business must be faced. His insurance plan, conceived after a lot of reading and his observations in the United States, was a good way out.

Private practice always bothered him: "I liked pediatrics but what I didn't like was the PRACTICE of pediatrics. What happens is that you would find a sick child who didn't have much seriously wrong and then the parents—because people here are so emotional and that was difficult for me—they would feel better if you would say, 'The child should be hospitalized; the child's life is in danger; I am going to save your child.' They felt happier if you said that instead of 'Don't worry, it's nothing serious.' People wanted you to do more things than were necessary. They were very emotional. They wanted you to live all your time for their baby because it was THEIR baby. . . . I could not adjust well to that situation." It went against the grain of his personality.

Ary Bordes is an emotionally suppressed person. His reaction to difficulty is action. He does not overflow with sympathy; he asks how he can help. Period. And he avoids what he cannot do anything about. He recoils from the temperamental and even more from agitation; has never placed an IUD in a woman's uterus in his life; and would be purring contentedly if he could sit forever and design programs and plan policies, free from people and details. What the driver is doing; how many IUDs are left; signing the papers; whether the staff is on time; blaming and punishing; the money; the discipline—he accepts the administrative hassles as part of the job but he hates them and delegates as much as possible. Private practice was even worse.

Ary Bordes was in a bind. When he went to his government office he was frustrated. When he went to his private office he was frustrated. "If I went to my practice and there were many people, it bothered me because I had to see all those people. And if one day there were not many people, then I would wonder why did I come here. So whatever the situation, it bothered me. And I think it was a time when I realized that this could not continue because dissatisfaction is very destructive and at some time you have to get out or it gets you."

The exit came spontaneously but really echoed all those years of hammering on a closed door to deaf ears. Ary Bordes was the pediatrician caring for the children of the new subminister of health, Lucien Daumac, a man more favorabe to thoughts about preventive medicine and public health emphasis. He bumped into Dr. Titus one day and asked, "Where can I get Ary? Tell him to come and see me. I need some advice." The message was passed, the word finally heard.

Ary Bordes was named director of the first maternal- and child-health facility in Haiti for which he would receive the "officier" award for health from the Haitian government—this time getting a lot done. Ary Bordes went to work to plan and create a program to help Haiti's mothers and children, to study their main health problems and develop solutions to alter their tragedy. He very deliberately chose to locate the new center at the downtown Port-au-Prince general hospital, a teaching facility for the university and entrée to influence students and the medical establishment in the direction of public health.

He had his headquarters, and the raised cement letters in black paint proclaimed the name—The Center for Maternal-Child Health. Everything was new. The chairs in the waiting room lined up as in a classroom—for a lot of teaching was on the agenda; three consultation rooms, another small room for group education; staff paid by the government consisted of two doctors, two public health nurses, an auxiliary, an auxiliary nurse, a health teacher, and two social workers. "We had what we needed," he recalls. Everything but money. His budget was $20 a month!

It was a problem. He had asked for $2,000. He was undaunted. "We had asked for a small amount and we were not able to obtain all of it. But the fact that we were able to receive even a little was something positive. Instead of seeing all that the government could not give me, I was happy with what they gave me and trying to find more. They could have given me nothing! We had to see what we could do ourselves to increase the resources."

He had an idea that worked immediately and overwhelmingly. A newspaper advertisement publicized the availability of a course on maternal and child health. The response was boggling—over 1,000 applicants, who paid $1 for the class and $2 for a certificate at its termination. There were young girls and grandmothers and a lot of noisy attention. Every six or eight months there would be a new batch of students and more revenue, as well as an important education function of the program fulfilled.

So much for the money. On to the definition of the problem. To determine what action should be taken statistics from 1952 to 1960 were studied carefully, as was the situation in the pediatric ward of the general hospital, coupled with Bordes's experience in private practice and his pediatric training. It was obvious quickly that the main causes of mortality in children were tetanus of the newborn, malnutrition, diarrhea, and respiratory diseases. All were killer diseases and unnecessary diseases.

Data from the pediatric service of the general hospital of the previous year indicated that 75 percent of the tetanus cases left the ward for the morgue, most around the eighth day after birth. Statistics from 1952 to 1960 showed that of a total of 19,036 infant admissions, 12,000 were for diarrhea and 2,438 died. In the same eight-year span, there were 6,049 deaths within a total of 19,000 children admitted, 31 percent from malnutrition. Maternal deaths at the Maternity Chancereles from September 1955 to August 1961 were 15.4 per 10,000, five times the U.S. figure; infant mortality was seven times the U.S. figure. Clearly there was more than enough work to be done—prenatal clinics, immunization of pregnant women and children, nutrition, pediatric consultation, education of the mothers and the population generally. These were the solutions in developed countries and in private practice in Haiti. Now they had to be applied for the benefit of the masses of Haitians. But how?

A methodology of work was established, to demonstrate how a health center might organize the needed services and reach the people in its area of influence. The plan proceeded slowly, on a small scale, constantly evaluated for strengths and weaknesses and limited by finances.

Each day a nurse would go to the crowded maternity ward of the hospital—sometimes two women to each bed. The goal was to get every woman who delivered at the hospital to participate in the services available at the center. The word was spread in individual conversations with the pregnant women, new mothers, and the mothers who brought their children for vaccination. There were group discussions and gradually, a home-visiting program into the surrounding neighborhood. The course in maternal-child health continued to gain momentum, plus there were lectures for medical students and a school health course at the National Teachers College.

As well as teaching, there was learning to be done, to discover popular ideas and practices about pregnancy, child health, and disease. As a scientist, Ary Bordes had always believed in learning as much as one could—both the bad as well as the good news. He was doing public-health medicine and wanted to know his public. He had read Benjamin Paul's famous book, *Health, Culture and Community*, and remembered

GETTING ACQUAINTED

the line—"If you are going to fight mosquitoes . . . you should learn to think like a mosquito." He read as much medical and social anthropology as he could find. But there was a scarcity of information on his people. Much remained to be discovered in these informal talks and group discussions, friendly inquiries, nonthreatening conversations, exploring folk beliefs and the spiritual world the patients inhabited as well as the "loa."

The people came. At year's end the December report recorded 2,121 people participating in the program; in April of 1963, the figure was 2,224 people; the next December, 3,251 people.

"It was like finding a new way and a new path," Bordes recalls, "like someone living in the desert and finding water or searching for gold and finding the mine." But not everybody saw it the same way. The center was autonomous and not really part of the hospital, while located within its complex. There was no open resistance, more a kind of background opposition. Absorption would have been death. The center fought for its patients. There was little referral at first. But then a thousand people wanting to take a course was a hard fact to ignore. The physical environment was good; it was the human factor.

A close advisor at the time, Dr. Victor Laroche, had returned from the States with a master's in public-health medicine the year after Bordes and was named professor of public-health medicine just about the time the center opened. Also a native Jacmelian, freckle-faced and a fierce mosquito-killer, with an appreciation for the ridiculous as well as for a good tailor, and the long-time president of the Haitian Red Cross, Dr. Laroche shared the same public-health perspective, in contrast to the clinical emphasis of most other doctors. They would work together for years, with Bordes making almost daily calls to the Red Cross office in his capacity as chairman of the organization's medical-social program and a board member.

"We had the same ideas and we felt we had to fight together, to start to work immediately to change the point of view. It was a problem of the training of the young doctors really. They were prepared to treat patients—and that's all. . . . They had not been informed of the role of the hospital in preventive medicine and education of the community. In the end it was accepted, but it took time." They worked at getting acceptance.

In addition to unsigned newspaper articles on maternal-child health, a year after the center was established Bordes organized the first Haitian seminar on maternal and child health in cooperation with the department of public health. "It was a very important way to get the doctors acquainted with this aspect of medicine and further the way for the concepts of public health," Dr. Laroche emphasizes.

"What we discussed in that seminar is what happened ten to twelve years later," Ary Bordes says. His paper, "Maternal and Child Health in Haiti," presented July 4, 1962, blueprints the current national-health policy of his country in that area.

About sixty doctors and nurses attended the four-day meeting, sharing the same frustrating problems, demanding better coordination between the hospitals and four existing health centers serving the capital's poor, talking about training midwives and being exposed to the population issue, remaining steadfast in the face of the catalog of problems ventilated with considerable anger.

Vaccination programs failed because of the "big discrepancy" between the first dose and complete immunization against disease, said one. Eighty percent of the pregnant women seen at one Port-au-Prince center had parasites, said a second. Another demanded adequate materials for his center, a refrigerator, vaccine and syringes, reinstatement of an obstetrical clinic shut down the previous year and fixed days for baby care and vaccination with a doctor assigned for that sole purpose.

The health center serving the Portail de Leogane section of the city where 60,000 lived in desperation was overcome with respiratory and gastro-intestinal cases, malaria, and most discouraging of all, tuberculosis. "We have so many cases with no solution because how can you isolate someone in a house where twelve people sleep in the same room on the average."

The comment of Dr. Louis Jacques basically summed up the prevailing mood of the participants: "After nearly a year of operation the Maternal-Child Health Center of Port-au-Prince organized this colloquium to explore among ourselves a point dear to our hearts. . . . In all honesty the problems are known; what would be preferable would be to approach solutions, which if not standard or definitive, at least are an attempt. . . . It is necessary to act."

The center struggled with this very matter throughout the first half of the 1960s. From experience gained came a change in style, particularly in administrative matters, more savvy about ways of getting things done, with Bordes growing in political maturity. Solutions were experimented with, and it became increasingly evident which ones worked. The objective became not so much a refinement of methodology, but extension of services. There was the will. There was the way. Always—there was no money. Then there was the National Seminar on Haitian Nutrition, Ary Bordes's paper, the impression he made, and a meeting.

"We had never seen Dr. Bordes. In fact, we had never heard of Dr. Bordes," Alice Sheridan recalls. "And that's one of the reasons I think this program is so unique in a way. It had to be a meeting. . . . And you

ns, our skills.
They seemed to merge. We didn't need any outside interpretations to
tear down the walls. We looked him up. He didn't look us up. Simply,
we were so inspired by his speech."

There was this strange kind of trust—people taking each other at face
value. Ary Bordes was nobody special at the time, beyond Haitian circles. He was not somebody they could look up back at the office. He
was simple in appearance, sincere, and not interested in showing off his
French. People spoke well of him; there were others the Service Committee duo was told to stay away from. "We knew there were the good
guys and the bad guys," Miss Sheridan sums up. Ary Bordes was approved of in a profession that does not characteristically recommend
highly without reason within its own ranks, while it is protective of its
own toward the rest of the human race. So they followed through.

Bordes took them to the hospital and explained what he was trying
to do. "There are so many things to be done . . . ," he said, all too obvious to his visitors, surveying the 101-bed pediatric ward, so over-
crowded, that sometimes there were two children to each bed. Seasoned
professionals though they were, Dr. Levine and Alice Sheridan felt deep
sadness at all this suffering.

"We saw one woman who had walked fourteen miles with a dying
infant in her arms, just dying from diarrhea—and there wasn't even a
bed! She just waited and waited! And Dr. Levine turned to me and said,
'Alice, that baby won't live long enough for a bed.' But then later he
noticed another infant, a dead baby. And that's the only way that
mother could get assistance because there wasn't a baby well enough
to be moved. It was all so desperate! Here this woman had walked miles
and miles!" She sounds desperate and distraught herself just at the
memory of that first hospital visit. "It was just so pathetic and heartbreaking to see the people standing there at the clinic and their hope
that by bringing their child to the hospital, the child would be saved.
When realistically, the chances were almost nil. The child was just too
sick! But if they had been educated to go earlier or had the transportation. . . ."

There were not that many visitors to the ward; too much death around
to take time out to stop and explain the program underway. Dr. Levine
looked closely at the children, thinking, "This one has a chance . . . that
one is not going to live." By and large the prospects were not hopeful,
he concluded. The ward was tiny and crammed with as many cots as
could possibly be placed, as close together as movement would allow,
but nowhere meeting the needs of a city the size of Port-au-Prince. The
people knew it and most didn't bother to come. Levine thought Bordes's

intentions were right; the Haitian mothers were right, but . . . the mechanics for taking care of what was needed were not in place. He listened to Ary Bordes's ideas.

Complimented on his speech, he replied it was no spur-of-the-moment talk, but something he had been thinking of for a long while. And he was off and running, his voice more and more excited, his words, rapid, his thoughts, staccato precise. "Our idea is to take the zone around the hospital, start by a maternal and child health and school health program, hoping in the future all other activities will be included, making the general hospital a complete health center with curative and preventive medicine." Adding, "This task accomplished, it could be expanded to sixteen other hospitals and clinics in the country."

Then he rattled off a list of objectives: 1) to follow the pregnant women throughout their pregnancy and delivery; 2) to follow their infants; 3) to examine all children of the zone and immunize them against diphtheria, whooping cough, tetanus, typhoid fever, small pox, and polio; 4) to decrease the mortality by diarrhea, tetanus, and malnutrition in the zone; 5) to find the most effective method of health and nutrition education for the people; 6) to become a training center for the medical students, nurses, and other personnel of the health and other government departments; 7) to study the approach to family planning.

"Our personnel for the time being can start the work," he wrapped it up with a gasp for air. "What we need is a budget to substantiate a bit and support the expenses. . . . " He was looking for $12,000.

Dr. Levine liked what he heard.

"Then we had another meeting with him the next night. He came to our hotel and what did he come with?" Alice Sheridan laughs. "One, HIS questions, and two, answers to some of the things we had asked him," she laughs some more. "He was really something. He wasn't going to let us get away. . . . He said he had a dream, and I'm sorry that phrase has been used so much because that's what it was with Ary Bordes. He always had a dream . . . he always felt it would come to something. And so that's the way we left it."

Ary Bordes was to write up his well-thought-through plan and submit it to the Unitarian Universalist Service Committee for discussion and possible funding. "We explained it couldn't be very elaborate because the Service Committee was not very rich, but it could mean the difference between a breakthrough and. . . ."

Bordes recalls, "The link came rapidly." While he had no firm guarantee, he felt "somewhat sure. It was an easy negotiation. We agreed pretty quickly," he says with a reminiscent smile. "It was a very, very happy meeting of somebody looking for funds and somebody looking for a project to fund." He repeats, "A very happy situation."

Conference coordinator Dr. Saldun was very happy with the conference results as well and wrote Alice Sheridan shortly afterwards with enthusiasm while conceding difficulties: "This seminar surpassed our expectations but it is a country where it is very difficult for international organizations to work—and this time things turned out well.... Haiti still needs much help and this time has demonstrated that they desire supervision and willingly accept assistance."

It was a thaw. Up to a few years earlier, the United States alone had provided Haiti with $12.5 million a year until the coffers closed because of politics. The U.S. could not even guarantee the security of its nationals on Haitian soil. Perhaps the situation had improved some. The work and recommendations of the seminar were to be published as a book, the cost shared by the institute and the Service Committee. The meeting itself had received wide press and radio coverage. And, of course, the president himself had presided at the opening session. Participants had visited points of interest throughout the country. The meeting had been well planned locally. Some of the papers were excellent. While the political situation had been discussed, the overriding factor appeared to be the obvious dependability of local health personnel and their associates, the effective programs underway, the desperate need for more. Yes, it looked promising.

Bordes detected the same atmosphere, and that September flew to New York for a wrap-up meeting at 405 Lexington Avenue, headquarters of the Research Corporation, representative of the Williams-Waterman Fund. He made his presentation, then repeated it before an informal meeting of the board of the Foundation for International Child Health, convened by Dr. Levine. In Boston, Miss Sheridan maintained telephone contact on developments. The conversations went very smoothly.

It was to be a threefold program: nutrition funded by the Williams-Waterman Fund; immunization by the Foundation for International Child Health; family planning by the Unitarian Universalist Service Committee. Dr. Levine was the key contact person, respected by all and related to all—a close friend of Dr. Sam C. Smith, secretary of the Research Corporation; on both the Service Committee and Foundation boards; a high regarder of Waterman; bringing together three organizations who had never worked in collaboration before, but desired to help. Each group seemed able to do something the other could not, but together....

That July, while the coordination was under discussion, Smith had written Levine, making a most fateful comment: "... if the results are good, a larger sum could be considered for expansion of the work. It would also be a good idea to try to involve the government to some extent. Eventually, the program would have to be self-supporting, and the earlier this idea is brought home the better."

That November, 1965, the letters arrived with the usual "sincerely pleased to join forces with you in this endeavor which will mean so much for your country" and "looking forward to a fruitful and pleasant collaboration," etc. And the checks: $5,500 from the Unitarian Universalist Service Committee; $5,675 from the Williams-Waterman Fund; $5,175 from the Foundation for International Child Health.

Total: $16,350 ... more than Bordes had asked.

5

PLANTING THE SEEDS

"People working in very difficult conditions should accept that they are working in very difficult conditions and not complain about them. Accept the facts; not be ashamed of them; accept them. . . . Learn about them the most you can so you better know the situation. Learn about your people. Why they act the way they act. What are their expectations. How to go along with them. Learn about your history because history teaches a lot.

"Then prepare yourself in order to cope with international organizations so in their presence you will not feel any position of inferiority because everything works to make you feel a lower position. . . . An expert that comes here might know quite a few things I don't know in science and techniques and I must admit that, and try to get from him whatever he can bring. But there is one thing I should have on him—the knowledge of the country. . . . It is not the latest techniques that are going to be applied in Haiti, so there can be a kind of equality.

"And I think it is very important for a person in a small country to maintain the highest level of competence he can for himself in his own situation. You can take a postgraduate course now and then, keep reading, go to conferences if you can. . . .

"Then, try to build a base for yourself so you feel secure. There are many ways to do that. You can build a political base by playing politics, but then your base is very fragile because politics is a very, very tricky type of thing. You can be with one group; it is powerful; then it is not powerful anymore—then you fall. Or you can build a base by working and everybody knows you do your work honestly, correctly.

It gives you a strong base. And I think if you want to be a technician and not a politician, working hard and doing your work well gives you a good base, a very strong base. To me work is as good a political base as playing politics. And I think that in my career my base has been my work because people know I do my work the best I can, to my full capacity, and they let me do it. I have no political trouble because everybody says—let that man do his work.

"Also, try to have a certain material security because it is very difficult to work when you have many material problems. That's why I am very grateful to the Unitarian Universalist Service Committee for giving me the opportunity to work and have a certain material stability."
—Ary Bordes

A sprawl of one-story white buildings with huge green shutters, the general hospital looked like a cross between an army barracks, outbuildings, and a plantation. Open doors and windows led off from the surrounding porches into spartan rooms with crowded beds and the infinitely high ceilings of the tropics. Family and friends gathered about the doors and windows to chat with patients, waiting hours or not, contributing to the leisurely, relaxed atmosphere.

The center was located off to the right of the central courtyard, sandwiched between the chapel, ambulance service, and the National School for Auxiliary Nurses. Its peripheral location was symbolic of its acceptance by an institution which fancied itself solely a treatment facility, a pervading attitude and major obstacle to health services for the masses.

Dr. Gerard Legros, a staff physician then and director of the center today, remembers those early days all too well. "I am ashamed to say," he responds when questioned about the attitude of the hospital to the public health center in its midst. While the ministry of health favored the center's preventive approach, the hospital continued its nonchalance, a kind of apathy and passivity which thwarted the work to be done. "For example, the pediatric service had need for preventive medicine," he begins, getting progressively more disgusted, a faint insight into what is beneath the tall, lean, precise and deliberate exterior, a style epitomized in his clipped mustache. "A child would arrive for treatment for diarrhea. He would be treated and then return again— because the causes remained the same in the family situation. The family should have been sent over here so we could explain the cause and measures to be taken for prevention of a further recurrence of the disease!"

His pompous facade starts to crumble. "But this was never done! EVEN, when we went over there and explained to them what we wanted to do. STILL, they would not refer!"

PLANTING THE SEEDS

In-house debilitation was one problem. Not too many people had seen the light. It was a beleaguered enterprise which now had been slightly beefed up by a nutrition rehabilitation center, so no longer using the hospital's; a small family planning component with the minimal objective of 100 women the first year; two new social workers added to the staff on loan from the department of labor to expand home visiting and education—a small program with limited objectives.

Another diffuser dampening take-off sparkles here and there was the lack of knowledge about modern medical care and theories of disease, an enormous problem. How to get people to come to a clinic for maternal-child health and family planning when they believed babies did not die of tetanus of the newborn, but were eaten by spirits called "lougarous." People got sick for sure, but were cursed by an enemy or harassed by an angry "loa." It had nothing to do with bad sanitation and infection. They were resigned. Women were always having babies as part of their female destiny; they had always been delivered that way; babies had always died. It was all part of life—and death. And this center was talking about things like immunization against diphtheria, typhoid, and polio? It measured a woman's abdomen during pregnancy and inserted a speculum in her vagina? It spoke against putting cobwebs on the umbilicus of the infant? And all this talk about food?

Babies were dying of marasmus and kwashiorkor and combinations of both, their systems weakened by poor diet increasing their susceptibility to respiratory infection and diarrhea, more illness, and eventually, death. But red hair was so common, it was considered normal in a baby. Malnutrition edema was due to worms, the people believed, bad breast milk or magic. They knew nothing about proper food groups, proteins, and vitamins.

An investigation of food and cooking habits told the sad tale. Nutritional behavior actually worked in reverse, with the head of the household getting the best, rather than the children, because he was the most vital person—the breadwinner. Regardless of how deficient his earnings, without him there would be nothing. Diet was well below nutritional levels because of poverty, plain and simple lack of funds to purchase food.

And what about this thing called family planning? Now that was really something to get across.

"I asked for four children, but God sent me eight."
"I asked for three children, but God sent me eleven."
"I asked for . . ."
"I will have as many children as God gives me."

Nobody had ever had much of a choice before, although they did try. Magic, that power that transcended all else in life, might intervene here too: a few remedies, folk brews, teas and potions that nauseated rather than interfered with conception; "devices" such as leaves and peelings that caused inflammations rather than prevented pregnancy.

Some were quite intriguing, albeit ineffective. After sex if a woman did not want to be a mother she should turn face down on top of a piece of money. A man who did not want to be a father should get a piece of crimson paper and make seven knots in it with different herbs, attaching the device to a fruit tree on the night of a new moon, intoning, "You there. You see this tree? It will continue to bear fruit but you are not to cause children—EVER!" Some of the women had sexual relations with the spirits, they said. It was unavoidable, twice a week with Urzulie Freda, every Tuesday and Thursday; or once a week with Erzulie Dantor, on Wednesday. And what could they do with the demands of the "loa" for their bodies? A good question. Sexual fantasies know no cultural limitations.

In short, contraception was a puzzlement on par with interfering with the music of the spheres in the Middle Ages. There were some things you really could not do much about, just as your parents, and your grandparents... that's how you had gotten here in the first place. It was brand new, unfamiliar and foreign.

In talks with the people, the staff did discover some information about human physiology and reproduction, analogies between humans and animals from observing butcherings, but the functions were way off. The lungs were called the "soft liver" and the people believed air circulated through their heads. Reproduction was linked to sex but the sperm came from the lower part of the back. Menstruation was an obvious loss of blood but why and how, unknown, and for sure, pineapple and sour foods were to be avoided by a woman during her periods. That's a hint at what the center was up against.

The tiny staff ventured forth into the thick of it each day, into the eighteen-block area surrounding the hospital, confronting these issues face-to-face, educating the people, inviting them to visit, obtain more information on medical care. They made their way through the labyrinth of Haitian slum life in microcosm. The one-room shanties and mini-storied buildings of precarious construction, seemingly held together by mumbled voodoo, elemental and compelling little boxes of human habitation, welcoming grins and crying babies. They walked along the footpaths threading through the urine, laughter, potholes, insanity, love, garbage, firewood. Past the constancy of commercialism, the tailors, barber shops, radio repair, stalls of sugar cane, sandals, suitcases, soft drinks and always—lottery tickets. On the East, a people's market was packed with vendors, the din of squabbling overhead along with the stench of garbage, featuring everything but good sanitation.

PLANTING THE SEEDS

A slaughtered pig bled into a basin, while food cooked nearby and a shoeshine man with pleading eyes and tinkling his hand-held bell tried to attract the attention of passers-by. There were intent domino players, vacant-eyed women in doorways, a coffin-maker preparing for the inevitable. There was little water, fewer sewers, a minimum of latrines, much unemployment, great poverty.

There were 15,398 people in the area: 3,224 families, according to a survey done by students of the National School of Nurses, organized into teams to blitz the neighborhood with assistance from a statistician from the Pan American Health Organization. They had defined the target group, so objectives could be set and evaluation made of progress. Their data showed half the people were sixteen to forty-five years of age—4,066 women of child-bearing years. There were about 500 children under a year; about 750 up to two years; over 1,000 in the three-to-five age group; 3,225 school-age children. They all had to be reached.

Madame Monique Souvenir was one of the social workers in the early days who walked into this black Brueghel of swarming life in all its body postures and facial expressions. Each day she would be given the addresses of women who had delivered babies at the hospital maternity, part of her quota. Her job was to know her area intimately well, to enlist the support of all institutions and everyone's collaboration with the program. To make contact with all the schools, clinics, pharmacies, hairdressers, dress shops, sports clubs, restaurants . . . . To seek out and recruit the pregnant women, lactating mothers, malnourished children, schoolchildren. To educate them, follow up their cases, keep an eye open for any birth and death statistics and other information such as attitudes on medical care and complaints about family planning. It was a huge job; she loved it.

A lawyer, she later had completed her three years of work for certification as a social worker; had spent some time as a radio broadcaster and a year in social welfare before she came to the center. Supervivacious and emotionally expressive, almost a floozy, she puffs passionately on cigarettes in a medium-length holder. Her flashing jewelry swings and her voice gets louder and louder and louder with excitement just remembering those good old days of home visits and group meetings in the neighborhood, the personal satisfactions of being asked for by name at the center, brought an orange or a fig in appreciation, spoken about affectionately in the neighborhood.

As were her satisfactions, so was her approach—personal. The staff emphasized informality, a relaxed friendliness, confidence-building, chatting, and joking. "Because it helped the women in the area who you were talking with understand why you were there, why you had come to their homes," she explains. "Not to pry into their private lives or personal affairs, but to help them . . . . In time the women came to see that we wished to ameliorate their situation." Thus, the warm and casual; also, the nontechnical. The approach was free of details on the esoterics of anatomy and physiology or reproduction.

Her typical family planning rap in the neighborhood went something like this. Brief, to the point, optimizing time. She would spot a house with four or five children of young ages. "I would say, 'Hello, how are you? Are these all your children!?' She would reply, 'Yes, it is good to have a family.' Then I would ask her whether her husband worked or not, because so frequently it was only a part-time job and an irregular salary and the woman might work, but clearly not sufficiently to care for five children. Then I would ask if the children went to school, because the people really want their children to learn to read and write. She would reply, 'Well, this year it is not possible but maybe. . . .' At that moment I would say, 'Look, I work and my husband works but I only have two children'—at the time I only had one so I lied a little." She laughs. "When I had one baby I didn't want to have another right away because you have to feed the baby and you must feed the baby well, give him corn and vegetables, beans and meat. This costs money. If the baby is sick you must be able to buy medicine. So if you have five children and you are going to continue to have children, you are going to bury them. Do you want to bury your children?"

The answer, of course, was an emphatic *no*! "Then, come to the center." Sounds like the hard sell. And it was. But the facts of the matter were all too true. It was the best way. Pragmatics. Living children. A better chance economically for everybody.

The work did go well and the people did come to the center for services and education. It was a noisy place, particularly during the pediatric clinic, with the perpetually crying children being immunized. There was a lot of moving around and evident apprehension about examination and treatment, particularly family planning. The people would sit in their bandanas and simple dresses, the children in their best clothing and shoes, if they had them, the men in a suit, if they had one. They would walk about, go buy a soft drink, return, talk, go to the chapel next door to pray, come back, talk some more.

The very first thing that hit them were the hyper-colored and giant drawings of the human reproductive system in the entry way by the center's staff artist, Ulrick A. Ambroise, as arresting a vision as a first high-school cat dissection and a source of wonderment to the visitors and education at first sight. This was what the human body was really like. Inside the center were other educational sketches—a proud Haitian peasant woman, very clean, in a dress and wearing shoes; a scene of milk taken from a cow and being boiled; fishermen netting their catch full of protein, a food not popular among the poor, and a loss; fruit being picked from trees and not from the ground, where it gets spoiled or infected with parasites.

There was a large plywood educational exhibit in the foyer developing the concepts of proper nutrition with lifesize figures following all the appropriate steps, and other pictorial messages of visits to the health center, vaccination, advice at the first hints of sickness, the signs of malnutrition.

Outside the center around 2 P.M. every afternoon could be heard one funeral after another across the courtyard in the little chapel. The shrieking. The moaning. Death. Two or three times a day.

In the pediatric clinic the pink-dressed baby screamed as she was weighed on the scale, face streaming tears. No, the grandmother did not know the baby's age, she replied. The baby was quiet now as Dr. Legros used a stethoscope, then examining eyes, ears, checking hair growth, sparse and orange and easily broken. He pointed to a chart on the wall with the picture of a marasmic baby, staring back, with the same look of lifelessness, hair discoloration, and hanging skin as this child. He pinched the baby's thighs, showing the loosened muscle texture from malnutrition. The baby's weight? Seven kilos, not the thirteen it should be. There was a respiratory infection as well. "The baby will always be sick," Dr. Legros warned, advising milk, vegetables, fruits and speaking of malnutrition.

In the family planning clinic, Filomine Ceavrier, twenty-two, all in black and serious-faced from recent grief, mother of one child, waited most apprehensively for an IUD insertion, while an auxiliary nurse placed the device in the palm of the hand, speaking quietly and calmly, trying to assuage her fears and demystify her upcoming experience.

In the prenatal clinic, Chritane Celestu, twenty-five, pregnant with her third child and wearing a silver wedding band on her hand, red ribbons in her hair, and a white dress distended by an eight-month pregnancy, received her second consultation. She giggled as she struggled to get onto the examining table and, directed by the nurse, advanced forward, her feet guided into the stirrups, clearly feeling she was about to fall off. Her abdomen was measured, the fetal position checked, the heartbeat as well. She had a slight vaginal infection, but everything else was normal, she was told.

It was going well and the enthusiasm and spirit of the staff were considerable. There was great pride, no conflict or intrigues; work was a pleasure. "Ambiance counts," says Madame Souvenir, "and Dr. Bordes is a man who likes to work and he rallied the staff. It was a nurse who named my first baby and the secretary who named my second. That tells you. We were really a family. We had a lot of work to do but it went along well."

There was this high regard for the head of the program—"a tremendous high regard," some say. While there was a recognition of the distance between the staff and the director, blatant in any Haitian situation with authority, it seemed more relaxed and freer. "Frankly," comments Alice Sheridan, "there was a relationship between Dr. Bordes and his staff that I had not seen in any other country . . . almost idolatry. It was as if this man says it is so, it must be right and I want to serve under him. That's the kind of relationship he had." She adds, "And I think the best nurses and the best social workers and anyone willing to do something, wanted to be with him."

It came from Ary Bordes's own example, as Madame Souvenir notes, rather than any domination or authoritarianism. He knew how to lead. He took a personal interest in his staff in his precise way. In the beginning Madame Souvenir thought he was an ice cube frozen in his office, an impression that did not persist. "I could see this was a very understanding man, a very good man, but a strict man." One day Bordes asked her into his office, noticing her usual jokes and laughter had ceased. He wanted to know what was wrong. Her first-born son had a gastrointestinal problem, ending up hospitalized every two months with a regularity that dispirited her. He immediately recommended a specialist and arranged an appointment. "I tell you this to show that he is interested in the people who work with him and takes care of them and helps them. And we cannot ask more than that."

While he supported, he also demanded, hammering away constantly at the need for data and reports, something not easily obtained in Haiti, instilling a respect for the facts he needed for proper evaluation of the pilot work underway. And he educated. There were frequent staff meetings with full participation, in-service training, and close and interested supervision. He brought out the best in people, nurturing strength and independence, distributing small assignments with a few guidelines, expanding individual capabilities and sharing the conclusions. All very, very unusual. "He gave me a thirst for work well done," Madame Souvenir sums up Ary Bordes's management, "inculcating in all of us this formation and training. I never felt I had too much work to do." The staff responded with a commitment to the program and to him.

Madame Souvenir often worked at a round table at the center, maybe gathering the women to talk about breastfeeding—"Mothers milk is the best . . . ," using the same familiarity perpetuated from home visiting, always emphasizing naturalness. She is said to have been quite a sight jubilantly launching into the specifics of certain sexual pleasures to a group of women—sitting in stunned silence. It was during one such round-table discussion that Alice Sheridan got her favorite story.

She had come to Haiti for an on-site progress report and with some of her usual reluctance. "I always saw such suffering as I had not seen in many other countries." There were always the hovels outside her hotel window, the stray dogs barking all night long, the bare spots on the hills of the capital where, she was told, an American furniture company had done its bad deed. Haiti depressed her. She would be brought to the department of agriculture, but someone forgot to say they were coming and nobody was there. She went to see Duvalierville. It hadn't come off. "And you got that feeling. . . . If you don't go up, you go down," she sums up the recurring theme of her visits.

But Ary Bordes cheered her somehow. He was different. As she arrived at the center she saw him talking with a group of women and watched unseen for a few moments. "And he was saying to these women: 'Give me your background, your age, your family, how many at home.' And then he began to explain to them what he was doing, why he was trying to be so comprehensive.

"Do you know what that means?" she says so emphatically, almost a threat. "Talking to women in a country where women had almost no say except to work a little harder than their husbands maybe and produce a family in between. . . . He had this rapport that was purely Haitian. Otherwise he could never get these women to come! He was just the right local person. The leader. A Haitian leader. He knew the temperament of his people and he responded to it.

"He was like a professor when I walked in with this group of women. I think he had a slate and a chalk . . . six women sitting like schoolchildren in a room and he had this chalk and was teaching them something, writing it in Creole. He was a born teacher and he was explaining family planning to them. And this one woman turned to me and said, 'Are you married?'

"And I said, 'Yes.'

"And then she asked, 'How many years?'

"I said, 'twenty.'

"Then she asked again, another question. 'How many children?'

"And I replied, 'I don't have any children.'

"And then she jumped up and down on her chair! Clapping her hands. Shouting, 'It works! It works!'

"I was a living example!"

She also took note of Ary Bordes's growing political practicality. No more irate letters to the minister of health. He had learned some of the rules of the administrative game, less self-expression/more accomplishment, demonstrated in incidents like the time Dr. Levine and she came from Santo Domingo. "We didn't plan to do anything except to confer with him, but some of the higher health officials saw us in the hotel and rushed over from the palace an invitation to a meeting the next morning. We had no intention of going, but we couldn't say NO! It was almost a kowtowing thing. We were very surprised when we got into the meeting and there was Dr. Bordes. The first thing he asked us when he got us alone was, 'How come you went to that meeting today? I didn't know you were scheduled to go.' We said we didn't know either until we got an invitation from the palace and we thought we had better go.

"And he said, 'I thought I had better go too when I heard you were going.' Just like that! He passed it off. . . . I don't think you can live by being devoid of politics in Haiti," she sums up. She sounds an ominous tone and spits, ". . . the medical school!"

Everyone and everything was moving along. The first year 312 pregnant women from the zone came for examination, immunization, educational sessions in diet during pregnancy, family nutrition, lactation; another 886 came from other parts of the city. Given the estimated birth rate of 45 per thousand, the center fell short of the first year's objective, only 58 percent of the goal. There was room for improvement but the results were encouraging. The second year, 1,232 women came to the prenatal clinic; the third year, 1,037. Total: 3,467.

In the pediatric clinic, 561 infants under a year were examined, about five percent of the estimated number in the area; 2,000-plus older children, one to twelve years, 40 percent of the estimated population. The second year, 2,106 infants and children were seen in the pediatric clinic; the third year, 2,004. Total: 6,744.

While there were discrepancies in the children's immunization series, the first year, 476 children did receive the first dose against diphtheria, whooping cough, and tetanus, preventing these serious and dangerous diseases; 1,245 against diphtheria, tetanus, and typhoid; and 800 against typhoid. The big breakthrough came in cooperation with the tuberculosis control division of the health department in September of that first year, something Bordes had nursed along. In the last three months of the year, 1,831 babies were born at the university hospital and 80 percent of them vaccinated against tuberculosis. The center provided cards to record the vaccination and an explanatory pamphlet for the mothers, presenting the protection just received against "the sickness of the chest which is treated at the sanitarium" and other medical advice.

"The facts are obvious. Never before have we attained such results in our vaccination program," the director of the bureau of tuberculosis control responded, with warm thanks for the collaboration and "eloquent" pamphlets which, he said, should be in every health center and maternity. They would be the next year at the second-largest maternity in the capital.

The mountain had gone to Mohammed. The center had tried both approaches and learned what worked best—its function. This way mothers did not have to think about walking the distance, be ashamed if they had no proper clothing for their child, or maybe concerned about missing a work day. The limitations of vaccination at a health center had been overcome. The following year the results were even more dramatic in every way: nearly 23,000 shots administered, over 90 percent of the children in the zone had been immunized against communicable diseases, including 96 percent of the newborn infants in the maternity. Again they had used a mixed strategy, not only clinic immunization but massive vaccination campaigns in the neighborhoods in cooperation with the Red Cross of Haiti and assisted by a bad typhoid epidemic arousing the fears of the people, the campaign well publicized in advance, with immunization available at certain fixed points visited by mobile vaccination teams. By the third year of operation the immunization campaign had more than doubled to 52,203 shots.

While the dose discrepancy persisted, the gap would close with education, Bordes believed. He wasn't worried. It was a natural phenomenon, with people unaccustomed to vaccination at all, to the idea of the number of doses and the specificity of vaccines. "My first concern is extension of the vaccination program, hopefully at some point, countrywide. There will be discrepancies—I know it. But in the meantime, we are building an organization to have immunization in a national program," he told the staff, repeatedly. "The first step is to have the children vaccinated, even if it is once, and then as years go by, to strengthen the organization to decrease the dose gap. We can never spread without gaps and what's the use of 80 percent third dose for just a small number of people?"

The first group of malnourished children left the rehabilitation center, created in cooperation with the bureau of nutrition, the week of April 15, 1966—beginning the second part of the project. They were visibly improved by combinations of 70 percent rice, corn, or sorghum and 30 percent red, white, or black beans. About 101 children would come to the center that first year for a four-month stay. Each morning, their mothers received person-to-person instruction in selection, preparation, and feeding of their children with proper combinations of cheap local produce. Basically, the mothers were being taught to keep their sick babies alive. They could see before their very eyes the changes better diet accomplished and how to keep their babies as normal as their resources would permit. That was the most important thing—to educate the mothers while their children were recuperating.

The core of the education effort was to insist on more good foods for mothers and children within what was possible on the average 10 to 40 cents available per day. Some had the money in the morning and others not until the end of the day's work. Economics was the major problem. The center struggled to do what it could. With 10 cents they couldn't do much; with 30 to 40 cents, there was a chance. Poor mothers had great ingenuity and the imagination to come up with some resources to satisfy the protein needs of their children once understood, they discovered. Like the "hausfrau" of Berlin during World War II, the maternal drive could accomplish the objectively impossible when children's lives were in the balance.

And the staff was not above using a little bit of guilt, frankly. Bordes was a firm believer that the people should be made conscious of their responsibilities in the promotion and preservation of health, countering disease and early death as most often beyond their control.

There were problems, of course. Lack of funds for the food. Difficulty in obtaining the mothers' cooperation in food preparation in the kitchen each day. Little human confusions, like the case of a missing two-year-old. But the most vexing and consistent hurdle was financial. The teachings about the importance of fruit puree and meat for children were understood, but often just not possible. POVERTY! Lack of food, illiteracy, poor sanitation, high rates of infectious disease were the main cause of malnutrition.

Inevitably, the question had to be asked: why rehabilitate a baby who in short order would be in the same malnourished and desperate condition? The causes were all so interrelated and manifold, the solutions so long term. Bordes would often speak of the "poverty scale" of multiple grades from partial lack of means to absolute misery, counseling the sometimes-despairing staff about their task. "We have to accept the meager daily resources and build on them." He was asking a lot. They carried on, recognizing the job was far more profound than could be tackled in four months of restoration. The families had to be rehabilitated economically.

The funding agency, however, was pleased. Malnourished children were an urgent problem, and throughout the world much had been done for such children in rural milieus, little for poor urban dwellers. While the weight gains at the center were not startling, the education program was considered more important than ounces. Bordes was thought of as a good organizer, a hard worker, with ideas of real merit, confronting the most difficult nutrition challenge. Yet, no matter what people on

PLANTING THE SEEDS

the outside told him—he was not satisfied. It seemed futile, an opinion that would eat at him and someday he would deal with it.

The second year another 101 children passed through the nutrition program—four died despite all efforts; the third year, 126 children—three deaths.

"I must say it was to me a rather devastating experience," confesses one visitor to the nutrition center in those days. Dr. Samuel M. Wishik, a member of the Service Committee's medical advisory committee, paid his first call in 1967. His assignment was to take a look at the project and see if it should be expanded further and whether Bordes might be put on full salary to give it his full-time energies. Service Committee program support had already expanded that second year to $10,000.

Wishik's opinion counted heavily. For years his field had been maternal-child health, clinical pediatrics, and population. A former dean and director of population studies at the School of Public Health of the University of Pittsburgh, an internationally recognized public health specialist with the expertise and the contacts, he would come to head Columbia University's International Institute for the Study of Human Reproduction. Most people called him "Sam" with affection, even though he was always running them into the ground to control everything and prove some pet theory. Not imposing physically, he was all inside his head, a well of knowledge and experience, someone who put a lot of stock in brilliance and background, the insecurity of the hyper high-achiever. To those who demonstrated the talent he so valued, Sam Wishik could be most generous and supportive, sharing all his resources and influence to help.

What Ary Bordes noticed most was his "sparkling mind. You'd talk with him and he always had so many ideas coming out all over the place all the time. Every few minutes! 'Well, we could do this . . . we could do that.' He was just like that"—he snaps his fingers rapidly. Also, Wishik's was a most rational mind. "When he sat down to work, he took a piece of paper and drew lines and organized in a very logical way." From the first, they liked and respected each other and in time Sam Wishik would prove very, very helpful to Ary Bordes. At the moment, however, he had big reservations about the nutrition center's utility.

"I was certainly impressed with how little they had to work with," he recalls. "Here were the children, just sitting on the floor. The bare cement. There wasn't much furniture because they were only daytime visitors. They didn't sleep overnight." He looked around with great scrutiny and also found some strengths,—making it all so complicated.

"He was trying to tell the mothers that babies just didn't grow because they were babies. That they really had to work at it to accomplish what they hoped for their children. The women knew that things were limited. They were doing the best they could. And Ary seemed to have attracted to his center from among the many, many mothers in Port-au-Prince, the small number of those who had the notion that maybe there was something they could do in the face of deprivation.... Without being able to make any changes in their economic situation, he hoped he could help them do the most with what they had."

He took note of that, also, the ease and interest of the women. There was not a constant turnover. Some of the women returned for further sessions so there was a chance to fortify the educational effort.

Despite the obvious strengths, Bordes's reservations would lead him to drop this component after three years of operation. There was disagreement without hard feelings with the funding agency. However, the shutdown would create long-term ill will locally, with those committed to continuing the approach interpreting Bordes's move as a criticism and rejection of their work.

The third component, family planning, began with the first IUD insertion in March 1966, with six more by the end of the month; eighteen in April; thirteen in May . . . by year's end 133 had been placed, beyond the very modest objective of 100. Four women were put on pills. Altogether 207 women had come for family planning information, and Bordes was encouraged.

At this point in time in the developed world, the pill was by far the most effective technique of birth control, but it did require a continuing financial investment and a relative amount of sophistication to calculate the twenty-day schedule. To help, when the pill program first began at the center, each woman was routinely given a three-month supply and a small poster of a woman taking a pill to put by her bedside as a reminder. By contrast, the IUD, a small piece of plastic inserted in the uterus, could be placed and forgotten, although it did sometimes expel spontaneously and had a higher failure rate. There was one pregnancy on the IUD recorded that first year. The basic purpose of the work was to study recruitment, the reactions of acceptors, and find the most suitable means of providing family planning for the Haitian people. Bordes himself favored a wide variety of birth-control methods and a forceful educational program regardless of the choice.

The initial reactions to the IUD were dramatic at times. The IUD was blamed for everything—headache, a toothache, any complaint. One woman came into the clinic clutching her throat, gasping, sputtering, like the death throes of an opera singer at Lincoln Center. It was the fault of the IUD. It must be removed immediately! She was dying . . .

obviously. She complained about EVERYTHING. She had pains all over; a headache; she moaned and groaned to prove the point and generally carried on loudly and at some length, scaring to death the other family planning patients in the clinic. It was getting out of hand. She screamed out for the doctor, "I do not want any longer this IUD!" She was examined, bathed, and treated. She had twelve children and no real difficulty.

Another had bigger troubles. The unfortunate sought out help, desperately! An uncommon side-effect of the pill, she was collecting milk in her breasts. That was not the real problem. Her husband was. He was enraged by her alleged pregnancy and abortion, since he could not have been the father, and vented his wrath and hurt male ego by beating her up daily. She arrived in the clinic after one such encounter.

"You have to help me!" she said, breaking down into sobs. "It is awful. You are the ones who got me into all this trouble!" True. "You have to explain to him that it is from the pill." The husband was called in and head nurse Madame Carmen Monpoint sat him down and gave him a long talk, requesting respectfully that he stop beating his innocent wife. Nature had these little quirks when trifled with a bit, she explained. It was nothing serious. But bruises and black eyes were. She did it in her inimitable style.

A short, stocky woman with a wide gap between her two front teeth, Madame Monpoint doesn't like to smile when she is photographed, self-conscious about this little flaw. But she smiles all the rest of the time in her indomitable spirit and constant energy, infinite dedication, and zest for work. In constant motion, she doesn't even have time to put her many wigs on straight before she flies out the door to her job. Her rapid-fire conversation proceeds in overdrive interspersed with expressions of emotion and bursts of vitality, feeding her tendency to run off chasing all the letters of the alphabet at once, occasionally forgetting the priority of "A." If she gets a piece of chalk in her hand, it's all over. She is a teacher, committed to community medicine with all of her rare being. Throughout her career she had so worked, including seven years of experience in a large, integrated development program backed by international assistance, where she had trained auxiliary nurses and midwives in public health, and in a variety of other ways had learned her stuff before she joined the center's staff. When the northern project closed down, she absolutely refused to be transferred to the capital in institutional health care, and had been working at a semirural location outside of Port-au-Prince when Ary Bordes lured her away.

A field worker as well as head nurse, she knew how to handle almost everything. Even the irate husbands who wanted the doctors' hands to stop examining their wives' breasts, and no way were her clothes to be removed! No need to lie on the examining table, the women would say, just give me the pills. "No. No. No," said one husband emphatically, "no need to touch her or do anything. She has just been taken care of," he maintained with confidence. She roars remembering the incident. One of her favorites. She gushes with delight at her experiences and the questions about family planning.

Was it expensive? No, it was free. How was it done? With big pieces of rubber? Or chunks of iron? Could it travel inside them and cut up their lungs or organs and pierce their heart? Would it injure their husbands during sexual relations? Would it cause worms to enter the woman? No, it couldn't possibly work. If it were the will of the spirits to have a child, the string (of the IUD) would lose its magic power.

The women's main complaint was that the IUD would "break their nature"—that it was unnatural and would disturb sexual rapport with their husbands. It was all new, the necessary biological knowledge lacking. There were human reservations. Very human, alas, even including male insecurity and jealousy. The men feared family planning would give their wives gynecological problems. They said. But they knew it would also give her more freedom for sexual relations in their absence without the possibility of detection by a pregnancy. It was a reservation never documented scientifically but heard often or clearly implied.

Despite the comedy and the tragedy, the program grew—with some very interesting implications.

The first year the women came largely because of home visits. The following year the center concentrated mainly on the prenatal clinic patients, the postpartum and pediatric out-patients, and a boosted educational program. The results were excellent: 2,692 women came to explore family planning—731 IUDs were placed; 89 women chose the pill. But by December, only 22 pill users had returned for their monthly supply, a trip required by the bureaucracy and generating a tremendous amount of paperwork.

The main difficulties, it seemed, were motivational. It was obviously an easy method, elementary for a motivated person. Humans know how to swallow before they are born. It had nothing to do with literacy. The IUD seemed more acceptable since it made no further demands once placed.

The trend continued. Of the 232 women on the pill during the three years of the program's operation, only 79 were still using the oral contraceptive by that final December, 1968. But 2,118 women were using the IUD to control births by that same date.

Nearly 8,000 home visits had been made to get the results. Experience showed it took six to eight calls for a woman to come to the clinic. About 10 percent of the women who delivered at the maternity came to the center for family planning by the third year. They had heard the short daily talk on family planning from a center staffer during their stay.

They were studied. In July and August of 1968, a survey was done of 200 women who had delivered their babies at the hospital and agreed to a rendezvous for family planning forty-five days after birth. All the women were from around the hospital's neighborhood, and poor. In addition to the usual family planning talk during their hospitalization, each had received a follow-up home visit, during which 68 percent of them had said they were very interested in planning and had agreed to come without delay. Another 21 percent were less interested but leaning; the remainder, basically neutral.

But what really happened? Fifty-seven percent of the women gave false addresses, a phenomenon that had meant an enormous waste of the staff's time for two-and-a-half years. Armed with their lists of postnatal women given out by the maternities for home-visiting, Madame Souvenir and others never could find them in the maze of the neighborhood. As it turned out, it wasn't all avoidance and subterfuge, either.

Many of the women simply did not know their exact address. They knew a crossroad or a landmark, the street maybe, but not the number. Others used the malaria-control number of their house rather than a street number. Still others gave the last two numbers of their address—rather than 2091, just 91. Why? That's what they used for their lottery ticket, the last two digits. Why should this be any different? Also, there was much transience. A woman might rent a house for a month, keep the landlord waiting for the next month, and leave it in the third when forced out for back payment—paying rent only four months out of the year. She would cover herself with a false address as well as a false name. And there was shame. Shame about where she lived and in what conditions. Shame about her unstable sexual liaisons which had led to her pregnancy. Also, some of the women came from the countryside to have their babies at the hospital and returned home after delivery, inaccessible for follow-up. And, as to be expected, many women did not want to participate in family planning and simply lied about their address, rather than risk someone's displeasure.

But two out of three women surveyed simply did not really know where they lived. The information was used immediately: the women, questioned carefully to localize their homes and the record forms revised to accommodate this new information, including duration of residency, adjacent landmarks, place of employment, or where a message might be left. It made a large difference.

Of the 136 women who said they were very interested in family planning and would come without delay, only 10 percent did. A mere eight percent actually began family planning. The rest simply were not interested, even after two or three follow-up visits. They only had two or three children and wanted more, they said. The methods caused pain, they said. Their husbands refused to permit it, they said. Never was religion cited as a problem, although eight out of ten women claimed they were Catholic.

Some of the reasons for failure had been established; what about the success? Another study was made of 150 women who had come to the center and begun family planning. Why? Economics, pure and simple—87 percent. Strong support from their husbands—66 percent. The majority of the women believed an ideal family size to be about two or three children. They didn't want huge families—85 percent of them thought four children was the absolute maximum family size. Also, the study showed the acceptors to be young, generally under twenty-two years of age. They had had their first babies and didn't want any more or they wanted a rest—"I would like a little vacation," was the recurring theme.

And how had they heard about the possibility of such a vacation? It was equally divided, among the maternity ward messages, word-of-mouth from other women, and home-visiting by field workers. All approaches worked as well, it seemed. It also was evident there was little point in trying to argue against the opposition. A half-hour's discussion simply did not pay off. They would listen; maybe they would fight back, maybe not; they would not come. Prolonged home visiting was out, too. A five-to-seven-minute chat was best. Otherwise you were wasting your time and limiting the people to be contacted.

And the men must be attended to in view of masculine authority prevailing in the Haitian family. Male acceptance of family planning or opposition to it made a significant difference in the decision of the women. It was an insight Bordes stressed, and gets Madame Monpoint off and running. "Everybody always says that family planning is for the women—but no! It is much more the concern of the men!" More excitement. "Everybody was doing education with the women, and trying to motivate the women. But Dr. Bordes said it was also important to motivate the men and have them participate in the program . . . . And with his system of work, Dr. Bordes made you love your work. He made you love maternal-child health!" She remembers the period fondly, the very best of her entire career, she says. "Frankly, it was

PLANTING THE SEEDS

extra ... very, very good." So, she went the extra mile—on her days off.

Saturday and Sunday afternoons she could be found propagandizing family planning amidst the cheers and gesticulating crowds of men gathered ten and twelve deep throughout the city for the traditional cockfights of carefully paired-off fighting birds, like boxers—weighing in before their confrontation, ready to let fly with a barrage of pecks and ruthless aggression. The men howled and cheered, given the fate of their favorite and the luck of their bet; faces intent, almost eager for the kill, their straw hats off at times in hip-slapping disgust or gleeful victory. There in the thick of it all, dodging the enthusiasm and the hats, just as perspiring and involved in pitching family planning, would be Madame Monpoint. The stakes were higher, often life and death or at least very serious concerns for the well-being of her people. She took community medicine very seriously, gushing with it like a water fountain of good will and competence. Divorced with two children, her work was her life, her comfort, and her expression of caring.

Another fact from the surveys, affirming the worst, always a very high hurdle—seven out of ten women were illiterate. How to best educate people about family planning given these unique circumstances? THE question. There was the searching and the trying. Just about every possible means. There were no hypotheses. It was virgin. Nobody knew.

From the beginning there had been the personal touch—individual talks and group discussions around the conference table at the prenatal, pediatric, and family planning clinics, the nutrition rehabilitation center.

There was the child health course that reached hundreds of people each year and was growing wondrously, double sessions on Saturdays now supplemented by a Wednesday afternoon class at Red Cross headquarters to meet the demand. The contents improved each year, expanding into family planning and marriage by 1967; mimeographed lectures the second year, soon published in book form at coauthors Bordes and Titus's personal expense.

There was the school health program in the eighteen blocks, a natural for the former director of school health services, and from the first, eliciting an overwhelming positive response. The center's nurses reached the teachers, who in turn passed the word on to the students and their parents; the schools pleaded for an individual nurse assigned to each. Impossible, because of the staff limitations.

There were films on puberty produced by Tampax Corporation in a French-speaking version. Plus, Bordes's own efforts, 8 mm, short, amateurish, and laboriously made productions, following the recovery of a malnourished child at the rehabilitation center, another on measles filmed during an epidemic.

There were little articles written for magazines circulated by Protestant groups and published in Creole; artist Ambroise's plywood exhibits; slides on mumps, tetanus of the newborn, breastfeeding, infectious diseases; flip charts on food groups, infant nutrition and growth; mimeographed pamphlets with line sketches by Ambroise and Creole commentary, always ending with a visit to the center.

Actually, Ambroise was a very good artist and two of his oil paintings still hang in Ary Bordes's office—but there was this problem with his aesthetic temperament, particularly trying for Ary Bordes, who had enough problems with the emotional demands of private practice in his afternoons. Essentially, Ambroise was driving Bordes crazy. He tried to police him.

"Don't you know I am an artist? I cannot be pushed," Ambroise would say. Bordes tried . . . and tried, and on April 10, 1967, put it in writing: "Dear Mr. Ambroise, I would like to inform you for the last time that your lack of discipline, your irregularity and your lack of interest in your work have reached their extreme limit. I will no longer tolerate your deplorable attitude. Hoping that you do not force me to take the required actions against you. . . . " He did. Ambroise was fired in a letter October 5 of that year. So much for oil paintings, plywood exhibits, and purple line sketches by Ambroise.

Enter Madame Edith Hollant. "I know you artists," said Ary Bordes, leaning forward threateningly with a sneer of contempt at her first job interview. "You don't know anything about discipline. You just want to do WHAT you want WHEN you want! I'm telling you in advance, I don't like the type," he concluded, leaning back in his chair in complete command. She was unshaken.

Madame Hollant has the self-containment of the true aristocrat, detached, disengaged, absolutely royal at times. Tall, attractive and fair-skinned, she is a fragmented woman, cold and hard as granite or as soft and fragile as an easily collapsed soufflé: someone who snaps at waiters and is rude to beggars, while working for the development of her country and capable of warm rapport with its peasantry. Trained in elitism by her father, a rare Haitian male who ironed his own shirts and exemplified equality to his impressionable daughter; held back from venturing into carnival crowds as a child and isolated from her peers by machine-gun bearing guards on the grounds of her home during his tenure as subminister of health; turning to solitary horseback-riding from the stock of the president's stable, solo photography and art lessons; never needing contraception nor bitten by mosquitoes; disliking bright sunlight and disruptive surrealism—she was a unique Haitian woman and a snob. She was not going to put up with this.

"I'm not asking you to like me," she replied with all her considerable dignity and style, as well as a hint of disgust at his bad manners. "All I am asking is for the job." That took him by surprise and he is Haitian and knows of the best families. "You are right. That's okay. We'll try for a month," he responded honestly to the appropriate rebuff, which in turn speaks well of him. They tried for a month. He was satisfied, but cautious. He put her on probation for another three months. This Ambroise incident had gotten to him. "But I was determined to get that job!" Fresh from course work in statistics and economics, she was desperate not to find a job in statistics and economics. Her father had wanted her to keep art as a hobby and have a "serious" profession. There was all this talk about banking. The prospects were horrifying. She wanted to do something with human relations and a social impact. She would.

To her work she would bring her far-ranging talents, taking pleasure in computer crisscrossing, testing the effectiveness of her educational materials, in turn demonstrating her artistic sense. Regal and vulnerable, always graceful, Madame Hollant's job interview was a fateful day for the program, albeit tense.

And there were other fateful events. Hurricane Inez. "Nature has been cruel toward my people," Bordes wrote Boston. Inez wrecked his plans and destroyed a great deal of his native city of Jacmel—and gave him an idea. While he was shaving and thinking about his work, as usual, he listened to the radio. For the first three days after Inez's surprise intrusion upon Haiti, only one radio station continued to broadcast, a small station near a power plant. Bordes had made a discovery, an educational station which broadcast in Creole, sponsored by the West Indies Mission. Maybe the project could make use of radio communication?!

The week of October 21, 1966, Bordes paid a call on Pastor Edwin S. Walker, the station manager of Radio Light, and a missionary of the fundamentalist southern school. His impeccable professional announcer's richness of voice intones in a French mélange of Southern drawl and a preacher's propensity to go on and on. . . . Bible-believing and a good businessman, Pastor Walker does not share his market survey results with the competition; that's confidential, as he goes about carrying out "God's cultural mandate." He is a nervous man. It is not easy to run a radio station in Haiti, though filled with people whom the Lord has called to follow the biblical wisdom: "How shall they be saved, except they hear?"

Evangelicalism and family planning were about to become bedfellows—no pun intended. Bordes proposed a weekly program on maternal and child health and family planning in Creole, the language of the masses, directed at the rural population with emphases on nutrition education of the pregnant and lactating women, feeding of children, malnutrition, tetanus of the newborn, diarrhea, and contraception. Clearly, not the kind of stuff you could get broadcast very easily over the other eleven stations in Port-au-Prince.

"Our first impressions were very positive," the pastor recalls. "His devotion, unselfish attitudes, willingness to give . . . " When Pastor Walker talks, Ary Bordes begins to sound like the Messiah of educational radio. It was agreed. The program was to begin the very next month and continue for a year. Then, there was this delay. "We kept seeing him and he would say it was not ready yet." Ary Bordes was planning, that's all. "He planned *everything* he did meticulously," the pastor discovered. "A year ahead of time we knew what subject matter would be treated for every broadcast—clearly defined."

Ary Bordes had no experience with radio with the exception of a few interviews while in the States. Suddenly, here he was responsible for the production, direction, writing, narrating, musical coordination, and delivery of a weekly broadcast. It was to require all the character Pastor Walker credited him with. He had a reel-to-reel tape recorder, a copy of a health song of the health department, and his tenacity. The program became a virtual Sunday-afternoon ritual from 2 to 6 P.M. It took that long for the ten to fifteen minutes of air time to come about, but, "His content was superior and his evident sincerity came through on the air," Walker says. Every Sunday afternoon's hassles ended with a tape dropped off at the station, then a sandwich and an ice-cream cone for gratification, and a drive-in movie to escape it all.

The format gradually began to evolve through the first few months; in time the prolonged musical introduction was dropped. "We finally convinced him," Pastor Walker laughs. So too was Ary Bordes the announcer, not for poor performance, but intensity: that one voice talking for ten to fifteen minutes at a time created a psychological pressure and a defensive reaction. He was talking right at people—they couldn't escape.

How about a dialogue? Two people talking with each other with the listener eavesdropping on someone else's conversation. So was born the team of Fannie and Ti Dio, and Madame Souvenir's gradual rise to national prominence. She was joined by a medical student, a program director at the station, Lovinsky Sévère. "It was a beautiful team," Pastor Walker recalls with satisfaction.

From the beginnings of basically expository material—the pill . . . how to take it—the program evolved into little comic scenes full of human nature and truth with more impact, and maybe two or three messages along with the entertainment. The couple argued, of course, the players looking for points of identification with their audience. A case in point:

TI DIO: "You left early this morning. Where did you go?"
FANNIE: "Well, I went to the Maternal-Child Health Center."
TI DIO: "What is the Maternal-Child Health Center?"
FANNIE: "There is a program of family planning there. I have two children. Do you think I am going to continue having more?" She was getting irritated.
TI DIO: "Why don't you want to have more children?" He was getting irritated. "You want some contraceptive method so you can have lovers." He was getting very irritated.
FANNIE: She was getting even more irritated than he. "You don't give me money and I have to feed them."

And they were off. The audience loved it.

A health-department survey of Croix-des-Bouquets, just outside of the capital, indicated that during the first broadcast year, 90 percent of the people listened to "Radio Doctor," while at that time only 60 percent routinely listened to the station. The program grew from eight talks in 1966 to thirty-seven in 1967 to forty-nine in 1968. The second year Station 4VEH beaming out of Cap Haitien in the north agreed to pick up the program in that part of the country. By the third year, two other stations were involved, and Bordes started thinking about the long-term possibility of every radio station in the country being involved in health education.

Sam Wishik's overall assessment of the radio broadcasts and all the other approaches and innuendos was highly positive, and he would recommend full-time funding for Ary Bordes. He found Ary Bordes's approach to be in the avant-garde of organized health services at the time, something nowadays called primary health care. He saw them operating back then in the center in Port-au-Prince—and in a rural village.

6

THE KHRUSHCHEV OF FOND PARISIEN

"There are so many different values. And when you come from a poor country, whatever happens to you, being poor, you are very impressed by the materialistic civilization of America. But we should understand that this is not necessarily the best type of civilization. Americans themselves are starting to realize that there are other values . . . ways of living. And I don't think we should be judged on only the materialistic scale. Is it the best scale to judge people by? I wonder. To me the greatest value of a country is its people because human beings are the best that a country can have. Even if you have material resources, it is the human beings who are going to use these material resources. . . .

"Now what are the greatest qualities of my people? I would say that we have a mosaic type of culture full of vitality. And if we use that vitality and put all the strength of that vitality into change and development, then, I think we will make it. I have seen the Indians of mid-America and they look sad. I have not seen their moments of joy. While here people are poor, but we seem to have a different type of vitality.

"And I think if we are given the possibilities, we can do great things. As you know, I am very interested in Haitian painting because I am proud of it. This is something we can show. We CAN do things! Things that can astonish people! And I personally encourage that movement as much as I can to create pride in us. . . . Usually here they say it is very difficult for Haitians to get together and not talk about 1804, our independence time. And it is true. It is something we are very proud of. It means that we stayed 400 years in slavery and under those very difficult conditions we made one of the greatest feats in history, the first successful slave revolt, the first time blacks ever became independent in recent history.

"I think that if we can get together we can do a lot of things. Our only problem is just to get together."—Ary Bordes

"I had a feeling of a very, very poor village," says Sam Wishik, shocked, despite his years of travel throughout the underdeveloped world. "I was surprised, frankly, by the extent of the misery because I had not seen things like that before. This was a desert! The ground was flat, packed sand! That's what it looked like to me. There wasn't grass. There wasn't foliage. And I thought, 'My God, how deprived this area is!' "

So felt the Haitians. "It was a most distressful village," says Dr. Titus. "Malnutrition, umbilical tetanus, and diarrhea . . . dry and dusty in normal times and muddy in rainy times. I remember there were a lot of very skinny and malnourished dogs. It seemed to represent the population." Elaborating on the so-called "dog index" when applied to the village of Fond Parisien, Ary Bordes would say that once in a while the dogs felt like barking, and in order to have the strength, they first leaned against a wall.

It was this village, about thirty miles away from the capital, that Alice Sheridan and Dr. Levine visited during that first fateful trip to Haiti, down the road which she had bounced along and ultimately onto. Fond Parisien had about every problem a Haitian village could have, beginning with just getting there, a formidable obstacle and during a tropical downpour, impassable.

It was a very, very poor village, filled with Haitian fatalism, a safety valve for mental health, but a hindrance to development. People were resigned to whatever happened. A hurricane came. The people lost their animals. Their families were injured. Their gardens ruined. Their homes lost. Everything lost. Hunger. The response would be—"I resign myself," usually followed by, "God is good." No point in prompting more anger; neither to seek change.

Arid, dusty, destitute Fond Parisien had been a Haitian disaster area since shortly after the turn of the century. Some say beyond redemption. In his research of old papers and reports at the department of agriculture, Bordes was gleeful when he discovered Fond Parisien had once been a most prosperous area of colonial Saint-Domingue. A fieldstone silo, moldy with lichen and the savage little plants that survive rooted in the cracks of rocks, still stood, a remnant of those glorious bygone days. Fond Parisien was renowned well into the early days of the Republic for its high food production and the excellence of its vineyards. The records up to 1890 showed considerable sisal, latanier, and red-bean production, but noted that this "privileged situation" did not survive the devastating rains that began to fall November 12, 1909.

They continued for eight consecutive days, primeval, torrential rains that flooded the nearby Lastic River, the water source irrigating the region. The accompanying winds were of cyclone force and the land trembled with earthquakes, filling the river with debris, forever altering its course, disappearing underground—altering Fond Parisien. Old people, now gone, but their words remembered, are said to have referred to that rain as the deluge, a mystical cataclysm and retribution for some great and unknown offense.

Twenty-six people were killed, and with the loss of the irrigation system, many families moved away. The heads of households that remained began the annual pilgrimage to the Dominican Republic to harvest sugar for six months of each year, a migration from January to July which still continued, periodically interrupted when relations between the two countries which share this island were strained. When 12,000 Haitian cane cutters were slaughtered by the Dominicans in the spring of 1937, the village church records of that March showed 350 refugees came to Fond Parisien for help. Living in such misery themselves, the villagers had no food to give, but did try to save some of the children by taking them in as servants. The next month, on April 26, forty Haitians crossing the border near the village, returning to their homeland, were killed by Dominican troops. Only one boy survived to tell the story. "From then on the villagers lived in misery," the record book says, "because they could not go into the Dominican Republic." There was nothing much for them on their own side.

Fond Parisien had been the object of some development efforts in the past, but each resurrection seemed doomed to another hurricane and a reversal once again to extreme poverty, charcoal-making and dry farming for survival, further impoverishing the already devastated land. Ten years after the first hurricane, a Roman Catholic priest named Father Peters and some German nationals began a cotton-planting project, but were soon discouraged. While many people worked for them and were well treated, the record says the project fell away and they had left in despair by 1923.

Most villagers survived on charcoal production, which got them through the present but insured more poverty in the future. Year after year the villagers, mostly the women, went up to the surrounding hills and mountains, often for weeks at a time, cutting down precious trees, chopping the wood, then placing the pieces in the ground, igniting a few and burying the hole over so the wood would burn without oxygen.

Those whispy ribbons of white smoke on those mountainsides year after year signaled more than charcoal-making on the job. It meant trees

THE KRUSHCHEV OF FOND PARISIEN

were being felled, root systems loosened, topsoil exposed. The land showed the strain: scabs of bare patches growing bigger each year, deepening gulleys, landslides, bone-dry earth redeemed by occasional scrub grass and a few cacti. The search for timber grew tougher and tougher, forcing the people farther and farther up the mountains.

The real coup de grace for the land came in 1937-38 when the Haitian-American Sugar Company put the villagers to work cutting down trees for railroad ties for four years. That pretty much completed the deforestation. More lumber companies came in 1943, and once again the villagers went to work cutting down more trees. That's the way it was. . . .

In 1947 the regime of Dumarsais Estimé came to power, purging the government of Mulatto officials, replacing them with blacks, and initiating a program aimed at improving the lives of urban workers and the agricultural poor. Clearly, Fond Parisien qualified for assistance, a recognition compounded by its strategic location along the Dominican frontier. The idea was to build an irrigation system from the Lastic River, about nine miles away. December 10, 1947, work was begun to divert the river's course, construct a dam and build a canal system. It continued to July 1, 1948, at which time 875 acres of land were being irrigated and Fond Parisien was on the rise.

The village even got a preparatory school, an agronomist, and an assistant assigned to the area. They trained the people in agricultural techniques and introduced new varieties of produce—fruits and vegetables. Since there was not enough good grazing land for cattle or goats, the technicians suggested raising rabbits and urged the people to fish in nearby Lake Azuey, the largest of the country's two natural lakes.

By June the following year, 1949, there were 25,000 feet of canals going from river to arable farmland of the village—and very visible progress. Regeneration is very evident in a place like Fond Parisien. It is literal. Things are growing out of the ground; people can eat; they can buy; they can trade. Fond Parisien started to look like an oasis in a surrounding desert.

The government provided transportation to bring the produce to the capital—ten trucks. Twenty-five children were sent to school in Port-au-Prince. When a typhoid epidemic struck, 1,800 vaccinations were given in five hours in a village which had never had a doctor, dentist, pharmacist—any medical care—in its history. The epidemic stimulated latrine construction and greater attention to sanitation.

While in 1948 only five of the villagers had an income of $20 a year, by the 1949-50 period, half of the people were earning $19 to $24 a year; another quarter, $25 to $40 a year; and the rest, in the $73 to $100 range. While before 1948 so little meat was eaten in the village only one steer was slaughtered a year, on the thirty-first of each December, by 1948-49, two steers were being slaughtered each month, two pigs every Friday.

Before the irrigation project, there had been no commerce of any kind in the village. The people raised what food they could and went elsewhere to market. But in March 1949, a little store opened with the beginning of the canal work, and was doing about $1,000 a month in business by 1950. It was so good that soon there were six other competitors, joined by a bakery, a slaughterhouse for cattle, another for goats, and two for pigs. Because there was more money, three tailors moved to Fond Parisien to join the two already doing business; next came a shoemaker; even a furniture maker.

Things were definitely looking up for the villagers of Fond Parisien. The water was flowing and the gourdes as well. The village began to flourish. The population rose from 1,270 to 1,873 by 1950. Their wealth was measurable in the also-growing animal population, one of the vital signs of development in an agricultural community: 89 horses, 217 cows, 547 goats, 140 lambs, 132 donkeys, 1,558 chickens. . . .

Abruptly, without warning, it ended on October 12, 1954. Hurricane Hazel. The irrigation system was completely destroyed, visible only in a few spots of parched earth, some stones, and an old man's memory of where the water pipeline had divided left and right, the foundations upon which the lifeline of this village had rested. Fond Parisien returned to its former desperation. All was lost . . . slowly but emphatically. The banana planting in 1950 told the story. It had been 65 acres; up to 312 by 1953; 350 acres just before the hurricane; plunging to only 150 by 1956. The drop signified a lot of sadness and hunger.

Following the disaster the government established a commission to once again study the problem of Fond Parisien. As a village church record puts it, "Many bureaucrats came to visit each week." A number of technicians worked off and on for two years, with many of the villagers joining the rebuilding of the irrigation canals. A threshing machine was brought in; a silo was built. But the effort was half-hearted and a preliminary report of July 1956 was pessimistic, emphasizing the extreme cost of the work and reconstruction and the lack of guarantees that it would not be entirely blown away in the future by whimsical climate.

In short, Fond Parisien was a bitch of a place to work; the problems were enormous, and it wasn't surprising that by 1959 not a single bureaucrat could be found. Their reservations proved correct.

Fond Parisien was struck repeated blows by the hurricane force of Flora, October 3, 1963, and by Inez, September 29, 1966, leaving in their wakes an epidemic of malnutrition and acres of flooded farmland. Crops were horribly damaged; houses destroyed; people killed. The crops were replanted; the houses repaired; the people grieved. They watched the sky for the next punch. It seemed to come with an historic regularity. Thus their fatalism.

Also, there were the droughts. Rather than a violent death blow, they were the slow but persistent killers of the life-giving growth of the gardens and daily sustenance of the people. Their food ebbed away to less and less, almost nothing, sometimes only sugar cane: more and more hunger, weakness to all the diseases, often death. Starvation and illness in fatal combination.

The droughts would persist for eight- and nine-month stretches at a time; sometimes, two and three years in a row. There was nothing to be done about it. Just that awful waiting, that watching of the skies for some clue of moisture, clouds, rain, the rains that were supposed to come twice each year, gradually getting more torrential and tropical, peaking in June and in September. It was expected that January and February would be difficult regardless of nature's moods the rest of the year. That was known. But now there was total insecurity for the rest of the year as well. Would there be water for the gardens? And if not . . . that must be accepted too.

It caused other problems. Everyone so beleaguered and miserable— and passive—but inside there was the rage. It oozed itself out now and then upon the minor mistake of a child, or maybe no mistake at all. Just anger and the need to attack someone, something. Neighbors quarreled, too. They had so little, and therefore, so little trust. It was difficult in Fond Parisien for a variety of reasons.

Dieumaitre Jacques had lived through it all. All his life he had seen the small market with little piles of mangoes, rice, plantains, and roots, sold for a few cents. A bag of charcoal for $1. If there were little food, the charcoal would last longer. He had seen the hungry dogs, the lean burros and pigs, the gaunt goats, the few cows, the stunted people, the red-haired children.

He was born here in 1926, the fourth child of his mother and the fifth child of his father, and his parents were also born in the village. Dieumaitre's father had told him there was virtually nothing here during his boyhood, either. They could only harvest once a year and when the rains did not come, there was absolutely nothing, his father said.

The poverty perpetrated in his generation; his family was so very poor that at about the age of two, Dieumaitre moved with them now and then to the Dominican Republic to cut cane, and finally for a long time. He still speaks the Spanish he learned there.

In 1932 the road to the Dominican Republic was built and Dieumaitre remembers that. Two years later, he started school, attending for the remarkable length of ten years, a very extraordinary education indeed, if it is so. He remembers too when the border was closed in 1937 and all the problems began with visas and shootings and slaughter, how the migration to the Dominican Republic stopped; how the desperation increased. He remembers too all the trees and when the companies came, how the people had no choice but to cut them down because there was no other work. "People knew the cutting was bad for the land but poverty made them believe it was not really going to happen," he says. Then, the flooding came in earnest, he remembers. He was told as a boy that five pounds of millet seeds would yield 2,500 pounds of food; now five pounds might give you 100 pounds if you are lucky, he says—perhaps an exaggeration, but a point.

His life was as the others. He had married in 1950 and he married well, with characteristic calculation. His wife's three brothers and three sisters all had big houses in Fond Parisien. Twenty-seven months later he had fathered a child that died at five months, then another child died. In time he would have six children from his two wives, four of them sons. He was a farmer like everyone else until he became a worker on the big irrigation project, his talents recognized, and was asked to organize the fencing off of parcels of land. The canal system was a big success, he says, until the hurricanes came. Then, not much really happened until Dr. Fougère came in 1964. It was in July, he recalls, and the water pump was inaugurated the next year. Dr. Bordes started his vaccinations then.

Every Friday he could, Bordes made the trip, trying to know the people and the area. Fond Parisien was a kind of people's university and he noticed the villagers practiced a lot of preventive medicine from a spiritual point of view. The cotton in the ears of the newly delivered mother, the bath towel around her neck, the socks on her feet, the avoidance of red foods that caused hemorrhaging, the Bible open to a certain page and appropriate quotation under the pillow of a newborn infant, and the voodoo beads around the newborn's neck. He would use the insight.

He learned more. One day he was taken to see a man living by the lake. "He was on a mat on the floor and had a bad case of diarrhea," he recalls. "He was very weak and the people around him were making preparations for his funeral . . . trying to figure out how they could meet the expenses of the funeral. That really struck me! They were preparing for the funeral rather than trying to save him! And I said, 'Don't you think it would be better to see if he could live!' "

He gets astonished all over again at the memory. The man did not die and Bordes had learned a very important Haitian lesson—the importance of fulfilling duties to the dead, sometimes more important than to the living. It was all too obvious that when illness struck, it more often than not ended with death. Thinking follows the pattern of experience, and this is the way it was in Fond Parisien.

Bordes had chosen to work in Fond Parisien for a number of reasons, including his volunteer association with Sister John and St. Vincent's School for the Handicapped in the capital. Each week the worst cases of malnourished babies were brought to the village's Episcopalian church to be taken back to Port-au-Prince for treatment. Bordes would help and then return the children to the village. Also, Dr. William Fougère, director of the health department's bureau of nutrition, had maintained a nutrition rehabilitation center in Fond Parisien since 1964, supported by the Williams-Waterman Fund. Bordes wanted to blend in some maternal-child health and family planning into that activity.

Fond Parisien had been chosen as the pilot location to attack Haiti's vast nutrition problems generally ending in death because here was just about the worst situation in the country, according to a team of researchers' conclusions in 1958. Eight percent of the children died of malnutrition; on any given day, thirty to forty cases of nutritional edema could be found among the preschool children. According to the Gomez classification, 46 percent of the children suffered from first-degree malnutrition; 23 percent from second-degree; 11 percent from third-degree. Only 20 percent of the children of Fond Parisien were normal.

A little house had been rented in the village, white with green trim and a long porch with three small rooms inside and a cement floor. It was a rural middle-class house offering a little more space for teamwork and protection of material and equipment but still in tune with the environment. The nutrition-rehabilitation center was quickly occupied with babies and mothers being taught food values and how to use their modest budgets to best advantage. It was the model Ary Bordes followed in Port-au-Prince.

Complementing this, Bordes conducted his vaccination program for preschoolers during his weekly visits. Also, there was an agricultural program jointly underway by the bureau of nutrition and the department of agriculture to raise more food of higher nutritional value. The program was very seriously hampered by drought, decimating winds, and the devastation of farm animals starved for food and wandering free. The Haitian-German mission also had helped build two new irrigation ditches for cultivation of new land; one worked well, the other not so well. In short, some cooperating groups were using Fond Parisien as a pilot program site. Dieumaitre knew everything about the work. He became involved and a prime mover, first in the nutrition project with Dr. Fougère, and then with Dr. Bordes.

Bordes wanted someone to collect data on births and deaths, and in October 1965, Dieumaitre remembers precisely, he offered this new doctor his services free of charge for three months. "Dieumaitre recruited himself," Bordes says with satisfaction. He had been working with the nutrition center, when he presented himself and said he was the man for the job, "I saw how easily he could fit into the situation," Bordes recalls. "We knew he WAS the man."

He was. Untrained in the formalities of community organization, Dieumaitre Jacques was a natural, a cross between the Mafia, the YMCA, and a guardian angel—all-seeing, nobly caused, and not to be messed with. He was systematic about everything, a virtual logician who defined his objective and moved toward it, almost for the kill. Asked a question, he sketched out little reports, charts, and graphs and had a habit of appropriating pencils and walking off with somebody's pen. He could clearly articulate his approach to his work, possessing the rapid-fire mind and retention of the highly intelligent. He was knowledgeable and precise.

"How many houses in City Rurale, Dieumaitre?"

"Forty-nine." Answered without a moment's hesitation or blink of those beady, foxy eyes always watching from under a perpetual, modern straw—not farmer's straw—hat. Probably hypo-manic, his energy was titanic, a veritable "type A." His stunted, hard, muscular body walked along, propelled by purpose and overdrive speed so at odds with his culture's "map venit" syndrome—"I am coming, but tomorrow." He absolutely could not sit still, bouncing about like a puppet; if restrained in one spot too long, his feet tapped nervously under the table, until he could finally spring free. He looked like the archetypal mischievous kindergartener, full of zest and smarts. He could help and he could hurt; his eyes smiling a greeting or becoming cold steel in a flash. Fortunately for the program, his considerable energies and capacities had been channeled into something constructive, the building of a program of maternal-child health and family planning in his village.

Dieumaitre reported to Bordes every Friday his jeep rolled into Fond Parisien. He would be there waiting, like a military aide on the alert for the general's wants—list in hand of house calls to be made. Alice Sheridan remembers him as "the little man always waiting for the car" when she and Ary Bordes made their trips out to the village in those early years. Dieumaitre was for real, but she wasn't so sure about some of the other things she saw, "obviously set up . . . people doing things, giving exams, gardening . . . but that little man. . . . "

At first Bordes went house to house visiting the pregnant women and postnatal mothers that Dieumaitre had found during the week. Bordes used a structured questionnaire to learn about their health practices and histories, vaccinating and checking the condition of the mothers and infants. His survey showed one woman in three had lost a baby to tetanus of the newborn. The death rate was 9.5 per 100 infants, 72 percent within the first ten days of life. "The name became known in November 1965, with the arrival of a doctor," Dieumaitre says of the dreaded disease, killing so many newborns in Fond Parisien.

By the second year, Bordes had expanded his work to a formal weekly clinic, but he still made home visits to check on the umbilicus of babies and the condition of the new mothers, guided by Dieumaitre's list.

His was not easy work, Dieumaitre says. The people were shy and not accustomed to having information collected. He needed help to overcome resistance. So what he did was find two or three people in each area of the village who had influence in their neighborhood. "Leaders," he says. He gave them a lot of attention. If they had a particular problem at home or with their family, he would visit and talk and make sure Dr. Bordes came to see them. Then, other people saw this and wanted attention too. They began to believe "in the program," he says, and he began to have fewer problems. When the people had problems their neighborhood leaders would tell them it was because they did not believe in the program. This is how the program started, he says. Ingratiation . . . jealousy . . . competition.

In January 1966 Dieumaitre began to be paid $25 a month for his work. His job expanded not only to record all the births and deaths and find the newly-delivered mothers, but to inform people about the medical clinic now available at the nutrition center, invite the pregnant women and new mothers to come, and the village midwives as well as the sick.

The first patient came. She had a vaginal infection; she was treated, given medication, and got well. She had gone to the "houngan" and despite all efforts, nothing had worked; now she was well and she began to tell everyone of her experience, advertising the glad tidings. A breakthrough. Dieumaitre's first clinic conquest.

From the beginning Dieumaitre seemed to understand the concept of priority groups. He would not simply go from house to house with his only and constantly used tools—pencil and paper—making lists for Bordes's visits. He was looking for the most vulnerable, those most in need of services—small children, mothers, the malnourished.

And he grouped the people in his lists, another extraordinary, intuitive phenomenon of his work methods in a country with few telephone books, a weakly organized mail system, scant vital statistics at a central office, and a mess of conflicting and unreliable names, dates, and facts, maybe kept in a church rectory. Dieumaitre understood the importance of data; and his data was completely accurate, not doctored to impress the doctor.

Each week he wrote a written report for Bordes's visit, actually two, since he made a copy and did not use carbon paper. He wrote in his supreme style, a flamboyant script, full of loops and rondos and other sundry acrobatics of the pencil. Dieumaitre was fanatical about his writing, and his lips would purse over his big teeth as he labored over his weekly reports.

In time Ary Bordes would know this village intimately well, week after week the facts flowed in on a pleasure cruise of Dieumaitre's handwriting. Births. Deaths. Marriages. Percentage of people of different religions. Lists of students. Lists of people who had been vaccinated. Lists of foreign religious missionaries. Lists of pregnant women. Lists of people with radios. Lists of midwives. Lists of leaf doctors and their specialties. Lists of the houngans. . . .

There was other information conveyed in these weekly reports, progressively more detailed, the virtual tons of written material Dieumaitre would churn out through the years.

Under the listing of deaths one week was that of the woman who died of "a jealousy crisis." She had been keeping two men dangling, apparently, and paid her dues. There were deaths recorded as poisonings, a ubiquitous fear in Haiti and not unfounded, since the subtle retaliations of slave days. Very importantly, and one of his main charms, Dieumaitre was a product of his culture, essential for his community rapport.

It showed up frequently.

There was his report on the two school teachers who did not like each other. Two students were allowed to fight one Thursday by these two teachers until all the students were involved in a melee and the people in the marketplace were forced to intervene, breaking up this battleground in the school yard. "These two teachers are a detriment to the progress of Fond Parisien," Dieumaitre wrote severely, "and when I contemplate the progress of Fond Parisien, I am not optimistic if we cannot have our schools run in a better way."

A recent drop in the birth rate was attributed to the fact there had not been many festivals lately and the young women had not had a chance to circulate very much.

And then there was the case of the four men just returned from cutting cane in the Dominican Republic, stopped by the local corporal, who demanded $50 from each. They refused, thinking he was joking, "so he took them to the commandant," Dieumaitre wrote, "who was at this point sleeping with Mademoiselle . . . in her house." It gets very

THE KRUSHCHEV OF FOND PARISIEN

detailed, but essentially the commandant was very disturbed at the interruption, came to the door, had the four men tied up. . . .

Ary Bordes was kept most well informed of each week's goings on in this Haitian village by Dieumaitre Jacques. Amongst the details and the gossip, he culled what he needed to plan his program of community medicine for the 4,000 people living in mostly mud-and-thatch huts in Fond Parisien.

There were 59 latrines for 790 houses. There was no electricity and no running water. There were two irrigation pumps and five small water sources. Only 6.6 percent of the people could read and write and none used a newspaper. There were two "houngans," four "houngan macoutes," six healers, nine "mambos," nine leaf doctors, of whom two were part-time midwives of the nine midwives serving the community. Medical treatment followed the traditional folk methods and cost from 22 to 42 cents, half payable in advance, when a leaf doctor was consulted. The "houngans" charged far more. Malnutrition and diarrhea were the major problems among infants. Infant mortality was 108 per thousand. The birthrate was 29 percent. The general death rate was 13 percent, newborns to six-year-olds comprising 54 percent of those who died. Only about one-third of the school-age children attended the village school. There were not enough cows or goats to meet the milk needs of the children. Egg production was inadequate. Produce was sold rather than consumed at home. A single steer was killed each month for the meat consumption of the entire village. There were ten radios.

There was a lot of work to be done. There were problems, many the same as those encountered in the city, only now compounded by the isolation and even greater poverty of rural life.

Dieumaitre's very worst problem in assisting Ary Bordes's work was voodoo. The village was full of black voodoo crosses and little one-room houses dedicated to the homage of the spirits and the dead, kept in good repair, lest a hole in the roof or the wall cause the residents to retaliate for the insult with illness. Rites were "owed" these beings and negligences punished. It was all in the family, a very extended family, right into the underworld and aboveworld, for the spirits were often ancestors, ever-distant relations who had lost their human personalities and become members of another world.

Then, there were the malevolent "petro" spirits, more violent and cruel, the villagers said in whispers. They had "taken over the region," some claimed, causing much more serious illness and more death than ever before. Their wrath could not be appeased with simple and inexpensive cornmeal, porridge, or soft drinks, for the "petro" loa demanded meat and blood and rum—in large quantities, the frightened people explained. It was difficult given the poverty of Fond Parisien to satisfy these inordinate demands and pay off their obligations and debts to these spirits, they said. This was not all. There were ghosts who could possess people, taking over their lives until death; "baka," the "djab," and "nam," evil spirits who changed shapes and could be purchased like a hired gun to do someone in, generally by inflicting illness.

And worst of all, the scourge of infants, there were "lougarous," living persons, usually female, who changed shape at night and gradually sucked the blood of babies each night until they died. Fond Parisien was said to be full of them. That's why so many babies died. "Lougarous" were particularly terrifying to the people because there was no appeasement, no protection against such a creature, maybe a seemingly harmless neighbor by day, someone who had become victimized by some malevolent spirit or sold herself for more success in life and had come to enjoy her nightly fate. The village seethed with suspicion and hostility toward those they considered to be such child eaters by night, assuming the shape of an insect or a bird, flying to a victim's house when the household was asleep, inserting a long, thin, strawlike tube through the roof, into the baby's neck, and like a vampire, sucking the child's life away. Each morning the child awoke more weakened than the previous evening. The powers of the mystical and the evil were everywhere in Fond Parisien, a most precarious world.

These were not the only causes of illness, however, for the people believed in natural forms of sickness as well: "gas"—air mixed somehow in someone's insides, not properly expelled and causing pain; "cold" which entered and harmed the body in much the same way; "blood" problems from sudden and strong negative emotions or too much time in the shade. The blood rushed from underneath a person's heart where it belonged, to the head and brain, causing fainting and skin problems, they said.

Given this flexibility in belief, what was the proper diagnosis? Spiritual or natural? The Haitian peasant was open to anything, demonstrating the country's saving grace, a fantastic ability to adapt to new ideas and try anything. Their culture and environment had taught them all along to seek out the innovative to survive their harsh lives without any feelings of conflict whatsoever. It was not a choice, really; they could move in tandem. And they would, just as smoothly as a late Saturday-night voodoo ceremony followed by a Sunday-morning Catholic church service—a visit to the "houngan" and the new clinic.

In time the villagers began to seek out the clinic after all ritual treatment had failed and the spiritual causes of the illness remained undetermined, or perhaps simply did not exist. And they gradually learned not to wait too long before making that move.

Dieumaitre understood the subtleties of the problem and courted the voodoo priests, visiting one particular priest every day, even assisting at some of his ceremonies to overcome his resistance to the new clinic. The "houngan" had his own practice to safeguard, of course. Dieumaitre became pals with the members of the priest's "hunsi"—the dancers at his religious center—ingratiating himself particularly with the "hunsi" who were members of the "houngan's" own family. He was always ready with a favor. When there was illness in the priest's family, Dieumaitre got him medicine without charge and the "houngan" saw that there were powers here too, curing beyond leaves and prayer. Given all the ministrations, it did not take too long to win him over—October to the following March. Dieumaitre was hard to resist; the "houngan" was sold on the program.

But the most powerful voodoo priest of Fond Parisien would continue to be a problem despite all of Dieumaitre's considerable tricks and tactics. He even tried becoming something of a godfather to the priest's favorite daughter, to use her as a go-between. As is the tradition, every January first, Dieumaitre would give the baby a present until she came to love Dieumaitre almost as another father, he says. He worked on the daughter as she grew, to get her to come to the clinic, to involve her in the program, to influence her father. But . . . she would be a "big Miss" before he succeeded in winning the father over. It took more than ten years, until November 1976. Only then did Dieumaitre succeed in gaining the cooperation of this voodoo priest, but he plugged away at it all those years with his typical tenacity.

Another one of his problems, Dieumaitre was constantly being pressured to get medical services provided free of charge, given the history of a great many sporadic hand-outs in Fond Parisien. But Bordes firmly resisted the idea of free medical care. A clinic visit was 20 cents, and payment was important, he repeatedly told Dieumaitre, who frequently badgered him on this point, looking for an easy way out of his difficulties. The services had value and if they did not cost anything they might not be perpetuated, Bordes would reply, adding, "The people manage to pay the midwives, the leaf doctors, and the houngans." This Dieumaitre could not deny. Bordes wanted the villagers trained to support the program. Hopefully, one day they could sustain the clinic, for one day international assistance would cease, and he didn't want the program to have the same fate. Dieumaitre had little choice but to carry on. The midwives also wanted money before they would come to the clinic for proper training in delivery, and he had to work hard to overcome their demands as well.

There were other little disturbances. The women did not like being examined by a man—they wondered what he was looking for?! They got accustomed to it. The children were afraid of the scale. That was usual in every country. Actually the situation was not too difficult because malaria, yaws, and smallpox teams had been coming to Fond Parisien through the years. Sister John had regularly cared for very sick children. There was some familiarity with modern medical care, although it was only now that permanent care was available.

Dieumaitre was given two assistants to help him recruit for the clinic, including a "mambo," the voodoo-priestess daughter of the uncooperative "houngan," and another man. A master supervisor as well, Dieumaitre personally went with his new workers to every single area of the village, training them in his techniques. Only after they had become accustomed to their work did he send them out alone.

He had some good ideas about supervision. It was not just discipline, he said. You encouraged. You supported. You never embarrassed an agent in front of a client. You go on visits once in a while and listen to him talk, but it is only after you leave the house that you tell him any weaknesses.

Those were the theories. There was the practice, harder for Dieumaitre, a product of his culture most intimately, with only those border crossings into the Dominican Republic for cane cutting to broaden his world-view. "I want you over to the clinic right now! We need you in five minutes!" he found it hard not to say, demandingly. Tugging somebody's lapels, he used the strong-arm approach, "Be there Sunday afternoon. Don't ask why! Just be there!" Nobody's perfect, not even Dieumaitre with all his exceptionalism. His name translates to "God is the master."

In addition to understanding the use of direct supervision albeit more in theory, he also used indirect supervision by counting the clients that came into the clinic to measure the success of his workers and his own efforts, keeping track of the qualitative and the quantitative.

Always there was a lot of hard work. Every day they worked. He would be at it by 7 A.M., making notes and organizing, proceeding by points one, two, and three, his alert, all-seeing, darting eyes watching everything all the time. He constantly received little messages which he read like a self-important delegate at an international confab, then tore into little pieces, too tiny ever to be reconstructed, and let flutter away to the ground, off in the wind. Then, he would be off to get the facts of births, deaths, sickness, problems. On Fridays there was his report to Dr. Bordes. Saturdays he walked all over and ultimately landed at the cockfights. On Sundays he went to different churches to see what was going on. He tried to know what was happening—everywhere.

Wherever the people were, there was Dieumaitre in their midst. He seemed inescapable. At church. At the Saturday night dances. At the cockfights. Burials. Wakes. Markets. Weddings. If people gathered in a group to gossip, his antenna picked up the tidbits: who was pregnant, who was sick, who had had a bad delivery. He would comment later that there were no political problems in Fond Parisien "... because I am the only politician."

He had the style. He walked along. He knew everybody. He chatted. He joked. He poked at little girls and commented on a dress tear, eliciting giggles and good public relations. He grabbed lapels and put an arm around shoulders like Lyndon Johnson on the Senate floor, on the rise under the tutelage of Sam Rayburn. He told the cemetery diggers— "save a spot for me." Everybody laughed. He saw a woman with two children, stopped along the fence and made his pitch. He led the calling at a community dance, in the flavor of a Virginia reel. He flirted with the women and had many girlfriends. At a burial, he spied a pregnant woman, not seen at the clinic, and gave her the rap. In organized groups he impatiently awaited his opportunity to add his postscript; running over to talk with someone, coming back to his seat, jumping up again to make another point. He had free access to every house without resistance or questioning by the men of the household—very unusual. As one villager said: "If he were here, you would know it."

In addition to the style, Dieumaitre had the contacts and he knew how to use them. Those rich in-laws. His cousin, the sacristan of the Catholic church of the village. He met with him each week for years, just to keep the cooperation going. Every time the cousin conducted a service, Dieumaitre would be given a few minutes to speak of the program.

When a new person came into the village, someone with authority, a new school teacher or a new corporal, he met with them immediately to see if they could collaborate, informing them of the services available at the clinic and asking their help with referrals.

Dieumaitre had an excellent strategy to ferret out leaders in unknown territory. "You go into a community you don't know very well. You contact everyone in a position of influence—the natural and traditional leaders in the churches, schools, politics; the "houngans," midwives. You explain your program and you ask them to convene a meeting so you can come and talk. Then, you see who was able to get the best response, invite the most people and what kind of people. Then, you ask them to give you candidates and you see how many candidates overlap, suggested by the different leaders. And then, you know who is the strongest leader and which followers are the most reliable. And you make a choice on who to work most closely with." Pretty clever. He loved it!

His greatest strength? His concern for the well-being of his family, he answered. His greatest weakness? He had none, he said, annoyed at the very suggestion. Well, he might have a bit of a problem turning a project over to others after bringing them to a stage of interest, because he is afraid that things will not be done well, that all the goals and the ideas he has for the program will not be fulfilled by others. So . . . this really is no fault, he concluded with satisfaction. No, he had no weaknesses, he repeated.

His arrogance of power had its justification. "Just as a barber is known in his community for his haircuts, so I am known as the man of the program," he explained. Absolutely correct. And without him, there might be a program in Fond Parisien, but certainly not as successful, the suffering much greater were he still a farmer struggling with water shortage. Dieumaitre Jacques really made the program work in Fond Parisien with his constant presence, his incessant talk, the sheer dominance of his personality—and the merits of his methodology. The epitome of the savvy peasant, in another society he could have ended up pounding his shoe at a session of the United Nations General Assembly.

Dieumaitre and his assistants impressed Sam Wishik enormously, and this was another reason he would recommend full-time public health work for Ary Bordes. Bordes was a man ahead of his time all the way, Wishik thought, as he watched the maneuvers of Dieumaitre among the clinic crowd. "The fact that Ary was willing to use a local villager with no particular previous background was to me a significant thing. It really struck me at that time. It is something standard now, but to think that he was doing it then! It is still not accepted practice in many countries. We still have a long way to go before we accept fully some of the things he was doing way back then.

"Automatically it occurred to Dieumaitre that statistics meant something . . . that he had to have a baseline census of the population. Otherwise he didn't know what the needs were and he didn't know what he had accomplished toward the ultimate achievement of 100 percent of objective. He had the notion, often missing in many programs, even under sophisticated public health people, that you measure unmet needs. The concept in most places is how much are you doing, not how much are you failing to do. And Dieumaitre felt that if he had a list of every person and every child and so on, he would know how many he had not yet reached. It is a very sophisticated concept in public health administration!

"On the same line, he had the concept of continuity of care, that it is not an episodic, occasional contact you make, but you have to keep on working at it. It takes time and he was quite concerned, I remember, at the drop-out rate, the notion that some people had started at the clinic and then been lost. So he developed the notion of the follow-up. He and his assistants would go out and make follow-ups and then in his meticulous recording, he kept track of those he had succeeded in inveigling to come back and those that he had failed to reach.

"He had the notion of high risk, that we must try to reach everybody that we can, and we must know who we have not reached. But he also had the notion that some of them had greater needs than most—even in an area of the deprivation there. Some people were in greater need than others and he made his more intensive follow-up efforts to recapture those for whom you could do more because they needed it more."

But the "tickler file" really bowled Wishik over: "He had this box with the different months so he knew he must be sure to contact this child or this mother during the month of February. So he would put in a little card with that mother's name on it for the February section. Then when February came, he would pull out all those cards and go after them . . . reminders, and the reminders were timed so when the time came, he knew the ones he had to see. And if he didn't get to do everything that needed to be done, he must make sure to see these."

This peasant's organizational abilities were incredible and his enthusiasm for Dieumaitre Jacques was so great, when a Canadian family planning conference came up, he tried to persuade Bordes to put Dieumaitre on the plane to Canada. Bordes did not think Dieumaitre would have very much to say in Canada, but he understood Wishik's high regard.

Dieumaitre Jacques was to become someone of great significance— the model for the "community agent." Under Dieumaitre's brand of leadership, the program expanded. The first year, despite Hurricane Inez and her clawing of the already bad road, Bordes made thirty-six trips to Fond Parisien. From the first, eradication of tetanus was the priority, almost an emergency. Nearly all the pregnant women of the village received their first dose of tetanus toxoid; meetings were called with the midwives to teach them about tetanus of the newborn, providing them with vials of antiseptic powder to replace the exotica they had always put on the umbilical cord. Over 100 tubes of powder were given to the women, midwives, and community workers. It worked.

In a survey made in the spring of 1965, the 9.5 per 100 births—the tetanus death rate—dropped to five percent by the end of the year; to 3.8 percent by the end of 1966. The following year it was .7 per 100— only one case out of 135 births. Neonatal tetanus had practically been eliminated from Fond Parisien: a major breakthrough for the program; a most heartening accomplishment; a development of incalculable value, achieved because the women had been taught at the clinic only to seek midwives educated by the clinic for their deliveries. Not incidentally, the tetanus decline rescued the reputations of a lot of people previously considered baby-eating "lougarous."

The one uncooperative midwife responsible for the sole death was severely reprimanded by Bordes in a very public confrontation full of the fierce psychological pressure he can muster. He wanted perfection; he was not going to tolerate a single death that was avoidable. He went to her house: "The baby died of tetanus and had you done what we said, that would not have happened." He spoke with suppressed, but most evident, anger, an awesome sight, given his usual relaxed, gentle, teasing manner. "We cannot accept this! If this happens again we will have to take some measures against you!" Exactly what, he did not elaborate upon, but he looked as if he were considering the very worst. The offending midwife was quite impressed, judging from her muteness and faint trembling—and shortly came in for training at the clinic. The last holdout of the nine, she was very important, since she was ranked among the top three in the number of annual deliveries in Fond Parisien.

With the elimination of tetanus, infant mortality dropped from 108 per thousand to 59 the following year, to somewhere in between the next year, at 75. Malnutrition and diarrhea had larger causes, social and economic as well as medical, and continued to kill babies, beyond the prowess of a medical-program impact. But with the success against tetanus, the people more easily accepted the new notions of prenatal care, in turn decreasing neonatal mortality, and boosting the prestige of the total health effort.

Prenatal care grew from 160 women the first year to total 482 women in three years. The immunization program for preschool and school children grew each year, with nearly 6,880 shots administered over the first three years of the project—reaching 90 percent of the children, with less of a dose discrepancy than in the capital because of a more captive audience. By the third year of the program, the nutrition center had been successful enough to push death from malnutrition and diarrhea down to two cases each in children under six years of age, and infectious diseases classified as "fever" ranked highest as the prime cause of death, followed by respiratory infections. In summary, child mortality had slowed down and there had been a swing in the causes of morbidity.

The family planning component was not started in the village that first year, while Bordes watched what was developing in the city, but the women did hear about the idea at the clinic. They appeared to like it, and many actually started to ask why they could not "do planning." When it was introduced, in March 1967, Dieumaitre put up a sign by the clinic fencepost spelling out the reasons why: "God says: have children in order to fill the earth, but he does not say that you should fill it up on your own. . . . " In addition, he pushed the economic benefits. The necessity for food, clothing, and education for the children; the inheritance laws and the amount of land diminishing with each generation.

It was a good pitch and ninety women came during that first year, seventy-two the next. Thirty women chose pills the first year. But their participation fell rapidly, to only six by year's end and a mere two new users the following year. It was the curve of the capital in miniature. The IUD was clearly going to be the favorite in Fond Parisien, just as in the capital. Whatever the method, the women now knew from experience that "planning" did not make them sick as opponents had claimed. It did not cut up their insides. Their husbands still desired them. Their main fears had been overcome. The success was obvious.

At the same time Sam Wishik noticed the desertlike environment of Fond Parisien and Dieumaitre Jacques, he also noticed "a very, *very* busy clinic. All the women in the village seemed to be out. It wasn't staged," he adds, sage enough to tell the difference. "Ary had not known that I was going to go out there. It was just a spur-of-the-moment thing. And the clinic was crowded, unlike the urban clinic, which I felt was underutilized, as many facilities of that kind are. The women of Fond Parisien, however, were there in large numbers with their babies." He saw the people standing around or sitting on the baked earth under a straw lean-to adjacent to the little clinic house. They looked relaxed, not seeming to mind the wait. It struck him more as a social occasion which they enjoyed. All those people under a "tonnelle" represented quite an accomplishment, transcending voodoo, human anxieties, and all the other problems that had so vexed Dieumaitre.

While Wishik did not notice malnutrition that trip, he says it was because he was looking for the wrong things—kwashiorkor and edematous babies with crusty faces or the little old men of six months. The nutrition center was doing its job. But . . .

"I saw that most of the people looked thin, small-limbed, including the children and the women, and all the adults, in fact. But only after I tried to assess the age of the children did I see what was happening. As a pediatrician, I had always prided myself on being able to judge the age of children within months—and I was years off! So they didn't look too bad to me because I expected less, since I thought they were several years younger than they actually were.

"The height of the children was so stunted!" he continues. "So reduced over what the standard of the American growth chart would tell you! They looked like thin, vigorous, active children with a lot of energy . . . running around. But they were so much older and had so little musculature on their skeletal frame! And their bones were so small! There wasn't much padding for sure."

There were the usual reasons which the nutrition project had been working to correct without much success. The elements were so overwhelmingly opposed; their efforts so hard hit by drought that year, 1967-68. The eighty-five carreau of land irrigated by the one pump had been devastated by roving farm animals, the sun, and the winds. Three new varieties of corn were introduced, but destroyed by the bad climatic conditions. White potato production fell from 472,000 pounds the previous year to 305,000 pounds in 1968. Milk production was off because of the lack of cow feed.

The facts were there to be faced. Fond Parisien was one of the poorest villages in the country, but down deep Bordes refused to concede defeat. He kept looking for some kind of a solution despite what his logical mind told him the case really was.

He saw the lake. Fish might be a solution. He researched and found about thirty-two fishermen in the entire village and only a spare-time occupation. He researched some more, this time at the department of agriculture. No sizable fishing history in the area ever. But in 1964 the lake had been stocked with tilapia from Alabama and Jamaica, and Israeli carp by way of Singapore no less, quite a trip for the carp.

He researched some more and found that on an average day in the Fond Parisien market, there was a small lot of tilapia, an occasional mirror carp, and a few other types of fish hustled by some pipe-smoking lady merchant for about 10 cents a pound. He went over to the lake and saw that fishing was done very simply with hand lines cast from shore or by a fisherman wading into the lake. In all of Fond Parisien, Bordes could discover only one multi-patched "seine," the large fishing net with floats along the top edge and two long poles to control its movements.

Bordes asked the department of agriculture to develop a minimum proposal to bring more fishing to Fond Parisien; more food to carry the people through the present and future bad moments. Because of the drought the people were living mostly on potatoes, beans, corn, sorghum, and plantains for their daily diet, and malnutrition was endemic. Something had to be done. It was a possibility. Fish was a complete food unto itself, cheaper than meat, even cheaper than milk and vegetables, and within the limited purchasing power of even very poor peasants. The subsequent proposal requested $1,240, with the objective of 2,000 pounds of fish caught per week. "The people will pray for those who will help toward the execution of such an important project," the proposal read.

They never did get the money for the two boats, the large fishing net and small nets, the hooks and the lines, and the salt for preservation. The Service Committee had found a sponsor, Alice Sheridan says, but it "hit a stone wall and I don't know why." They could not get the project through "to the internal parties concerned" is all she knows or says, while lamenting the loss of the fish protein potential to this day. The Service Committee had wanted to follow through with some kind of economic development component from the very start, and fishing in the lake seemed to be one of the better ideas for expansion of the program.

"The Service Committee had never thought of maternal and child health without an interdisciplinary kind of assistance," she begins. "We saw the greatest need—high infant mortality—was just fanatical and we started when we found Dr. Bordes. But he didn't have to be a doctor, he could have been an agronomist. Maternal-child health was the pivot from which the other disciplines could work. Our idea of interdisciplines was not an afterthought, but there originally, and Dr. Bordes always concurred. . . . His interest, number one, was the nutritional problem—the biggest problem. . . . And he believed that a country that doesn't have any health is not going to get anywhere without improving—and eliminating the causes of malnutrition."

Wishik agrees: "He talked about fishing in the lake and he talked about small industry, maybe making bricks or blocks, almost as long as I can remember." It was obvious what was needed. They tried. It didn't happen.

More of the same with efforts at improving literacy. The national literacy organization had planned a program in nearby Ganthier, twelve kilometers away, but with all the activity underway in Fond Parisien, switched to the village to teach adults, fifteen years and older. The plans sounded great—again: a regional committee and community counselors directing five action groups to work on recreation, rural economics, health, road restoration, as well as literacy. It was to be a demonstration project so the people could learn modern work techniques and have a social center as a community focal point.

It began in January 1966. The people were all set to provide the labor for a center, but the literacy agency was never able to come up with the cement, the wood, all the materials necessary for the job, and the food for the workers, since they would be doing the building at the neglect of their fields. Once again, Fond Parisien's hopes rose and fell—hard.

Literacy classes did begin, finally, in April of the following year—ten classes offered in different neighborhoods from 6:30 to 8:30 P.M., Monday through Friday, with 339 local residents eager to learn to read and write. They did not last long: no lights, no benches, no chalk, no blackboards, the people too poor to purchase the books costing 50 cents each. With no money available from headquarters, the project continued for a while at a very slow pace, ultimately failing for lack of funds—not interest.

Fond Parisien was a small village without much political importance. It just could not get the help it needed. Economic development and literacy did not make it. But nutrition and maternal-child health and family planning were underway. Health education continued on the clinic porch and through the field workers and the radio program.

To the ten radios in the village upon Bordes's arrival, another twelve had been given to certain families active in the program, a reward for their participation and a ploy. The so-blessed families were picked for their strategic locations throughout the village, in order to be overheard by the largest possible numbers of hangers-on. Given Haitian village life and its total absence of similar distractions, it took no time at all to entice an audience for Radio Doctor broadcasts. Dieumaitre often grabbed a radio and went for a walk in different sections of the village come 7:20 P.M., program time.

But Bordes discovered the people were so amused by the experience of listening to a box that they did not hear what was being said. The illiterate villagers did not have the habit of learning, especially through a medium that was a novelty—in most cases, their introduction to radio. It took months before the radio program became effective education.

That's what Bordes's careful and consistent research in Fond Parisien had indicated. His methods really impressed Pastor Walker. "He conducted the most constant evaluation of the effectiveness of the radio program in Fond Parisien . . . one of the most backward places you can find in all of Haiti. And if you can make progress in Fond Parisien, any place in Haiti has tremendous hope because he chose as his test area one of the most difficult he could find."

[PART III]

7

NOT QUITE WELCOME

"*I know there are two ways to look at things—internally and externally. Some criticisms are justified; some are not. Some criticisms may be correct scientifically, but incorrect without sufficient knowledge of the country. But a program to be fairly judged must be judged both ways, scientifically and according to the level of the organization of administration of the country. Very often programs are criticized only on a scientific level. For instance, this is the problem . . . this is the solution . . . but the solution is not applied . . . there is criticism.*

"*But besides scientific problems, there are many human and administrative problems. I imagine in all countries politicians say quite a few things before they are in power. 'We are going to change this . . . we are going to change that.' But when they have the power, they don't make the changes. It is not because they are dumb. There's the establishment. Even if you want to change quite a few things, there's so much you cannot do because everywhere there is a type of establishment, a kind of brake, a mechanism to halt change. . . .*

"*We know the solutions. If they tell us to solve our health problems we can give them a very beautiful plan theoretically, on paper. We know most of the solutions! But the problem concerns the application of the solution and the forces that prevent that application.*"—Ary Bordes

"I think the family planning label was avoided," says Alice Sheridan, who remembers walking into the center just as Bordes was about to demonstrate 'the equipment.' "He was very careful."

Discretion was called for. The Schweitzer hospital was not using contraceptives, because, as one old-time humanitarian put it, "We didn't want to get into a situation where we couldn't hold our hospital open." He is secretive to this day. "When you go into a country that maybe is opposed to something that you think is better than what they think is better—they have every right in the world to ask you to leave," he sums up the concern.

There was no formal opposition; there was no formal favoritism; there was nothing—which is what made everyone so nervous. Miss Sheridan maybe captures best the spirit of insecurity of the time in her analogy to an urban walk along Boston's historic Beacon Hill, the area where she lives in her retirement. "Nobody tells me that the man in back of me with the sneakers may pick my pocket, but my own good sense tells me that I have to watch my step."

She took some chances in her Haitian career days when most were not interested or just plain scared to get involved for, "I feel that I was sort of privileged to be the person who got the opportunity to start from scratch and sort of dig away. We dug and dug and dug . . . . "

On-site inspections were part of her job and she remembers them well, in particular getting off the plane one trip with a suitcase filled with "equipment" that had been donated to the Service Committee. There was always the man with a white stick at the airport, indicating who could leave and when, and who should be detained and how long, maybe forever. She did not fear the medical people or the health centers or the high government officials, she says, but she feared "little customs men like him who could get the ear of some lieutenant of Papa Doc . . . I feared the petty politicians." She admits to being very nervous that particular trip and when she stepped off the plane, she felt about as awful as she ever had in any situation abroad.

"The manager of the airport said, 'Oh, is this your first trip to Port-au-Prince?' 'Oh no, I'm coming to see Dr. Bordes,'" she replied—"but immediately I thought of what I had in my suitcase! And he TOOK my suitcase! Then he said, 'I know him well. He is waiting for you!'" She was hustled through customs and the suitcase was given to Bordes with the words, "Here is your guest. You may go, mam." That was it. "They didn't even open it! And as we passed through clearance I saw everybody's bags being opened, with things strewn all over the place. I think Dr. Bordes had arranged somehow to have me met; certainly the IUDs would have been all over the lot had my bag been opened!"

While she is not categorically certain that Bordes knew what was in the suitcase, it was her impression he did. He says he does not recall any such incident. It was a time when a lot of people would have been willing to supply contraceptives to Haiti if it were open . . . and it was not? "No!" And Ary Bordes needed those IUDs for his work.

Alice Sheridan was noticed. She felt that too and the importance of prudence. "I didn't get mail from home the ten days or two weeks I was staying there once, and I complained at the hotel desk," she recalls, worried since her husband faithfully wrote her every day she was abroad in any country. She noticed someone using the telephone. "And I asked if the phones were working, because sometimes they were not very good, but today they were very good and I said, 'All right, I'll put a call to my family.' Oh, they hustled around fixing things up . . . I was waiting in the lobby . . . the bellboy came in and said there was a car waiting outside for me. 'What car? I'm not waiting for a car! I'm waiting for a phone call.'"

She started to feel angry, confused, and—very anxious. "He said they had tried hard, but could not get my call through so they wanted to get me to go to the central telephone office and had arranged a car. I said, 'No, thank you! I'll just wait here for the phone situation to clear up and get the message here.' I thought they might be trying to get me. Wouldn't I have been a fool to go down to that central office!? They could never have gotten me into that car unless they tied me up and dragged me out!'" Next morning, like magic, with lots of smiles, she received a big accumulation of mail without any explanation as to why it had been delayed. "It was the last time I tried to get a telephone call through—ever, I assure you!"

There had been a few voices hoarsely imploring for more attention to the need for "equipment" and Haiti's growing population through the years, but no real figure until December 1957, when a small research study was undertaken in Port-au-Prince by Dr. Felix H. Laraque. He would be a coauthor of the truly revolutionary article in the July 10, 1959, issue of *Science* magazine—"The Effectiveness of an Oral Contraceptive." It would be Dr. Laraque who would have many, many conversations with Ary Bordes about family planning, an interest logical for someone so involved in maternal-child health.

Dr. Laraque is an old man now, frank, open, with nothing to lose, a gutsy style which he has maintained for many of his years and which doubtless got him into family planning long before it was fashionable— some say dangerous. Semiretired but still researching and publishing, he is a nervous man, jumping about abruptly, almost scatterbrained as he leaps from one idea to the next, searching through a mess of papers with incompleted thoughts, spilling ashes from his cigarettes all over them. Sensitive to public health very early, Dr. Laraque was trained in the United States in 1944 and participated in the American Sanitary Mission in Haiti during World War II, working on a variety of disease-control campaigns. He hates politics and loves science. A panda-bear-eyed photograph of Dr. Gregory Pincus has a hallowed place on his office bookshelf.

Laraque became interested in family planning through a side door. In 1959, Dr. Lucien Pierre-Noel, a specialist in obstetrics and gynecology and number-three man in the Haitian health department, attended a conference in endocrinology in Buenos Aires, Argentina. There he met Dr. Pincus, who wondered whether Haiti, given its overpopulation, would not be interested in some birth-control research and Pierre-Noel responded with an invitation. "But at this time," Dr. Laraque says, "because Haiti is a Roman Catholic country, birth control was something entirely taboo. The Catholic Church was entirely opposed, so when Dr. Pierre-Noel returned he wondered what would be the reaction of the Church, the Haitian government, and also, the Haitian people.... Dr. Pierre-Noel was not afraid, but as an official of the Haitian government, he didn't want to get involved," he explained the caution.

Basically, Pierre-Noel backed off, but not before he had contacted his personal friend Laraque, who as a private practitioner might be in a better position to respond. Subsequently, Laraque met with Pincus and did agree to work on a study of the efficacy of the oral contraceptive, using 100 Haitian volunteers.

The first test group were mostly middle-class women recruited from a semiprivate hospital in the capital, where Laraque worked. He would ask candidates to come to his private office, where they were interviewed, screened, and studied. The women came for a checkup every month but the dropout rate was high—50 percent that first year—due to side effects, but effectiveness was 100 percent. Still, it was not conclusive enough because of the dropouts, and the following year Dr. Pincus asked for a test group of 300 women for a study which would continue for ten years. In December 1961, Laraque began another study to compare cancer incidence with a much larger test group—5,000 participants.

"At this time I had a lot of advice from my fellow doctors, my friends, everybody; all of them told me to be careful. You don't know the reaction of the government! You don't know the reaction of the Church! But I was convinced," he continues, "that I was doing something good for the women and also, that I was doing a scientific work. As a doctor I thought that I was entitled to test something that might be good for the health of the people. That was my conviction, but except for my assistant, Dr. [Raymond P.] Borno, everybody was trying to discourage me."

While he had never encountered any governmental pressure, indifference might switch in an instant. He explains: "Haiti is a country that when you do something, you have to look and to think about it; then, to look at what the government is thinking about it. But I was very confident because Dr. Duvalier was a friend of mine. He knew what I was doing." Laraque never met with the president or talked with him about his work, but he was convinced of Duvalier's toleration by a series of delicate insubstantialities indicating the president's awareness and a hands-off policy.

A big wave to Laraque watching through a window the inauguration of a new technical school across the street from his clinic . . . very subtle but something, and seized upon. A handwritten note of regards in 1960 brought by a friend who had talked with Duvalier. The scenario went: "By the way, I have a note for Laraque. Give this to him." It read: "To my brilliant colleague and excellent friend, my feelings of admiration and friendship and affection": interpreted as "the president's way of letting me know he tolerated the work," and treasured to this day. In April, 1964, a regional conference of the International Planned Parenthood Federation (IPPF) was scheduled in Puerto Rico and Laraque wanted very much to attend, but could not obtain the necessary exit visa because so many physicians were emigrating. A friend in an official position who had a meeting with the president mentioned Laraque's difficulty and a telephone call immediately went out from the presidential palace to the police department on Duvalier's direct orders. While he had anticipated some opposition from Church officials, nothing ever materialized, even following Pope Paul's encyclical opposing birth control. He continued his work.

As early as December 1960, a representative from the Western Hemisphere Region of IPPF came to Haiti to begin a family-planning project in the country. Dr. Laraque did his best to rally support, contacting several people who might be interested; very few showed up, typical of the lack of enthusiasm at the time. A few years later another try was made, this time more precisely calculated, with supposedly $35,000 available. Laraque began thinking about the possibility of some kind of official government policy on family planning since there was a difference between working with 300 women in a private study and operating a public clinic. Caution seemed justified.

He visited a government organization called the Haitian Institute for Social Welfare and Research, headed by director general Dr. Jacques P. Fourcand, a neurologist and neurosurgeon by medical training, a longtime Duvalierist and the president's personal physician. Imposing in appearance and smooth of style, too impeccable, Fourcand was born in the same town as Laraque and they knew each other well. Laraque talked to Fourcand.

"I'm going to encourage you, but I'm going to give you some kind of cover," Fourcand replied. "We'll have a committee," he said, basically to receive and administer the funds. Thus was born the National Council of Family Planning in October 1964, with $500 a year operating expenses from IPPF and hopes of expansion of influence. A government statement favorable to family planning had been issued with the official blue seal of the institute along with the announcement of the committee's formation. In a letter to Pincus only a month later Laraque could report: "So far, with the new attitude of the Haitian government toward birth control, it has become less hazardous to recruit patients at the government-sponsored clinics and hospitals. . . ."

But the IPPF program per se would be a failure—in a way. The clinic opened in April 1962, serving different areas of the city, without charge. "The first month, people were swarming all over the place," Laraque recalls, the demand great, the response to five field workers out home-visiting, excellent. But there was not enough funding for oral contraceptives and vaginal methods were being used—the drop-out rate was an incredible 95 percent after one or two cycles. After three years of operation Dr. Laraque recommended the program be stopped unless pills could be provided.

Meanwhile his cancer study proceeded. By August 1963, 1,355 women had been recruited, later rising to the 2,000-user mark. Interest was so high, Laraque complained of the "disturbing number of patients hanging all around the place." He also told Pincus of the considerable interest in family planning expressed by poorer women, but the project concentrated on reaching the middle class because their literacy and stability were necessary for research purposes. Poor women were able to get IUDs, an estimated 3,000 women, through a program of Dr. Maurice Armand at the Maternity Isaie Jeanty clinic starting around 1966, also very cautiously; the Albert Schweitzer Hospital served women in the Artibonite Valley beginning in 1965, also with a very limited and careful approach.

There were problems with family planning, and Dr. Fourcand says he was more than a little helpful to Laraque behind the scenes. "They wanted to close him down," he says simply. There was a lot of confusion about abortion and family planning, for one. There were rumors about financial rake offs—"any time money is involved you hear that." Fourcand also met unofficially with Church leaders, he says. The upshot was a tacit "Do it, but don't talk too much." There was fear, concern, and an effort to be fair, avoiding a confrontation. There were "big fights," he adds, although he categorically states President Duvalier favored family planning, recalling a conversation in which the president agreed: "Yes, that is the only way. If the socialist countries agree to it and need people to work, a country like Haiti should go ahead." But

Fourcand adds, "The government is not the president, the government is all of them . . . some members of the government didn't know where to stand because they didn't know the problem very well."

Laraque would never be able to get a strong government position favorable to family planning. In addition to not having the temperament for the political process and the necessary political connections, the timing was not yet right. Very few people really understood the importance of the issue. He was a pioneer, a man ahead of his time, who accomplished a great deal of the groundwork.

What was most significant, the silence had been broken, and it is obvious from 1964 onward that Haiti was awakening to the problems of population, the trend internationally. By the mid-1960's over half of the world's countries, containing over three-quarters of humanity, had instituted public and private programs to hold down their birth rates. Their moves reflected the growing realization of the consequences of overpopulation on individuals, families and societies, as well as the intolerable pressures on food supplies, employment opportunities, housing, transportation, health and social institutions. It was too obvious to ignore: where population increases were highest, so were poverty, hunger and unemployment of the masses of nationals, swamping any strides in economic development. India would launch the first major population program on a national scale in 1964-65. The vigor of the Chinese success would create astonishment. Both in turn influenced Pakistan, Korea, Malaysia, the Philippines, Taiwan, Tunisia, the Arab Republic of Egypt, Colombia, and Costa Rica.

By the middle 1960s, seventeen facilities were providing family planning in Haiti—with the exception of Dr. Laraque's clinic, the vast majority since 1965. Most had a doctor or nurse in charge and offered services once or twice a week, generally without charge, reaching by 1967 a little over 7,000 women in the capital—a dismal one percent of the estimated number of the childbearing age group of fifteen to forty-four years.

The IUD was by far the method most widely employed. Recruitment came through regular prenatal and pediatric consultations, group meetings with women, and by word of mouth from satisfied users. Conditions for participation did vary but most required that the women be married and already mothers. The clinics were supported by a number of international organizations, including the Unitarian Universalist Service Committee, Worcester Foundation, Pathfinder Fund, Population Council, and the family planning sector of World Church Service, which funded a variety of small efforts by missionary groups involved in health care. Ary Bordes's center was by far the most successful program, not only in numbers, over 1,000 clients a year, but in visibility through its educational program, particularly radio coverage and health courses, and a fully functioning program including staff training, ongoing study, and evaluation. Only Dr. Laraque's Maternal Center served a clientele in the 500 to 1,000 range; three had 250 to 500 clients; four, 125 to 250 clients; the rest, less than 125 clients a year.

Family planning had become an increasingly important component of Bordes's health project at the general hospital as the years passed and nutrition declined in emphasis. Always, however, family planning was a part of a total maternal-child health package. Its position was typified in the schedule of radio broadcasts that very first year, covering a range of health issues and winding up in the final month with a program devoted to family planning. That had been agreed upon from the very beginning of the discussion, despite the delicacy of the issue.

Radio was intrinsically public, reaching all age groups and all social levels, all families and all their differing codes and levels of sensitivity. The station did not want to offend. "We realized when we began a program dealing with family planning that even the majority of the Protestant pastors would be offended with the idea," recalls Pastor Walker, just a little nervous all over again at the recollection, an insecurity even more pronounced as an international operating on foreign turf—just a guest, easily uninvited. "They were not prepared for it. Hardly any teaching had been done in this area. And we knew the traditional policy of the Catholic Church on family planning. We knew the majority of the people were Catholic and even some Protestants had strong objections to family planning. Others were uninformed and it would come as a great shock. So we had to make a decision where we stood and how far we were willing to go and how much risk we were willing to take in going in this direction.

"Dr. Bordes never once made a statement that was embarrassing to us—never once," Pastor Walker says, almost relieved. Oh, there were a few people in the beginning who objected to family planning per se . . . one letter even accused Radio Light of being "radio dark," but they weathered the few clouds since there was little reason for complaint. "When Dr. Bordes spoke about family planning," says Pastor Walker, "he did it in such a delicate, wise manner. . . ."

That was to be part of the success. Ary Bordes proceeded cautiously and avoided mistakes. He moved in a preventive rather than reactive way. In weekly staff meetings, during consultations, he always checked against being too pushy, jamming things down people's throats; constantly emphasizing rumor control among his people, keeping their ears open for any bad vibrations.

"I had a sense he was going slowly. . . . He knew there might be a potential problem somewhere and he didn't know where or what it

NOT QUITE WELCOME

might be. And better to be cautious than to find out after the fact that he had made a booboo." That's what Susan F. Klein felt during her months of research work in Haiti around that time, the first of a series of graduate students from Wishik's institute who would spend time in Haiti connected in some way with Ary Bordes's work.

Young and attractive, assertive and outspoken, most of all eager for international experience after a stint in Jamaica, Sue was ready to do everything and go everywhere in Haiti. She would have many adventures during her months on the job, including hiding out in a closet so as not to get shot one particularly harrowing weekend of experiential living as the house guest of a high-ranking government official with a lovely home along the coast and a drinking problem. She would catch many diseases given her American immune system, the worst, rashes on the soles of her feet so each step was an agony. She would spend her evenings and nights and weekends collating data, week after week, in a project that took far longer than she ever imagined, typical for Haiti. She would brush against the intense human warmth and authenticity of this country. She would watch Ary Bordes constantly with wonderment, including his remarkable deliberation.

"What he always said was that we will not rush into anything because a mistake means the ax; that we really want to test things on a small scale to make sure they work ... that was the way to prevent getting into problems later. He described his role as the private sector project that would do all the testing and find out the right ways, then turn it over to the public sector to be carried out and spread throughout the country."

Newly arrived in Haiti in 1967, Dr. Gretchen Berggren, a research associate of the Harvard School of Public Health and on the staff of the Albert Schweitzer Hospital, experienced in public health medicine in Africa as well, does not go so far as to say there was risk involved in family planning in those days; but she does say, "There was legitimate concern." The private clinics persisted in providing family planning as a necessary part of treatment for ill mothers: "Family planning was begun to help the mother with tuberculosis or heart disease or diabetes ... at very high risk both for her own life and the life of her child. Then, when other mothers asked for it, they cautiously felt that perhaps this could be done.... But there was this caution...." She comments with her characteristic intensity.

Summing it up: "It is a Catholic country and in 1967 there was a great deal of unsureness on the part of many people," as well as "an interesting confusion" between abortion and family planning and other misunderstandings. In time they would be clarified by international press reports on family planning; by the World Health Organization's growing recognition of the family planning part in a total maternal-child health package; and by more local familiarization with the various methods of family planning. "I think Dr. Bordes himself played a very important role in the things he was writing in the newspapers," she adds. "This was very much welcomed by most of the educated people and it gave a certain respectability also to the discussion of family planning."

In addition to his trips to the radio station every Sunday before a drive-in movie, Bordes for many years had been a newspaperman of sorts without a by-line, had taken a French correspondence course in journalism, and even had thoughts of starting his own newspaper. He wrote anonymously, but in the late 1960s adopted the pen name "L. Bambou"—the initial for his wife, Lillian, a severe editor and his rewrite person at times, and Bambou, a plant which easily and widely multiplies—what he wanted for his health concepts.

His column was well received by the public, and generally placed on the front page of the Wednesday issue of the Port-au-Prince daily, *Le Nouvelliste*. Bordes wrote long-hand on his weekends after wandering around the streets of the capital searching for inspiration—trucks full of oranges leading to a discussion of Vitamin C; flamboyant trees, red like blood, onward to the problems of anemia . . . and family planning, of course. The articles later would be compiled in a book, *Reflections of a Doctor*, and published with a grant from the Williams-Waterman Fund and distributed without charge to physicians, medical students, student teachers—for their information. Always the effort was to sensitize the professionals.

Then there were the speeches and the conferences and the meetings and the contacts, ad infinitum, year after year, no opportunity passed to propagandize maternal-child health integrated with family planning—an exhausting record even to itemize, let alone live.

The word spread and physicians and other professionals began to visit the center for more information. They came from the Southern Peninsula, and Gonaïves in the North, to be informed about the program. Correspondence was received from harried medical residents seeking assistance with vaccination programs and problems in the field with nobody else to turn to for support; or informing him of their efforts to develop a course in maternal-child health or a radio program patterned after the center's broadcasts. Meanwhile the maternal-child health class continued to burgeon. "The center was literally assaulted," he reported in a letter to Boston in 1968. "We registered 500 students in two days and had to send away a flock of unfortunates because of the lack of space."

Marveled Sue Klein: "His productivity was absolutely incredible! I mean he was holding down four full-time jobs! And he was doing them so casually, doing everything in stride. It was amazing! He would go off to lunch, come back having written and taped a radio program, then between leaving the center and something else, he would have written a newspaper article. He wrote ... a couple of books. It's just incredible the amount of work he turned out...."

Requests came for information from the outside as well. Development circles were definitely interested in what was happening at the center and contacts were established with the Ford Foundation, U.S. Agency for International Development, International Planned Parenthood Federation, Population Council, World Population/Planned Parenthood, Population Reference Bureau, American Friends Service Committee, Pathfinder Fund and many others.

That's the way it was, agrees Dr. Berggren. "I shall never forget the day the head of the Pan American Health Organization (PAHO) mission in Haiti said to us that PAHO was going to take a much more favorable stand on family planning. He said with a big smile, 'We have someone in Haiti who is Mr. Family Planning himself, and it's so wonderful that there is a Haitian doctor who is so willing to take such a strong stand. And particularly a Haitian doctor who is so highly respected and who is a pediatrician and obviously interested in the health of mothers and children as well.' This was rather an accurate expression of the feeling of many professional people in Haiti at the time—Haitian and otherwise," she says.

By the summer of 1967 three Haitian doctors, with Ary Bordes taking the lead, decided it was time to develop more coordination among the various family planning efforts in hopes of a rapid and orderly expansion of family planning in the country. Some kind of umbrella group. Joining Bordes in that initiative were Dr. Armand, the distinguished gynecologist on the medical school faculty who directed the early IUD clinic at the Maternity Isaie Jeanty, and Dr. Carlos Boulos, a former public health minister and director of the Haitian American Community Help Organization (HACHO), supported largely by CARE. They wondered: were they reaching the neediest mothers? Who were they reaching, anyhow? What was the influence of child mortality on family planning? What about voodoo? What was the people's ideal family size? How were they finding out about family planning? Nobody knew.

On August 10, 1967, fifteen people showed up at the Church World Service office to talk about family planning. "We are here to have an exchange of ideas," Bordes said. "Each year the movement spreads and we would like to have a central office to inform everyone of the progress made and learn of the experiences of each other. This meeting is not official," he stressed.

"We would like the doctors present to present their opinions. We would also like them to consider the type of reports that should be made. We know that is not easy," he added, and the freewheeling and conflicting discussion that would characterize the group for years to come began immediately with Bordes's suggestion of the importance of a uniform reporting system for proper evaluation, quantitative and qualitative.

A second meeting took place October 5, 1967, where Bordes made his now-famous points: "We are trying to see if family planning can be a national program. We are not ready now because we are not prepared for the following reasons—money, personnel, extension with administration."

To comments that they should extend the program now by distributing certain methods of contraception to clinics and hospitals, Dr. Boulos of HACHO strongly disagreed: "You cannot have a national program unless you have people trained for it." Bordes concurred with gusto: "First we have to coordinate our actions rather than extend them. So far, no clinic has really extended the idea of family planning," he said. To the suggestion that an official committee be formed to accomplish such a task, Bordes vehemently differed, with characteristic deliberation: "No committee should be formed now; because as soon as we create a committee, the work stops."

Later in the meeting he made a fateful prediction: "Before the next ten years are over we will have a national program. Now we are reaching three percent of childbearing women and within ten years under normal and existing efforts, we should be reaching two-thirds of childbearing women." This time Dr. Boulos disagreed: "If we made a good effort this could be reduced to, let's say, a few years," provoking a response from Bordes which would be a major theme, drummed . . . passionately: "If we go too fast, the program may lose its importance. The family planning program must be built to stay." This would be a running argument between Ary Bordes and many people for many years to come, his go-slow carefulness—test scientifically, educate, build an infrastructure that will endure—in opposition to family planning enthusiasts pushing for quick distribution of methods to the masses of Haitians right now.

Bordes was very excited about the new group, and two days later wrote Alice Sheridan the good news, adding, "I also had a meeting with the minister of health and we talked at length about family planning in Haiti. He seems ready to cooperate with the already-existing services."

Everyone agrees these informal monthly meetings were a milestone in Haiti's family planning movement—opening up the issue to discussion and legitimizing activities taking place in a still-insecure vacuum. "I considered it [the group] very important and we encouraged other organizations that were involved in family planning to come . . ." Dr. Berggren comments. She participated as an interested observer and kept Harvard informed on the progress of the group and its setbacks, "documenting the early beginnings of what we hoped would be a family-planning movement in Haiti."

The International Planned Parenthood Federation had the same idea, active in Haiti during its association with Dr. Laraque. On two occasions, Bordes had visited with the executive director, in New York, describing current Haitian family planning activities, and hopes of consolidating existing services and expanding comprehensive maternal-child health nationally. About the same time Bordes visited family planning associations in Puerto Rico and Jamaica, just taking a look and talking things over. Nothing special. Curious. Bordes had been told the federation was very interested in exploring the possibility of renewing its work in Haiti, creating a voluntary family planning organization—a definite agenda item for 1968. This could have advantages . . . and disadvantages.

At a meeting of the informal committee, January 10, 1968, Bordes stressed that IPPF "wants to give funds for their program only" and subject to the conditions that a voluntary committee be formed, government approval obtained, and the group request IPPF affiliation. Strings . . . IPPF would have a great deal of control. But maybe worth a few tugs. The next month the group began taking preliminary steps toward obtaining government authorization, in short, official existence, something they had talked about frequently but always hesitated to request expressively, lest the answer be "no!" Then, what would happen to the group? Could they continue to meet informally as before? Maybe not. They could be worse off than with their current nebulous status but nonetheless actual presence. There had always been a great deal of hesitation about seeking official status as an organization, but much behind-the-scenes discussion with the revolving-door health ministers, sounding them out, keeping in touch, maintaining a connection but not pushing. Bordes generally held the diplomatic portfolio.

With IPPF requiring government approval, the troops moved out . . . very gingerly, concerned about even the direct use of the words "family planning." Bordes was directed to draft the letters seeking official recognition in which he referred to "voluntary procreation." But a formal request would never be made, and, of course, never be denied. The secretary of state for the interior, Dr. Aurele Joseph, told Bordes about a proposed government program, he reported back to the group. "In view of this we felt that we should wait so as not to cause any difficulties." They agreed.

That's the way it would go for years. Comments Dr. Laraque, "Dr. Bordes is a very careful man. He never forced it. He always acted very carefully and waited. Because, at the time, I don't think he believed it was the moment to pressure the government into it. But he succeeded ultimately."

It appears to be a question of the maturation of an idea—Haitian time. There would be many discussions with the minister of health ... who would change with each cabinet shuffle ... talk of a government program would get more vivacious ... the idea of a private association would quiet down. ... And on it would go, like a herringbone, the two ideas, private and governmental, proceeding along, one gaining more momentum one moment, the other the next, but both heading toward some organized movement of Haitian family planning, neither making it. Why?

"There is something called bureaucracy," replied Dr. Laraque. "When you present a high government official with something new, he doesn't say 'yes' and he doesn't say 'no.' He is neutral, and very careful not to take a position. You present a project and discuss it and if he should say 'yes,' then it is 'yes' but 'wait, wait, wait.' We never asked to have a formal association," he continues, "and we never had a formal association. Because we were always waiting for the approval of the secretary of health—who would never, NEVER, give his approval." His flying cigarette ashes emphasize his point. "Even when he knew the president tolerated family planning, he would not take a position. This is what you call bureaucracy! The man simply does not want to be responsible because he does not know the reaction of the Church, of the people here. ... Haiti is a very closed country and you have to think about your neighbor's thinking, what the government is thinking. ... It's just bureaucracy!" he says, with very evident disgust at the entire situation, grinding out his cigarette butt. Grumble. Grumble. Grumble.

More contained, Sam Wishik pretty much agrees with Laraque, with a few additional implications. "There never was any strongly antagonistic solid group ... I visited the ministries and they were very receptive to the notion of family planning in Haiti and thought it would be a good thing to do. I think the go-slow attitude of the ministers of health would be because a minister keeps his head on or keeps his position by not rocking the boat in anything. And it wasn't family planning only. It was anything.... Most ministers didn't start any new programs ... just carried on whatever there was....

"I took it for granted that this was just the way the Haitian government does its thing," he continues. "In other words, you do not permit any organization to be developed. You do not permit any twenty-odd different groups in the country to form a society. That just isn't something you encourage in Haiti...."

Wishik also make the point that he was not sure the informal family planning committee was as cohesive as might appear on the surface. "There was considerable rivalry within the group, and more than rivalry—independence of action. They were willing to get together toward some general direction in a general way, but not in a structured way, where they would become subordinated to anything." He sums up: "Clearly, the leading force in the group was Ary Bordes. He was the outstanding one person who stood head and shoulders above anybody else. There wasn't even a second. There were all those people, but there was not one of them that stood out the way he did." Bordes was envied, resented, disliked by some—the usual and not-uncommon price and predicament of superiority. Throughout the late 1960s the informal committee continued its work with very frequent meetings taking a lot of Bordes's time. He did the group's writing and much of the organizing with assistance from Church World Service Pastor William Lloyd Shirer. "We were trying to assure that there not be a lot of disparate activities, but a PROGRAM with norms, education, personnel—something organized!"

Bordes was in New York in December 1967, where by one of those curious chance happenings, an offhand suggestion, almost fate at work, the title "Mr. Family Planning" would become even more appropriate.

His New York stop included the usual talks with Sam Wishik, who called him the morning of December 23 and said he had made contact with Dr. Charles Williams of PAHO in Washington, D.C., and it might be good for him to drop by the next day as he winged his way home to Port-au-Prince for Christmas. Wishik explained how to take the shuttle and Bordes made the trip to La Guardia in the wind and the ice of a vicious Northeastern winter day. He would slip and fall on the way to the PAHO meeting, but everything else would proceed smoothly. It was a casual preliminary discussion and brief, but in retrospect—essential and consequential. Also present was Dr. Ruth Comacho, an American, the light-haired, chunky, lively chief of the population service of the World Health Organization. At that time PAHO was a little skittish about family planning and Dr. Williams probed Bordes carefully, testing acceptability and whether or not the moment was opportune for some action. Bordes said it was because the job could not be done with Haitian resources, prompting Dr. Williams to suggest the Haitian government make an official request for a consultant. Maybe something might be done or at least begun. . . .

Bordes returned to Haiti and reported to the minister of the interior, Dr. Joseph, who was his usual neutral self—"That's okay. Let's continue," Joseph said. Dr. Fritz Audouin, the minister of health, took the same position. They talked at some length about the suggestion and shortly made an official request for a consultant to Dr. François Dresse, the PAHO representative in Haiti at the time.

The consultants came in March 1969, on a two-week investigatory mission announced in the first major newspaper articles on family planning ever. President Duvalier reportedly suggested a pilot project beginning in an urban and a rural zone and gradual extension of family planning around the country while developing the necessary infrastructure. Bordes had prepared the government's position paper, which also recommended that family planning be integrated into maternal-child health. It was a brief paper, a basis for discussion only, something he had not labored over. "It was easy to prepare because I'd been thinking about that for the past two years." While not difficult, it was enormously significant—the first official position to be taken by the Haitian health department in favor of a national family planning program with President Duvalier's expressed interest. "He was receptive," Bordes says of the president's position vis-à-vis the mission. The talks were published as cordial, vital to the socioeconomic development of Haiti and to be continued . . . the impression.

A few days after their departure Bordes again enthusiastically wrote Alice Sheridan: "The pace of the family planning movement in Haiti is increasing in speed and depth. The government through the public health ministry has taken a formal, favorable position . . . I had the opportunity to meet with the consultants and it seems that in the near future, a government program might be instituted in the form of a pilot project. The other programs will by no means be hampered and coordination will be sought from the onset," he assured her.

It definitely looked promising, even more so on April 2, when Wishik wrote Bordes: "I had a long visit with Dr. Camacho . . . she enjoyed seeing you in Haiti and is very optimistic about the prospects of the development of expanded family planning activities." Then he casually presented his bombshell. "I have agreed to visit Haiti for PAHO and to begin the organization of a national family planning scheme. . . ."

It was a rapid-fire and exhausting time for Wishik, including meetings in every part of the country, with sixty individuals representing many sectors, moving around the circles of Haitian geometry, poking about the opinion makers, the powerful, the not-so-powerful-but-the-dedicated, the bureaucrats, the technicians, the soloists. Not the least of his many contacts were members of the informal family planning group whom he met with May 16.

Back home Wishik wrote a twenty-seven-page report incorporating many of their suggestions, but what was very important about Wishik's report to PAHO was stated early, on page four. Basically he said the best way for Haiti to organize its national maternal-child health services and family planning activity was to follow the model of Ary Bordes's center in Port-au-Prince in all its related elements and implications. "It presents numerous advantages," he wrote of the center, "notably liaison with the School of Medicine and other activities of the ministry of health, immunization and nutrition and work in a defined geographical region with a determined population permitting precise evaluation." Late the following month the Haitian government formally applied for World Health Organization assistance for a national family planning program.

While things appeared to be progressing with the national program, Mr. Family Planning might be out of a job. Wishik's most favorable report on Bordes's work, recommending full-time salary in October 1967, had not been grabbed at with enthusiasm in Service Committee talks through its many funding channels over many months. Wishik also had recommended expansion of the project as the nucleus of a phased and unilateral countrywide service for all those who wanted it, strengthening the present demonstration project in the capital and in Fond Parisien in particular, given the opportunity they provided for education both of the public and of the professionals at the medical school. The program was an example of "effective family planning for possible ultimate support by the Government of Haiti," he had stated flatly.

So was born the idea of a family planning field laboratory, to evaluate methods and conduct pilot projects to get a national program off the ground on a sound basis, with speedy expansion of services when the time came. The centers in Port-au-Prince and Fond Parisien had been a beginning but much more was needed. For one thing, even if the national program reached all the women who delivered their babies in the hospitals, it would fail to reach the vast majority of women who had their babies at home. How to reach them? Then, what distinguished a satisfied user from an unsatisfied user? Why did some women continue for years with an IUD, while others demanded extraction after a short period? If they knew, maybe they could help the women maintain a method. Then, there was the problem of educating people about family planning and motivating them to participate; more communication methods had to be developed. Another obvious need was to find the best way of training and using the Dieumaitres—the outreach workers. Then, there was the ultimate question—how good a job had been done? Was the program really succeeding in controlling fertility? They figured it would take about three years' time and $50,000 each year to figure it all out.

Money had always been a problem and had caused Bordes a lot of grief since the program's inception. It seems that 1968 was a particularly difficult point because the three-year project was drawing to a close, yet the idea of a field laboratory had been making the rounds of the foundation circuit without any success. A number of organizations had been tapped—no word. Things were getting embarrassingly red as the thirty-first approached and then March 27, 1968, in a letter from Dr. Levine, the magic words: "I am glad to inform you that the board of directors at its last meeting approved the renewal of your grant. . . ." Three days to spare. Torturous, but okay. April 1, 1968. Funding was assured for another year from the Unitarian Universalist Service Committee as well. But what about the new dream—the field laboratory? Very bad news, June 12, 1968. No money from Rockefeller. A blow. Maybe a delay.

Wishik had an idea. He knew the rich Mellons from his days in Pittsburgh; in fact, just before he had gone to Columbia, they had offered him a very large sum of money to set up a program at the University of Pittsburgh, a Mellon pet. He reopened some old contacts . . . just maybe. . . .

To be precise, Wishik started courting, calling, writing one Robert E. Willison, the representative of Cordelia Scaife May, a daughter of the late and oh-so-rich, the very one, Andrew William Mellon. Her annual income required unloading much money to avoid paying same to the U.S. government; she had funded family planning proposals in the past, and if caught at the right moment, might be receptive to this one. Wishik worked on Willison: "I told him how special I thought Ary was," and he pumped away at the project's possibilities for exponential affect, something all the foundations loved. Wishik also had some ideas on how the proposal might be revised to please the Mellons more.

Meanwhile, the pressure on Bordes mounted; the field laboratory he so wanted was in limbo; Alice Sheridan was retiring at this very tense time; her successor—an unknown quantity.

Richard A. Steckel arrived in Haiti in late June to shape up the field-laboratory proposal to touch the spots of Mellon pleasures with hopes of a seduction ahead. Bordes went to the airport looking for the usual Service Committee elderly representative, given the ages of Miss Sheridan, Dr. Levine. . . . He found an old, fat-stomached, bald-headed man. He waved. No recognition. Steckel was young, muscled, curly-haired.

He waved. They met, Bordes concealing his astonishment, and rapidly developed an understanding, working swiftly together on Wishik's suggestions, as they would work for years, with Steckel writing Bordes lengthy and virtual stream-of-consciousness letters, enraging him by taking Lillian's side in the perpetual home debate that he worked too much, and charming him during his visits to the States with home hospitality—Uncle Ary coming to call on Shelley and the children. Their relationship would be a demonstration of the pros and cons of the personal within the professional and Steckel's constant capacity for high-intensity enthusiasm. Basically, Steckel thought Ary Bordes was the best thing since the invention of sliced bread and/or the eraser on a pencil.

The proposal was submitted to the Mellon connection. Bordes and Steckel waited. The grant was supposed to come up for review between August 19 and 21. Steckel wrote August 5—"sit tight and wait as painful as it is. The amount of anxiety generated in this waiting period is probably equal to 100 first-time fathers outside a delivery room! Any word from the Mellons or Dr. Wishik will be passed on as soon as received."

More pain. The weeks were very trying on Bordes's equanimity. To Steckel, August 27, Bordes wrote he felt "stretched to the outmost limits of tension. . . . If I were a fan of tranquilizers, I would be taking quite a few pills these days." He expressed the hope that Willison would come back from vacation in a good mood.

Wishik wrote Bordes counseling caution, sharing impatience but mostly realism—"some matters just cannot be pushed too fast."

The Service Committee executive director wrote Willison a p.s. letter August 27, following up on another most-friendly letter August 12: "I have just learned that there is a strong likelihood that a national program of family planning will be undertaken in Haiti in the near future. While we have long suspected such a development, it now seems quite imminent. This simply underscores the fact that the kind of proposal we have presented. . . ." He would keep him abreast of those fast-breaking Haitian developments—not all that fast-breaking, alas.

Wishik wrote Bordes August 30: "The present situation is unclear." He would keep him informed. Finally . . .

A date was set for a meeting in Pittsburgh, September 23, 1968, from 11 A.M. to 2 P.M. in Willison's office. Bordes was jubilant, writing Boston the week before the fateful day: "After having gone through a period of doubt, I am sailing now on the sea of optimism. . . ."

The meeting was held in a big, modern office, stark and conservative, yet posh, befitting the size and state of the coffers. Willison had a poker face. They talked and explained and Willison listened and maintained his poker face. Nobody knew what he was thinking when they left three hours later. Bordes was new to the game and at the moment all he noticed was this man's remarkable containment. He began making plans for the eventuality of failure, "not that I do entertain unpleasant and black thoughts," he hastened to reassure Steckel, "just realistic considerations."

December 24 . . . telephone call from Boston. It was a very, very Merry Christmas. The Mellon money had come through. . . . The Christmas present arrived in Boston in little coupons—stock valued at $140,860.01: 690 shares of INA Corp.; 1,400 shares of Coca-Cola; 50 shares of General Motors, to be used over a three-year period to support the family planning field laboratory. "Ary certainly sold the program," Wishik says. "His sincerity came through, his honesty and his integrity and his good sense. I think Mr. Willison felt this was a person who could be trusted, who was going to try to do what he said he would like to do."

8

WARMING UP

"The first programs fighting tetanus of the newborn were to train the midwives. This was really started some years back by the educational branch of the agricultural department . . . then the second step was organized by the Albert Schweitzer Hospital. They trained midwives around the area of the hospital and started to give shots of tetanus antitoxin and became quite successful with a wide program of vaccination of pregnant women around the time we started in Fond Parisien. But the main difference is that the Schweitzer group is a private group outside the lines of influence of the health department while we were within the organization of the health department. So I can be a member of the health department and take what is successful and try to make it become policy and infuse it into the health department.

"This is why I say a good experience in the private field has a great deal of difficulty reaching the decision-making level and being fully utilized for the benefit of the country without that strong government connection. And that is also why I believe that private help or international help that is channeled through the proper establishment ways is more beneficial, than when it is separated from government. For instance, we work here, but in full cooperation with the health department. What is bad, they might not even know except if it is necessary to say—Don't do it, it was done already and the results are bad. But the good parts can reach the decision-making level and I can bring it to the top of the health department . . . and also since I have a definite function in the health department, I can try to obtain authorization of the health ministry and extend it nationally.

"This is why I believe that in order to give maximum results, help must be walked through the proper channels. But what happens sometimes is that the proper channels can come from above. The organization can say this is the proper channel, can choose the channel, and impose things. I don't think this is right, either. To me a good program is not one that necessarily has good results in the present and then collapses after. A good program is one that is able to make lasting improvement within a country, not just show what can be done and then move away. I believe that even though the results are not the best, but if the local capacity is increased, that is a better index of the worth of a program. So with the experience in Fond Parisien and knowing it was the same at the Schweitzer Hospital, I was able to bring it to the attention of the ministry and then push toward national extension. So it was a matter of experience with good results and being in a position to make them known, and then, ask for extension. It was a combination of a situation and an experience. And again, the Schweitzer Hospital had the same results, but no connection with the decision-making people."—Ary Bordes

The very first thing he did was give up private practice, for fantasy had turned to reality with Coca-Cola *et al.* He was on full salary now and free to tackle the larger, more demanding issues he had wanted to take on since his return to Haiti—17 years back. "This is the last time you come here," he would say, sounding severe, almost a warning tone, informing his patients of his decision to devote himself full-time to public health. The second thing he did was buy a jeep. No more dependency on the much-in-demand and sole vehicle of the bureau of nutrition to make his weekly trips out to Fond Parisien. The next step—to have the flaming-chalice logo of the Unitarian Universalist Service Committee painted on the jeep door—a little pat on the back to the funding agency was always good form. Next came Rivière, the jeep driver, almost a logo himself in time.

Virtually Cro-Magnon, erect and primitive of feature, Rivière would wear the fatalistic determination of a kamikaze pilot about to go for a drive across the South Pacific as he approached, what he called, his "jet." He would pull on his red-checked crew hat, adjust his silver-rimmed sunglasses, and press down on the gas—unrelieved—all the way to Fond Parisien, bludgeoning his way through the capital's streets, scattering people, chickens, carts of fruit in all directions, horn blaring, bullying, pulsating along the rockbed of road to the village. Rivière was a simple man without an education, but with a driver's license, a wheel in his hands, and a vehicle under his control—there was $6,000 worth of bouncing engineering that appeared doomed for an early trip to the jeep burial ground. He would destroy, then nurture the jeep for eight years as it progressively declined in power and stamina, mellowing with premature age, use, and Rivière's abuse until it was probably the most seasoned vehicle in captivity.

Next step, more planning as Bordes critically analyzed the program that currently existed, putting on paper the precise organization he needed to carry off most efficiently the laboratory's goals. From the beginning the idea was to concentrate on studying the basic organization, methods of motivation, evaluation of education—not enlarging upon what existed; a true experimental project, the forerunner of something bigger, controlled and qualitative.

They moved to their new offices the afternoon of April 30, 1969, the so-called Family Hygiene Center—again the family planning label was avoided. The aqua, two-story building at 10 Impasse Lavaud represented many things to Ary Bordes. While continuing to direct the government-run operation at the general hospital—for which he was paid a whopping $2,040 a year—his new private center and full-time salary permitted him to pursue his own ideas, uninhibited by bureaucracy; the opportunity to exert more influence on the health department by coming up with some solutions and presenting them for discussion in government circles as accomplished facts; the ability to speak his mind more freely as a government representative in contacts with international agencies, since they were not providing his income. Ary Bordes was nobody's man but his own now . . . very important to him.

Another happening concurrently with the new laboratory headquarters . . . a national attack. The health department announced the launching of a nationwide campaign against tetanus of the newborn with the goal of immunizing 35,000 women around the country, along with a massive educational program. Bordes was named a member of the planning commission charged with coming up with the human and material resources needed to do the job rapidly and satisfactorily. He wrote Boston, "I am all excited about it . . . a direct consequence of the Fond Parisien program." The bigwigs were atwitter as well . . . the press full of coverage of the May 8, 1969, planning meeting in the office of the health minister . . . all the heads of all the different government departments present . . . a major initiative for maternal-child health in Haiti.

Some written material was needed; Bordes saw an opportunity to tie the fight against tetanus to family planning. He began thinking about preparing some booklets with that double objective, immediately having his private center contribute to a public enterprise. The timing was perfect.

The calabash concept was about to be conceived . . . a simple and attractive way of presenting family planning . . . Bordes's idea.

In the village, when a woman was pregnant, the saying went, her husband had filled her calabash, the name of the ubiquitous gourd found throughout the country with innumerable uses. A pregnant woman was full—with child; at delivery, she was—empty. The symbolism seemed perfect for the knowledge that needed to be conveyed, precluding the presentation of sexual organs or physiological information to get the message across, confusing people at the grassroots who did not know the basics of biology. They knew about sex—shown by a man filling the calabash of his wife with water. Now they had to know about family planning—the calabash with a cork blocking the opening so nothing could be placed inside. With an empty calabash the woman and her husband could make the decision at which time they wanted to fill or keep empty—her uterus. It sounded like a terrific idea . . . The Pathfinder Fund agreed to finance it.

Madame Hollant went to work, her assignment to do three booklets: one on family planning; another on pregnancy and the newborn; and the last on care of the baby. Each was to end with a plugged calabash keeping the uterus empty, a happy family, a healthy baby, and a two- or three-year wait before having another. Sounds easy enough.

It wasn't. Each booklet contained about twelve to fourteen illustrations, together thirty images . . . Madame Hollant did 268 to get them, later writing a paper on the experience entitled "Pictorial Illiteracy in Rural Haiti." The first booklet alone, "The Syllabus of the Baby," took four months of constant work to get twenty-four pages of illustration and very simple text.

Madame Hollant would do a series of drawings, a little bit of text, go out and survey the response, return, modify, test some more. At times her insides were in ferment, "I grew up in Haiti . . . these are my people! And I didn't know enough about them! My frustration did not come from the misunderstanding of the drawings, but the misunderstanding of my people!" She was shocked.

"When I first started, I tried to draw a calabash all by itself. But the people would say it was everything but a calabash . . . everything! One lady even told me it was an apple?!" There are no apples in Haiti. Finally, she got the idea of drawing a calabash tree, with a calabash next to it, and a woman with a calabash on her head. Then . . . they saw it was a calabash. This is the way it would go all along.

There was the infamous illustration of the sewing machine, a mother preparing the layette for her coming child. The people saw a woman listening to the radio—an object with higher status value. How could it be a sewing machine, the people told Madame Hollant, when it was on the side of her and not in front of her . . . so she changed the angle of the drawing to a full-frontal view. Still they did not understand. Not that many people had sewing machines, a luxury item to the peasantry, so on the next run-through, she added the woman holding a needle and thread in one hand and a little shirt in the other. The people said the woman was smoking and listening to the radio—the thread, the trail of a cigarette.

"Then, I *really* didn't know what to do!"

And how could she be sewing anyhow, they added, if there were not thread on the sewing machine and she didn't have a pair of scissors nearby? So she drew a woman with a sewing machine in front of her, threaded, a shirt, needle and thread, and a pair of scissors. . . .

Thus proceeded the story of pretest. . . . Bordes insisting on a trial run in the field for material which was so perfect, exciting, and clear to everyone on the staff and ready for distribution—they had thought.

About 5,000 of the calabash booklets were printed, the first of their kind ever done in Haiti, and widely distributed through the clinic and in Fond Parisien . . . impressing a lot of people, eliciting many compliments and a lot of attention. While the public relations were good, a follow-up study would prove disappointing. For one thing the women were not pleased with the idea of being plugged—at all! An IUD, yes, and contraception, yes, but none of this plugging! Symbolism was not understood; the pictures, taken literally. Family planning was interpreted as robbing the women of their sexuality, rather than postponing their maternity; the calabash concept turning out to have a very negative connotation, completely defeating its purpose of popularizing family planning.

Six months later Madame Hollant did a sample of two hundred homes in Fond Parisien where about 800 booklets had been distributed—she found only fourteen; only six people could tell her what they were about. The booklets had been lost or given away or used for their precious paper. Most people could not read and would not even try to understand anything published, particularly in French.

Family planning was considered controversial enough without getting involved in the French-Creole debate too, so they had chosen to write the text in French. "It was really because of me," she confesses, "that Creole was avoided." A mistake, and very naive it turns out. The people who were literate often had learned to read from missionaries whose hymn books and Bibles were published in the folk language. They could not read French, or if they had some facility, it was an enormous struggle.

"I would not put money into booklets again," Madame Hollant reported back to Bordes, survey results in hand. On further consideration they determined that the material did give a guide on what to say to the program staff, standardizing the family planning message in some way; and the limited numbers of people who were literate should have access to some written material. But the results had surely not justified the cost.

The national tetanus campaign the booklets had been designed to assist did not come off, either. Not enough syringes, cotton, and logistical supports like jeeps and refrigerators. There was the will and the planning and the people, but not the money—that most formidable Haitian obstacle. "It is not a negative thing," Bordes told the disappointed, "just one of the steps toward the realization of something. ... " He figured at this point that ideas took from five to ten years from development to realization. And the planning had been some of the impetus for the origination of new educational materials, one of the main reasons for the laboratory's existence.

More ideas were about to be tried. How about a little newspaper? The goings-on of Fond Parisien—a little bit of news, a little gossip, maybe; who had had a baby, who had gotten married, who had died, what big feast days were coming up, events at the Saturday-night voodoo dance— not to exclude health, of course. Tucked in with the personal tidbits and juxtaposed with the frivolous could be the facts of agriculture, commerce, sewing, child rearing, family planning, maybe even a little press pushing fishing in the lake.

News of Fond Parisien debuted March 6, 1970, a four-page, diminutive mimeographed publication, with colored-paper cover and line sketches by Madame Hollant, the editor. It read . . . A son to Louise Celestin, February 19; where to listen to the now thirty-two radios in the village and catch Radio Doctor; the national lottery—a major event of utmost importance—would be drawn on the 17th and 31st of April; the feast of St. Joseph was celebrated in great style, unique in the annals of Fond Parisien, with a major clean-up for the occasion, the young girls singing at Mass, civil and military authorities attending from neighboring localities; Philistain Bresil and Madeleine Fleurius were married on the feast day, after twenty years of communal living, with their three children present, all in school. "The father, the mother, and the three children— that's a good example of the ideal family," the newspaper commented editorially.

Bordes eagerly looked forward to his trip to the village to check on sales after publication of the first number. If it worked maybe other villages. . . . About 175 copies were sold the first week; 220 by the end of the first month. The run was reduced to only 400 copies, a ratio of one per forty villagers . . . still, it did not sell out. *News of Fond Parisien* was published monthly throughout 1970—and folded, unable to support itself despite its low budget and cost of only two cents.

Dieumaitre Jacques reported to Bordes: "The people want it and want to know who has had children and those who have died, but there are not enough intellectuals," he summed up the problem. Not enough people knew how to read. Only 1,317 of the 2,000 copies printed were sold. "Some of the people were very frank with me," Madame Hollant comments. "They said it was written in French—'We can read it, but that doesn't mean we can understand it.' "

The laboratory was not having too much luck with adults; it turned its attention to the schoolchildren. Some backup was needed to bolster the fledgling school health program, which was so enthusiastically received in the capital, Madame Monpoint continuing to conduct classes with teachers and parents—now about the students? Here was Haiti's next generation, too young to compound the population problem at this point, but pubescence was right around the corner. Family planning might not be appropriate in the raw for young schoolchildren, but the concepts of the small family and the population problem could be presented, a little preventive medicine.

Another challenging assignment . . . both concepts were complicated and not easily presented to children with very limited horizons . . . no trips to the museum on rainy Sunday afternoons, no magazines around the coffee table enlarging their world view. Just being in the classroom with shoes on their feet had been a sacrificial achievement of their very motivated parents.

Madame Hollant decided to find out what the children thought about family size and work from there. She went to four schools in the capital, two for boys and two for girls, and talked with ten children from each, individually at first, then later, in groups. Did they have brothers and sisters? How many? Did they like having brothers and sisters? Was there any good reason for a lot of brothers and sisters? The answers smacked of sibling rivalry in their naked and primitive truth. No, a lot of them replied, they did not like having many brothers and sisters, because . . . if there were fewer of them around, they would have more. There were a few who liked the idea of many siblings so they could grow up and go off to New York and send money home.

"When We Grow Up," a little mimeographed booklet of twelve pages with a calabash tree on the cover—they were still trying—was about to come forth, perhaps the single most important printed material to emerge from the center, ever. It was Bordes's idea. The children in its pages, having a conversation, lounged under a calabash tree in a village, situated interestingly, by a large lake likely packed with fish. It was a cute story.

"When I grow up," said the first little girl, "I will have two children: a girl and a boy, Monique and Jacques." "When I grow up," said the second little girl, "I will have two children, two sons, Paul and John."

"And when I grow up," said the little boy, "I will have two children, two daughters, Michelle and Nicole." And on they went. Their children would attend school and learn a lot of things out of big books; they would be given good things to eat so they could run fast, jump, and play; they would be sent to a doctor so they would not become sick. As the children spoke, all the animals gathered round—donkeys, pigs, goats, chickens, all skipping, jumping, singing, congratulating them on their good sense, on "two children, two children!" It had a happy ending. The children all grew up in a well-developed village, one of the most prosperous in the country with green fields and happy kids, joyful and healthy—singing the song of their parents, the song of the two children.

It was a story to be read and understood, hopefully retained deep in the back of their minds, and one day prove useful—when they grew up.

The Fond Parisien village school got the first batch of booklets, distributed to children up to ten years of age. Given the unfortunate tradition of rote education in Haiti, the children memorized the text in the usual singsong intonation, exactly what Madame Hollant did not want, but a mistake became a breakthrough. In no time at all the text of "When We Grow Up" had become a song, a very popular song. Dieumaitre Jacques knew a good thing when he heard it, seized the opportunity, and went around teaching all the children of Fond Parisien "the song" at every opportunity. Wakes became a veritable family planning sing-along. The children in turn taught their friends and family and on it echoed. . . . Madame Monpoint heard it on her trips out to Fond Parisien and began teaching the song in the schools in the eighteen-block area of most intense concentration in the capital. It worked there too . . . the song repeated and repeated . . . sing, song, sung in an ever-burgeoning chorus of Haitian children, growing and growing each year, to become the first song created especially for the children of Haiti. When Rivière pulled up to the clinic in Fond Parisien he was generally greeted by a full chorus from the schoolyard across the way.

The population problem was harder . . . reaching eleven-to-fifteen-year-olds, never easy. Many ideas were talked about and discarded; finally a statistical approach was decided upon, resulting in "By the Year 2,000." The cover sounded the main theme, a scale of unsmiling faces on the weighted-down low side; a black cloud of Haiti's outline on the other side of the scale, a country outweighed by its citizenry.

The facts were impressive: Haiti in 1804—500,000 people; Haiti in 1950—3 million; Haiti by 1980—7 million, 14 times 1804; Haiti by the year 2000—at least 10 million. Row after row after row of unsmiling stick figures, toppling over each other, a very gloomy sight, indeed. The scale was out of balance, the children were taught; there were more babies born and fewer people dying; population growth more rapid than food production and manufacturing; the number of students growing while the number of schools stayed static—something they lived with each day; the number of workers increasing faster than the number of jobs, something they knew from their families. By page nine of the eleven-page little booklet, Haiti had righted itself. Two pages later the reason: a linesketch of a father, a mother, and two children.

The booklet would not be as successful as "When We Grow Up," studies later would show. It was a try, and "By the Year 2000" would get a lot of use for years, beginning with Madame Monpoint's now-routine Friday-afternoon meetings at the center with groups of twenty and twenty-five students, generally in the eleven-to-fifteen age group. From time to time local educators were brought in to advise the staff on how best to reach schoolchildren, a continuing priority of the program. With the assist of the booklets, the children were taught about human reproduction, the concept of the small family, and the population problem, without discussion of family planning methods per se.

Sexually active adults, however, had to understand the different methods, particularly that family planning was not synonymous with the IUD—a constant problem—the first and most widely used form of contraception at the time. To present the cafeteria of choices, Madame Hollant developed more materials, similar to slim-Jim greeting cards, long and narrow little mimeographed flyers on the IUD, the pill, rhythm, the condom, and vaginal foam; others pushed family planning per se, using the calabash concept. Over 17,000 of them were distributed.

"The people are using the brochures for the paper . . . wrapping up cornmeal . . . sugar . . ." the field staff reported back. She would fix them and that, Madame Hollant decided, as she cut the eight-and-a-half-inch brochures in half—not much space for much cornmeal. Regardless, they were printed materials and in French. Limited.

The best way of teaching the merits of family planning and the choice of methods was not the printed but the spoken word. There was a lot of talking going on.

Way back in May of 1967 the program was so clearly a success in the eighteen-block target area, it had been extended to include the entire city. Port-au-Prince was divided into three zones—yellow for the North; green for the center; red for the South, the farthest from the hospital and Madame Monpoint's territory. Each zone in turn was divided into twenty-two subdistricts with a team of a nurse and two auxiliaries circulating daily in each, changing zones every two months to keep the program lively, the faces new to the people, the style as unique as each individual imagination. It did not stay professional very long. Soon, the nurses trained home visitors in the program's goals and methods—four for each zone. It didn't stay paraprofessional very long. The neighborhood wanted to join the action. Natural leaders surfaced, volunteering to help spot the pregnant women, send people to the clinic for vaccination, propagandize health and sanitation; one for every two or three blocks, greatly expanding the human resources for outreach. Next came another category of volunteers, "explicators," one in each block, a permanent propagandist in residence, speaking about the program to families they knew so well, people they lived with every day, repeating the information presented by the professionals and paraprofessionals, reinforcing the message, collecting birth and death data, plugging the radio program, countering false rumors, organizing group discussions . . . enthusiasm was high. "There were so many of them, we had to choose," Madame Monpoint says of the crunch to join the program. They picked students and people with some basic education, equipping them for the job in evening courses at the center and frequent evening meetings to discuss their experiences and exchange opinions.

"The natural leaders and the explicators performed a huge service," Madame Monpoint says, "because the staff was restricted for the size of the city." She laughs at the obviousness of her comment—three nurses and twelve workers at one point, for half a million people.

Did she ever feel overwhelmed? "NO!" Most emphatically not, is the tone. "Once the program was enlarged, we had the afternoons to work, from two to six. We had the time to work." That's all she wanted. Her only problem, she says, was transportation. Her red zone was quite a distance from the center and there was only one jeep and one Rivière. It took time to go out by public transportation. But the staff did its best, even providing the women who lived far from the center with a ride to the clinic for care and, whenever possible, a lift back, maximizing their retention in the program. It was in the red zone that Madame Monpoint first became involved with the midwives, all doing a thriving business since the hospital's delivery wards were so distant—with a direct ratio of umbilical tetanus. "It was just natural to train them," she says with the same modesty with which she assumed responsibility for weekend cockfight attendance. In time, her initiative with the midwives of the red zone would grow into something very large in scope.

To reach even more people, large group meetings were organized in the neighborhoods, so-called "Kola-Sips" for the national soft drink, to provide the proper party atmosphere and attract participation, like a be-in in San Francisco in the same time frame a few thousand miles away, only "Kola," not pot; family planning, not rock; a huge crowd of men, women, and children, gathered about for a universal sip of soft drink or juice . . . the streets packed with people, attracted by bullhorn

WARMING UP

announcements from the jeep beforehand and rapid-fire word of mouth
. . . the staff and all the workers of all levels moving among them . . .
inquiring about their well-being, listening to their problems, providing
advice on health, arousing interest in the clinic, hammering away at the
need for prenatal care, vaccination of children, family planning.

It grew bigger . . . users of family planning—satisfied customers—were
brought into the program's outreach. "You should be the ones who
expand the work," Bordes told them. "Bring in at least two friends to
the center . . . help organize group meetings in your neighborhoods.
. . ." They were briefed in classes and duly recognized for services rendered. To maintain interest, they were given a coupon for every two
women who came to the center at their incentive; the coupons were
collected and every six months a sewing machine was raffled off to a
winner. In time, the coupons became something of an admission ticket
to the clinic and a signal for preferred treatment of sorts, encouraging
the satisfied users to work even harder, since they had connections—
status. In short, a total community strategy.

It was studied to determine the most effective of the three basic recruiting techniques being employed. Data showed that in the first year
of the field laboratory's existence, home visits accounted for 59 percent
of all new clients; talks in the maternity wards brought in 30 percent;
the satisfied users, 11 percent. The following year, the order had reversed itself with marginal discrepancy, satisfied users accounting for
31 percent of the new clients; the maternity-ward talks, 29 percent;
home visits, 26 percent. The satisfied users had definitely paid dividends,
the high percentage of women bringing their friends taking the center
to the take-off point with the capacity for self-perpetuating recruitment.
Now the staff could concentrate more on the vital areas of follow-up
and education.

While thousands of people were contacted each year and 94 percent
of them agreed with the family planning idea, only 10 percent actually
put the information into practice. There was one family-planning client
for every eighteen home visits. Still, nearly 5,000 visits were made to
the clinic for family planning each year the field laboratory developed.
The second year, work was again pulled back to the original eighteen
blocks around the general hospital for better evaluation, but it was
gratifying to everyone that women from the entire city continued to
seek out the center's services.

Simultaneously the program expanded at its rural location extending
into two areas adjacent to Fond Parisien, to Ganthier in 1969 and Bas
Boen in 1970, both villages with populations of about 1,250 people.
Ravished by drought, Ganthier had had a little house with a health
department representative from time to time, but never a real health

center and regularity of care. Now it was being served by three "community agents" like Dieumaitre Jacques, and by a weekly clinic. Bas Boens, a scattered grouping of houses without any central core, had two agents. All were paid staff, responsible for the day-to-day operations of the program, rather than volunteers, as in the city. All had received in-service training, the goal always the same—decrease the number of births and number of child deaths with a solid maternal-child health and family planning program. A team of a doctor and a public health nurse went successively to the new locales, vaccinating the pregnant women, the babies, and children; educating the mothers about prenatal and child care; trying to control tetanus of the newborn, malnutrition, diarrhea; introducing family planning.

Both villages were along the connecting route between Port-au-Prince and the Dominican Republic, and Bordes began to entertain some very pleasant thoughts, indeed. What about a trail of services along the road, public health spreading out laterally into the Cul de Sac Plain? . . . "If health is a human right," he mused to himself many a time as he proceeded along the road, "all citizens should have that human right, not only those living near a hospital or a city." He continued to think about that . . . a lot.

Studies showed that any clinic had a certain sphere of influence; a good ratio was about five kilometers, an hour-and-a-half to two-hour walk for a Haitian, more difficult and longer for a child or a sick or pregnant Haitian. Unless people were desperate, they could not be expected to make a longer walk, and generally, their condition actually precluded making the trip. Now the people did not have to move . . . the clinic was coming to them, the new jeep being put to good use.

The program was expanding . . . what about the results? Something very interesting was happening. It seemed that the center in Port-au-Prince had spent a few years placing IUDs and was destined to remove nearly all of them. The complaints were the same as with women everywhere—discomfort, hemorrhage, discharge, vomiting, abdominal pain, dizziness . . . the word and fear spread. Hardly unique to Haiti, the phenomenon appeared part of an international trend, very evident in other Caribbean islands, notably Jamaica and Puerto Rico, where similar programs were being pursued.

Bordes's family planning work had coincided nicely with the IUD's inauguration around the world. The literature was full of it. The IUD had been considered "the solution" and had quickly become the most easily available method of contraception. The center had found a certain degree of acceptance and had begun to build upon it—but now the structure appeared ready for demolition. Apparently, the women were really afraid of the IUD, but had confidence in the physician or nurse and so tried the method—creating a curve of acceptance/withdrawal at the least discomfort.

There also were difficulties with the pill . . . drop-outs were exceedingly high. And they were getting nowhere with the men. There was only a scattering of male users of condoms in the capital and one lone participant in Ganthier in 1970 out of nearly 1,000 men informed about family planning. Many of their wives would become involved in family planning, but not them.

They couldn't even give it away . . . literally. The program started out with two dozen condoms in Fond Parisien, priced at a very reasonable four cents each. No sales. They went down to two cents. No sales. The men said the women didn't like them; the women said the men didn't like them, Dieumaitre reported the buck-passing underway. Whatever, nobody wanted them—even free of charge!

All in all, there were problems, always very interesting for a family planning field laboratory to study. In 1969, of the 1,640 new clients seen at the center, 57 percent chose the IUD and 22 percent, the pill; a marked pill increase over the previous year—13 percent. Plus, the rate of extraction of the IUD had jumped from 20 percent the previous year, to a whopping 34 percent. But . . . when seen by a social worker, more than half of the dissatisfied women continued with the IUD, and another fourth, with another method—IUD, pill, foam, (depoprovera) shot. Education seemed to be the key.

The following year the pill trend leaped even higher—66 percent of the new clients chose this method, compared with 22 percent the previous year. Drop-outs were still high, however—about one-third of all new users, the vast majority after only one month—63 percent. Again, they had the same complaints; again, the answer seemed to be more education, motivating the women to come back to discuss their problem with the staff rather than just abandon contraception completely, never to return. It was a difficult job, but the program was growing in service delivery despite all the ins and outs. About 14 percent of the fertile women in the eighteen-block pilot area were practicing some kind of family planning—the objective had been 20 percent . . . close.

"We could see the drop in birth . . . it was really special," Madame Monpoint recalls in a tone of real contentment. They were succeeding in cutting away some of the suffering of Haitian families. The word was spreading, the services, the geography, the rewards.

It was coming along very nicely in the countryside as well, student intern Sue Klein was discovering while doing a household survey: about 20 percent of the fertile women were practicing family planning, an exceptional record in so short a time with something so new, having to overcome the deeply ingrained value system and religious beliefs of

Haitian villagers. Also, project figures showed a decline in the birthrate from 39 percent when the family program began to 26 percent three years later. The people of Fond Parisien clearly wanted to limit their families.

The choice of method followed the same trend established in the city: a growing preference for the pill over the IUD ever so surely; but with a higher IUD retention rate than in the capital. There were 218 IUD users and 84 pill users in Fond Parisien. Why?

Sue Klein had her theories. "It was just a nice combination of people who cared," she sums up her view from her house-to-house calls. "In the beginning, I think it was Dr. Bordes's own charisma and interest in the village. He exuded empathy, yet also authority, very, very quietly."

Additionally, Ary Bordes seemed to have a gift for wise selection of staff and for training. "I'll never forget on the way out to Fond Parisien one day," she gives a case in point. "We stopped to pick up something or someone and a poor woman came up to the jeep and begged money. One of the nursing auxiliaries gave her some small coin and began to talk with her about malnutrition. She explained to the woman what she should buy with it to make the red hair of her baby go away. There she was with a baby in her arms and a baby standing next to her, clinging to her skirt. Then the auxiliary went from nutrition and hopped right into asking how many children did the woman have, and what was the space between them. 'You know, of course, your babies are malnourished because you had them too close together,' she told her. 'Do you know there is a way not to have them so close together? I'll tell you exactly where to go so you won't have another one soon . . . so your next baby won't be sick as this baby.' I listened to this and was absolutely amazed! Everything so very reasonably ordered, so well-integrated, and it wasn't even part of her job! Here we were on the street . . . but they had been trained so well. They had been taught how to relate all the different physical conditions to family planning. It was just part of having gone through Ary's training program."

The auxiliary's approach also indicated an adjustment in the family planning pitch—away from child limitation as a selling point, to child spacing. If the staff were to tell people to have only two or three children, they must be able to assure them that these few progeny, their psychological perpetuation and security in old age, would be there for them. Haitian children died—often. Permanent basic health services were a necessity if the concept of the small family were ever to have any validity for the people. Bordes was mulling that over, too.

What he learned, he wrote up . . . a thirty-nine-page procedural manual defining everybody's tasks, beginning from point one. It was widely distributed among medical professionals to influence how public health medicine might be done and done well. Although his charisma created the program, the unit could function by itself. There was a system. Everything that had been done could be replicated because it was all written down to a point of almost absurd detail.

Besides the yellow manual making the rounds, about every medical student, nurse, auxiliary, social worker, health worker of any variety Bordes could get his hands on was brought to the center for training. He was justifiably proud of the work and did kind of like showing international visitors around in particular. Occasionally there was embarrassment, like the time he wanted to impress some distinguished guests with his system of family-planning education and brought them over to one man seated on the clinic bench who had just been briefed by one of the auxiliary nurses.

"Do you understand everything she has told you?" he asked, friendly and smiling; the visitors beaming away cordially as well. The man smiled happily too. "Oh, yes, " the man replied, still smiling.

"And what method will you employ?" Bordes asked him, just a little testing now.

"I will take my condoms home," the man replied, still smiling, "and everytime I have sex with my wife I will swallow a condom." He smiled broadly; Bordes frowned; the visitors tried not to smile. Bordes learned a lesson.

While there were those memorable moments, generally the program moved forward in a slow, deliberate, efficient pace. "Radio Doctor" had gone daily in 1970, broadcasting at 6:20 A.M. and again at 7:20 P.M., judged optimum times to reach the rural area. A government survey of 854 people in the slums and markets of Port-au-Prince indicated an incredible 98 percent awareness of family planning. Most said they had gotten their information from "Radio Doctor." Bordes carefully examined each radio script with a blue pencil, making notations and changes, maintaining very careful control over content. Gradually the program became more direct in its description of the family planning methods to its audience, more secure in their reception. Sex was natural and not to be embarrassing, and there was talk of erections and extravaginal ejaculation.

Saturdays a new radio program began, directed this time at schoolchildren. Called "Health Class," it was a series of twelve lessons for children of the fifth and sixth grades, teaching the basic principles of health and talking about the concepts of the small family and the population problem, what Madame Hollant had presented in printed form in her two school booklets. There were an estimated 40,000 Haitian children in that age group, and the program hoped to reach 10,000 of them. For that extra push? A contest, of course. The schoolchildren were quizzed on five questions, the top student to receive a bicycle donated by a Port-au-Prince merchant. The first year 444 students replied from nine different localities in the country. It would expand.

The course in child health had gone into double session in 1969 because of the overwhelming demand. Sessions were held on Saturday and another at the Red Cross during the week, reaching 1,131 students in 1970 alone. Dieumaitre Jacques and the paraprofessionals and the neighborhood workers were all very busy. The data system had been improved, with a consulting assist from Wishik's Columbia contacts to boost the lagging record keeping, always a problem. The children of Fond Parisien burst into the family planning song every time they spied Rivière. The number of family planning visits was holding steady at about 5,000 a year.

In short, the family planning field laboratory had pretested several approaches and the services upon which a national program could be initiated on the sound basis Bordes was always preaching. And Bordes could accurately write in his annual report in 1970:

"The family planning field laboratory has again, this year, functioned as the main family planning program in Haiti. It has created a pattern: the integration of family planning in maternal and child health, developed educational trends in the use of radio and printed material, and tested the response of the public to the different methods of contraception. The way is paved for the national program," he said with great optimism, "and other private organizations to expand the activity throughout the country."

Discussions were underway this very moment with United Nations representatives who had settled upon the Bordes approach as the nucleus of any future family planning effort in Haiti. The quality and maturity of the organization and effectiveness of the program had made it the logical choice for geographic extension of services now being negotiated around the conference table.

It had been very slow going getting there, awfully quiet, in fact, since Wishik had made his report recommending a national family planning program and a World Health Organization consultant to assist the minister of health in the development of such a program. It had taken months before the Wishik report even got into Haitian hands. No real organization existed responsible for family planning, no actual structure or authority to maintain a dialogue on developments, or their lack . . . a definite problem, and recognized.

Finally, the Haitians started to move. A blue-ribbon committee was formed to report on the present status of family planning to the country's highest policy-making body, the National Council on Development and Planning (CONADEP)—which in turn reported directly to the president. Bordes was a member of the committee which issued its report July 7, 1969.

That summer Dr. Octavio Cabello came to call. Director of the population program of the World Health Organization for the Antilles and Latin America, he was visiting a number of Caribbean islands, an area of the globe chosen by the United Nations to assess how best to provide worldwide assistance for family planning. Bordes and four others were charged by the minister of health with preparing detailed information outlining what the experts could do to help Haiti. Incorporating the work of the health department committee, they were back two days later with a seven-page statement, indicating the United Nations could do a lot.

There were only two government clinics in operation in the capital, Bordes's center and the Maternity Chancerelles; six private facilities in the capital and its environs; fourteen others around the country. Most of the nongovernmental clinics were supported by World Church Service and used the IUD method, with the exception of Dr. Laraque's work with the pill. "Their activity varies and many of them function only in a sporadic manner," they summed up. Over the previous twelve months about 11,000 women had been reached.

What might international experts provide for Haiti? Public health doctors could help Haiti expand its current facilities and increase the coverage. Sociologists could study the structure of Haitian life and determine the favorable and unfavorable factors affecting family planning. Communications specialists could develop ways of spreading the family planning idea and health education generally. Demographic experts could help organize a statistical unit in the health department. Most importantly, the committee recommended a structure "to know, plan and organize these programs." They called it a Children's Bureau, the forerunner of a development to impact significantly on the mothers and children of Haiti.

Keeping Boston informed on developments as they emerged, Bordes wrote July 29, 1969, "The department of health had several meetings about a family planning program.... Dr. Wishik's report has been distributed for a coming discussion ... the discussions continue in all-day sessions...." The talks waged on ... and on ... and on ... Dr. Cabello came and went.

Then, big news, six weeks later. October 22, 1969: the national planning agency formally declared itself in favor of family planning as Haitian policy.

November 21 to 26 more U.N. consultants came to Haiti for discussion of a concrete plan to be submitted to outside agencies to fund family planning. More talk. Six days later Bordes was chosen to be on an ad hoc commission, with technical assistance from the World Health Organization, charged with preparing a plan for maternal-child health and family planning. More committee meetings.

"Up to now there are day and evening meetings," he wrote Boston December 1, "but for us it is a great satisfaction to see that our program in the capital and in Fond Parisien constitutes the basic experience from which the thinking evolves. Our laboratory is playing an influential part...." While time-consuming, the discussions were advancing, questions qualified, local support on the rise, motion definitely forward. The newspapers were full of it—"Round Table in the Department of Public Health on the Problem of Family Planning"—"Haiti at the Hour of Family Planning"— "Haiti Attacks the Scourge of Overpopulation"—"On the Start of Family Planning."

The Haitian working document would be revised a few times during 1969 and 1970, but basically held to the concept of the Children's Bureau attached to the ministry of health; the creation of several clinics in the Port-au-Prince metropolitan area, all in existing government health facilities; and another at a rural site outside of the capital.

Then, that strange silence again. Nothing. March 9, 1970, Bordes wrote Wishik, "The national program is at a standstill pending PAHO's answer." There was no answer.

In June Bordes received a surprise house call from a Dr. Richard Prindle, chief of the health and population dynamics section of PAHO. He said funds for a national program might well be provided and work begun by year's end, and he wanted to talk about what was necessary to get this thing moving again. "We keep our fingers crossed," Bordes wrote Wishik after his visit. In September Bordes met another PAHO consultant, Dr. Gerard F. Rolland, who returned again in December to continue the contact and see if family planning could not be pushed out of the paperwork phase into reality. He was to study the technical feasibility of the Haitian proposal and help with any necessary modifications, as well as prepare a detailed plan and a budget.

There was a lot of maneuvering underway ... on a number of fronts. In the end, Bordes would come out with a lot of clout but in 1970 he was taking a lot of soundings as discussion of a national family planning program intensified. Basically it was all in the last line of his 1970 annual report, "... looking ahead, the most important and necessary [next] step: the full integration of family planning into comprehensive health services and economic development."

The latter had continued to be a problem. Unsolved. More moves to organize irrigation improvements and get those protein-rich fish from the lake had failed miserably. Maybe the reasons were best explained in a little bit of scolding contained in the December 1970 issue of *News of Fond Parisien.* The article on the last page of the last issue was the last word published in the little paper, which folded on a note of irritation/discouragement: "What constitutes a serious problem in Fond Parisien is less the lack of water, than the absence of a spirit of collaboration among the different members of the community. There is no understanding, each is opposed to the other. Nobody has confidence in anyone else," the editor (Madame Hollant) chastised.

Meetings had been organized and sometimes attendance was quite large. On April 7, 1970, many men of Fond Parisien had come for a session on developing a savings association to accumulate the capital for irrigation development. It looked promising but nothing came of it. The same with the revival of that old idea of fishing in the lake. A team of experts from Auburn University did visit Fond Parisien in March 1971, enthusiastic about the possibilities of Lake Azuey as a fishing site for the entire Cul de Sac Plain, not just this one shore village. But their estimated cost for a thorough development job was $17,400, and the money was never found.

Still, the idea of a multi-disciplinary development approach plugged in his annual report had been growing in the back of Bordes's mind with every jeep trip through the Cul de Sac Plain. What he really wanted was to bring the entire project out from Fond Parisien into an area delineated by the three main villages in the Cul de Sac: Thomazeau in the North, thirty-five kilometers from the capital; Fond Parisien, fifty kilometers to the east; Croix-des-Bouquets, eight kilometers to the west of the capital. They formed a triangle when linked by lines on a map, and he called it the "triangle" project. The goal would be the integration of family planning and preventive medicine, already tried and tested, with all kinds of health care, including formal midwife training, improved sanitation, communicable-disease control, maximized health education, nutrition information and rehabilitation—everything reaching all ages and hopefully making some inroads into all the crying needs. He wanted even more . . . activities to raise the standard of living, a very definite and determined economic component . . . what had failed in Fond Parisien and never even been tried in Port-au-Prince. In short, working toward that small, happy, healthy Haitian family on the final page of the calabash booklets.

Bordes knew the educational material implied a falsehood. "Because if you are poor and do family planning—you still stay poor," he corrected. Improvement only came with income growth, and he wanted that for the people of the "triangle."

Bordes started talking up the "triangle," trying it on for size. What the World Health Organization thought of the idea; what the health department thought; what the private assistance organizations working in Haiti thought; what some of the public-health-minded physicians thought; what the international development and embassy circles thought; what the.... Exploring, testing, pushing, listening, reacting, waiting ... the usual quiet calm before the storm of activity.

Money, of course, was a necessity, and when Sam Wishik with his Mellon connections visited Haiti in December 1970, Bordes did not avoid the subject of the "triangle." He reported back to Steckel, "After meeting with the other programs, he became all excited and enthusiastic about the 'triangle' ... suddenly submerged with ideas about the potential of the project," adding, "He seemed quite interested in the search for funding." A revelation postscripted by a little suggestion, "You may desire to sustain his enthusiasm."

A few days later into the new year Bordes wrote again with calm and confidence: "The third year of the field laboratory has begun with serenity and a steady desire for progress. It should pave the way for the 'triangle' ... to nourish a dream keeps up drive and enthusiasm...."

Less than three months later, March 17, 1971, the minister of health, Dr. Max A. Adolphe, and the director general of the health department, Dr. Lauvinski Faucher, issued a communiqué. Bordes chanced upon it while routinely reading the afternoon newspaper, his habit around 5 P.M., a period of concentration not to be disturbed, except by the very brave or foolish.

The final paragraph: "... the functioning of all centers, clinics, offices, and others involved in conducting family planning services is forbidden."

Shut down.

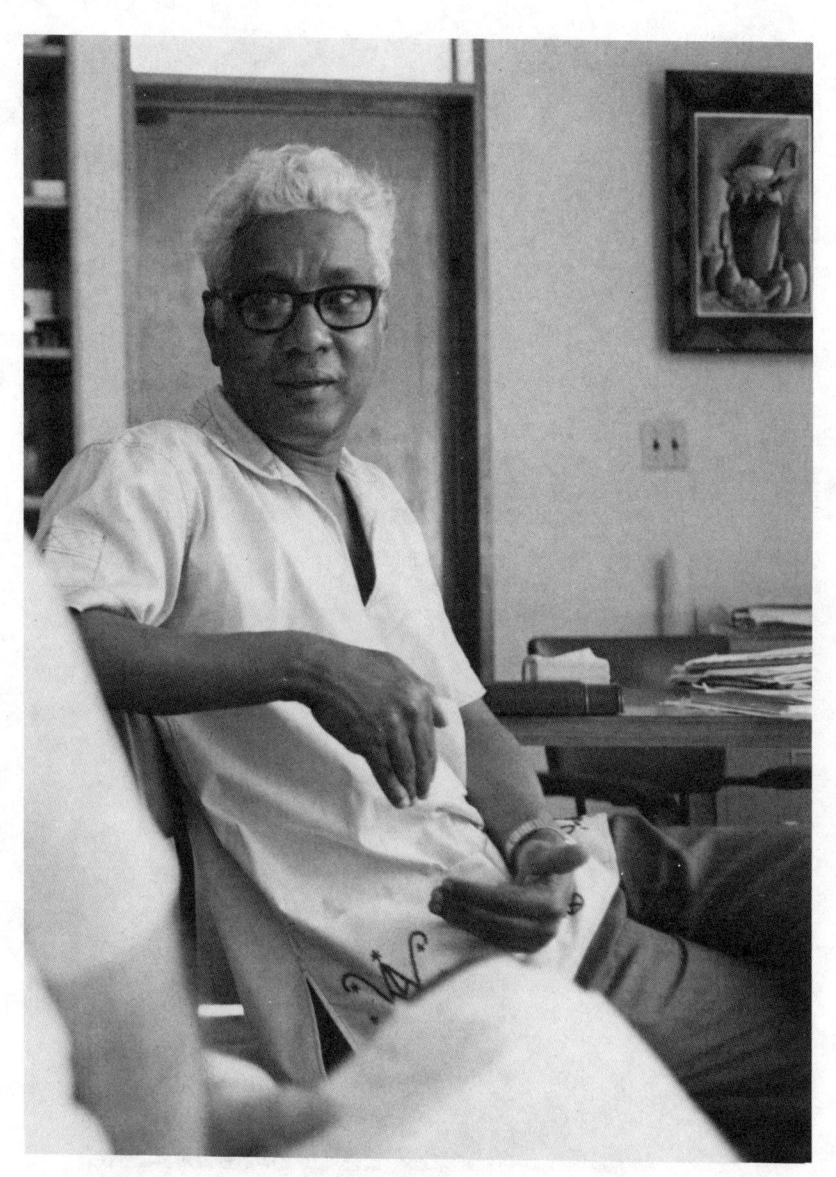

"Underdevelopment is a lack of administration and a lack of organization. . . . This is the heart of it. It is also created by all the surrounding forces . . . the big countries. Overdevelopment can only exist because there is underdevelopment of others."—Ary Bordes.

FOR THE PEOPLE, FOR A CHANGE

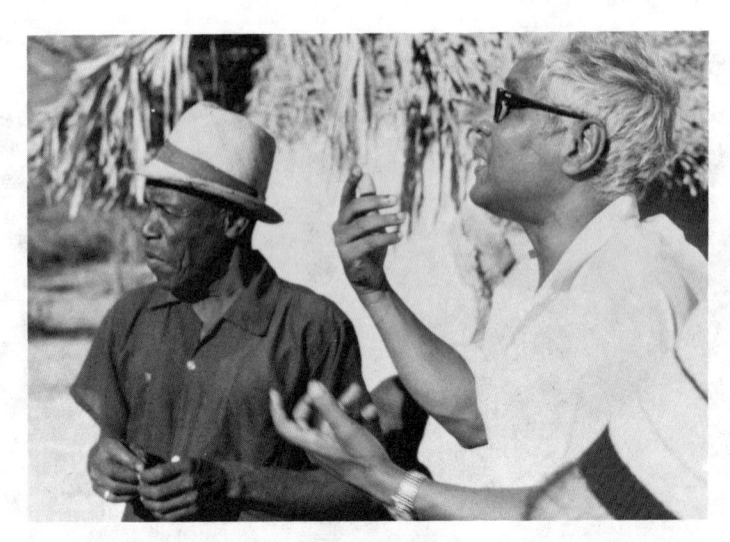

Bordes was always off in a beanfield someplace, coaxing. "Your future depends on uniting your efforts," he would say, his arms thrusting upward, index finger characteristically pointing up.

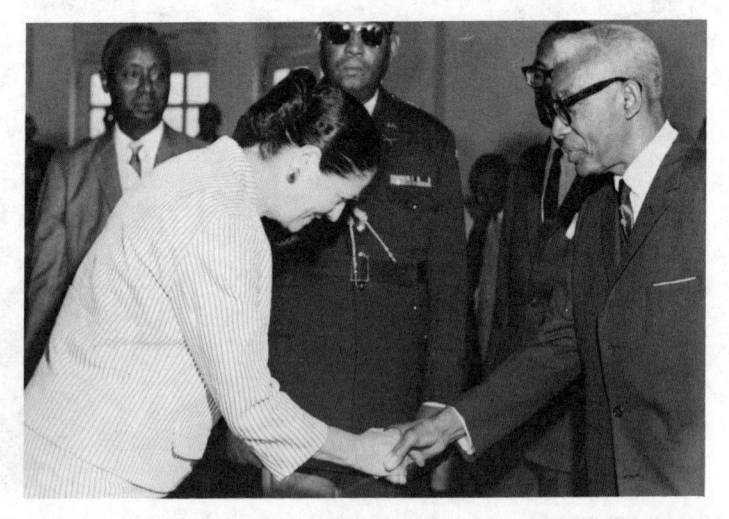

The conference began with a formal reception in the presidential palace, where seven hundred screened guests waited an hour for the appearance of President François Duvalier. "It was carried off with great aplomb," Alice Sheridan recalls.

WARMING UP 155

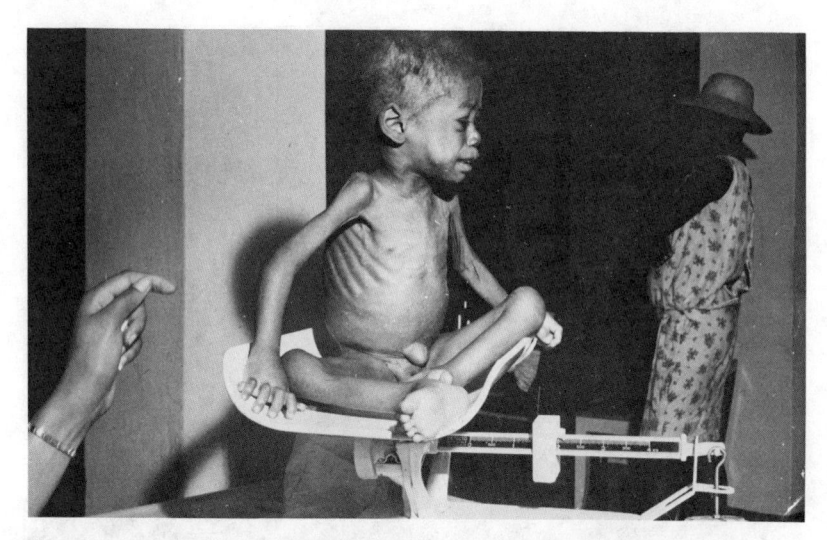

Kwashiorkor, a protein-defiency disease, and marasmus, caused by lack of calories, and combinations of both are endemic. Health is the exception—not the rule.

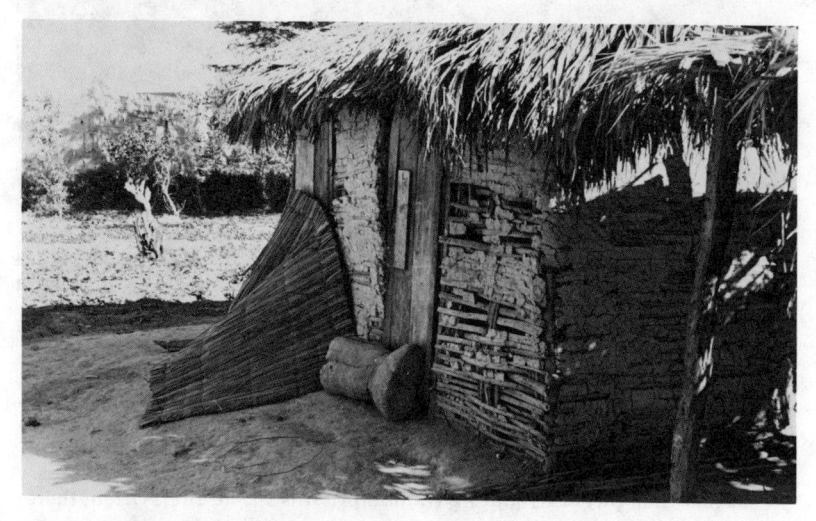

Like a solitary line of poetry there is a fragile beauty about this village which the starkness of poverty cannot intrude upon.

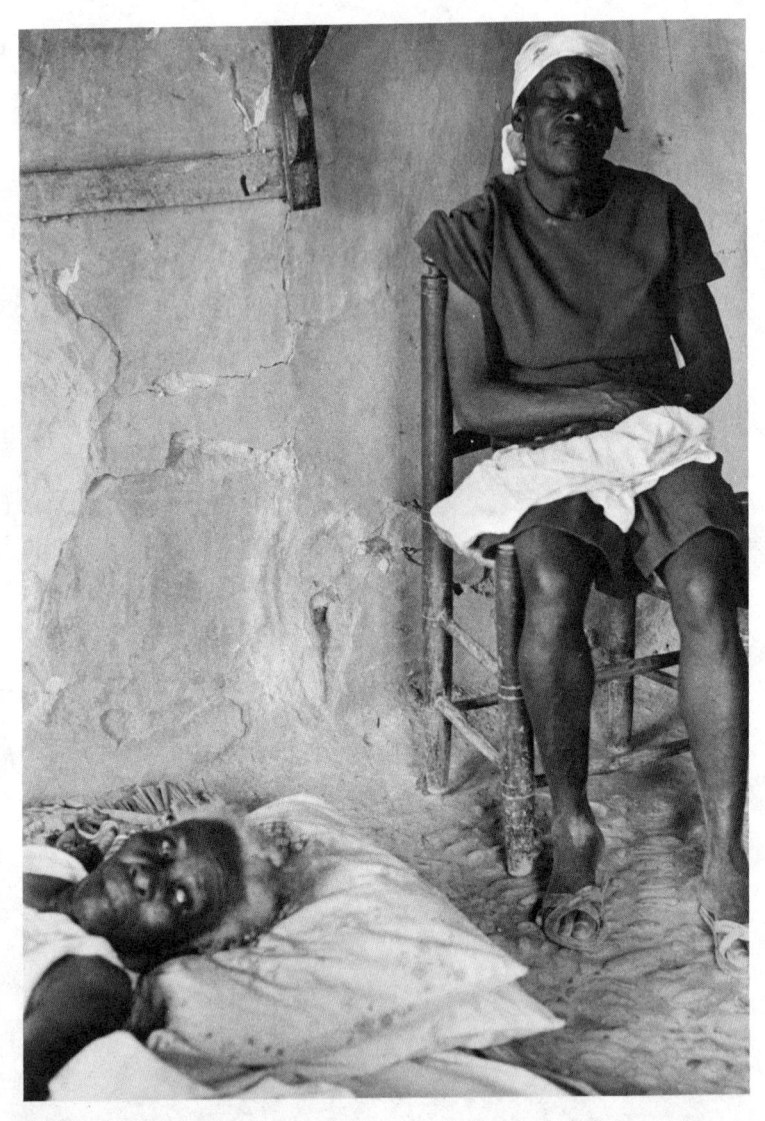

Sickness and disease are considered supernatural in origin, spiritual rather than physical, and the voodoo priest is visited first. Often, there would be no alternative anyway, given the scarcity and distance of modern medical care—as is the case with this deathwatch: ironically, the guardian is dozing while the dying maintains the vigil.

WARMING UP 157

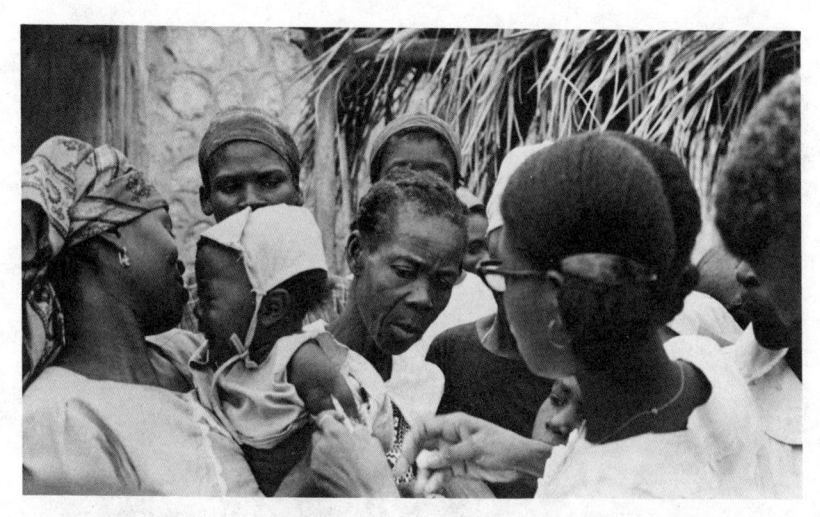

"My first concern is extension of the vaccination program, hopefully, at some point, countrywide. There will be discrepancies—I know it. But in the meantime, we are building," Bordes told the staff repeatedly.

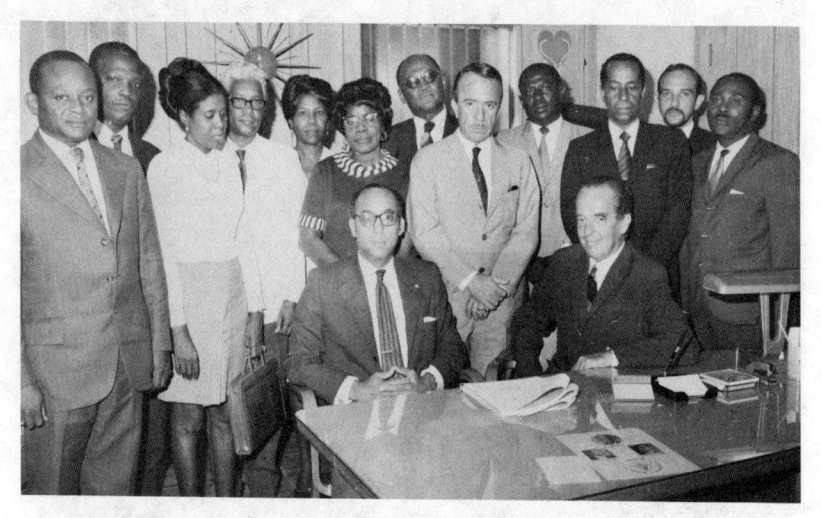

It would always be a struggle, with Bordes maneuvering constantly to keep the Haitian government in control, from the time of the signing of the agreement with the United Nations Population Fund Activities on April 13, 1972.

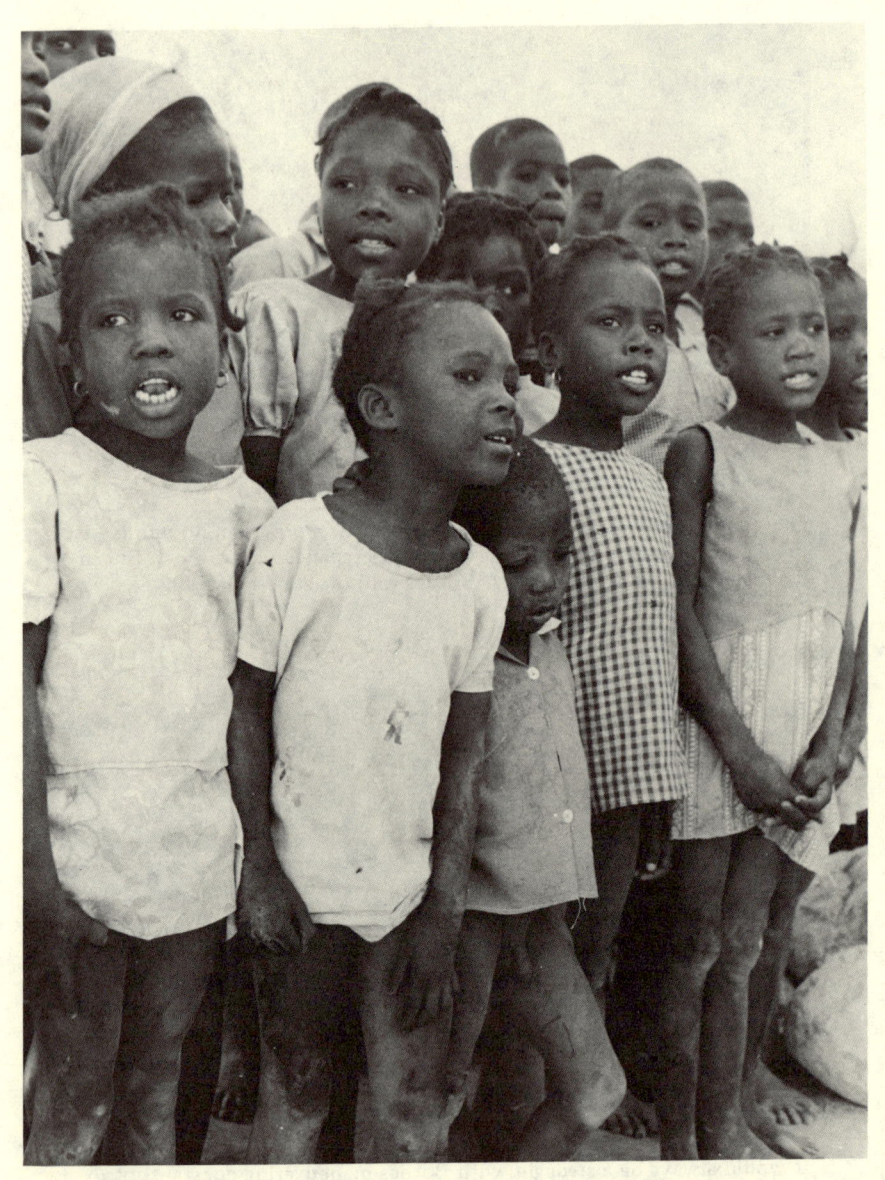

In no time at all the test of "When We Grow Up" had become a very popular song. Dieumaitre Jacques seized the opportunity, and went around teaching it to all the children of Fond Parisien.

9

WELCOME BACK

"The fact that I have been looking quite a bit at the past of Haitian medicine has helped me quite a lot in my work. It has given me a greater understanding of the difficulties previously met by people. Many men tried hard to change the situation. Some of them were more successful than others; some of them were more prominent than others.

"What were the main difficulties they faced? There were the financial difficulties as usual because the country was poor; then there were a whole lot of human problems, attitudes of certain groups towards others....

"And finding out the many things that have been tried that we are still trying to do—organizing mobile clinics, dispensaries—has given me a better perspective and a better understanding of the reasons for failure and the position we could take to be more realistic and make more advances."—Ary Bordes

"I stayed quiet and slept well," Dr. Laraque claims was his reaction to the communiqué, but promptly at 9 A.M. next morning he had a visitor at his clinic. Ary Bordes stayed until noon, discussing all aspects of family planning . . . what might possibly have motivated the government's drastic move . . . maybe if the government knew more precisely what they were doing . . . perhaps monthly reports?

"What's happened!" Bordes demanded rhetorically of Laraque, who clearly was completely in the dark himself. "We've been working on this for six years!" He was incredulous and bitter—not himself.

It was a stunning event . . . a complete shock. Just when the years of superhuman, patient dialogue seemed to be heading for some kind of climax, and now this!

Madame Monpoint came to the center as usual, found everyone on the job as usual, and routinely began a family planning education session around 10 A.M. with some mothers in the waiting room. She was quickly hushed up. "You cannot do that," she was told. She was stunned. One of her children had been sick over the weekend, and preoccupied with mothering, she had not listened to the radio or done much of anything. People did look a little chagrined, she had noticed when she first came in, but she hadn't payed too much attention, too involved in what she was doing. She was told of the communiqué.

"It was really sad . . . it was a blow for us," she recalls, sounding sad. Madame Monpoint had only reached half of her objective and there was so much more work to be done. She was exceedingly disappointed. "The staff were somewhat discouraged," she recalls, "but the ones who were really frustrated were our poor clients!"

Madame Souvenir shared the frustration: "I was not only surprised, but distressed . . . because we were working and we could see we were doing something valuable. We could see the program had an impact. The women were coming for family planning in great numbers. . . . And when we had to close down the activities—we didn't know for how long!"

The communiqué had referred to "dangerous consequences upon individuals and groups from the thoughtless use of contraceptives of certain types." It spoke of restraining the activities of an uncontrolled proliferation of groups—"groupuscules"—at work in a confused fashion in this most important area. Only the government's own facilities would be authorized to provide family-planning services until the government had met with representatives of the World Health Organization and the Pan American Health Organization "to establish the bases" of a sound program responding to the health needs of the Haitian people.

Speculation, protest, gossip, disappointment, all swirled round and round, causing a commotion commensurate with a cannon blast in a wildlife sanctuary. Everybody was atwitter.

A few days later Bordes commented to Madame Hollant, "When something like this happens in Haiti, it is usually for someone or against someone." He would not know how insightful a comment he had made until many years later.

At a soccer match featuring the great Pelé the previous December, Bordes had had a physician's look at François Duvalier, seated not far from him in the stands. "I could see he was a sick man." Plagued with diabetes, hypertension, a history of heart attacks, a few weeks later he would place his hands on the shoulders of his son, Jean Claude, and in a January 2, 1971 television address, with noticeable speech difficulties, he would appoint him his successor, preparing the transition of his government in view of his declining health. Politics was thick in the mild air of that Haitian January, monumental decisions being made to affect the atmosphere and everything else for years to come. The president evidently had more important things on his mind than family planning, and Bordes believed the decree must be from the ministerial, not the presidential, level. "But, I don't know why!"

There had been resentment over the family-planning proposal of a private foundation, which had had strong backing and pressure from U.S. Agency for International Development officials. "This is our country and we were told this was our plan, but it was the first time we saw our plan. . . . I think this was the last straw," comments one participant in discussions at the time. Maybe it was a factor.

Around the same time, at the routine Wednesday evening meeting of Haitian doctors who met for discussions at Dr. Titus's clinic, Dr. Paul Boncy, a prominent bacteriologist, had complained about what he called "groupuscules" the proliferation of small foreign groups at work at family planning without any local supervision or guidelines governing their activity. Dr. Titus recalls the meeting and the commentary Boncy generated and "hurt Haitian feelings that anyone could come in and openly just start work under no control, one group here, one group there. At the meeting, the question had been raised." And the communiqué had included reference to the necessity of "restraining 'groupuscule' activities, most often operating in a confused manner within this important domain."

It was a legitimate concern, and a year previously Dr. Armand had raised the issue of indiscriminate distribution of contraceptives at a meeting of the informal family-planning committee, protesting that pills were being bought freely in Haiti—a danger. "The majority of women buying them without doctors' orders have no idea of how to use them and no previous education," he had warned, strongly suggesting some action to restrict sales to doctors' orders only.

Also, there were rumors of foreign groups involved in family planning without any medical background or supervision, unconfirmed and very exaggerated, but, doubtless, damaging. There had been speculation about the placement of IUDs unknown to women patients in both government and private clinics. Bordes himself had had such a conversation with one individual in his office and been horrified. Since he knew of one case, perhaps others were aware of more.

Dr. Berggren, however, gets very irate at the charges of foreigners behaving so irresponsibly. She particularly fumes about one missionary wife, accused of IUD insertions unknown to the women—"she's never even inserted a speculum in a woman's vagina, let alone an IUD in a uterus!" She says categorically, "I know of no documented abuses of IUD insertions by private groups."

The same charge was leveled at a government-operated maternity in the capital and believed by several people.

There were many different rumbles: one theory was the simply obvious—the government just wanted to control the private sector's involvement in family planning as literally as the communiqué expressed; it was a way of putting the screws to PAHO and getting them to loosen up on the funding and get moving for a change; the reverse—it was PAHO's doing; just another example of antiimperialist acts by national governments, a trend throughout the Americas; intrigues and politics to control private foundation money; every other possible explanation.

But what appears to have been the single most significant factor was completely personal. There was animosity between the present minister of health, Dr. Adolphe, a dentist, and a predecessor, Dr. Boulos, a physician, who wanted to do family planning within his Haitian-American Community Health Organization working in the North. There were rumors of irregularities, patronage, vehicles used to commute children to school . . . and thwarted efforts to obtain accounting to the minister who wanted reports, who wanted "to supervise." He simply retaliated and used his power to make trouble . . . the kind of thing Bordes had speculated about.

"It was a side way to undercut Boulos," comments one physician in the know, confirmed by another high government official, "It was personal." Flatly. "You have to be in the milieu to understand certain things," adds a third confirmation. "You know, when you have a former minister of health and a new one, they become competitive. It was a personal dispute . . . I am sure of that. The government was not involved in this thing. I am sure."

The communiqué was abided by, even in the case of chronically ill women, some of whom would die with no access to contraception; others would be severely weakened by the strain of pregnancy and childbirth; some of the babies would die.

There were a few exceptions to the letter of the law.

Laraque charged into Adolphe's office the following day and demanded to know "What's going on . . . what about my clinic?" Adolphe replied: "Don't be concerned about it. You open your clinic. You see patients. You give birth control pills. You don't have to worry." Laraque's research continued without interruption, and in addition, he helped about five hundred patients a month with family planning. In time, the Albert Schweitzer Hospital approached the ministry with

WELCOME BACK

the emergency need for family planning for mothers with tuberculosis and other serious cases, and got the go-ahead.

By and large the communiqué was respected, including by Bordes's center. In a sense the staff circumvented the directive—but legally—by continuing to go out into the neighborhoods but referring the women on pills to pharmacies for resupply, and those who wanted an IUD, to the authorized facilities. They simply pushed other sources . . . and waited. The communiqué had said that family planning would resume in time when properly organized. "And this is what we told our clients," Madame Monpoint says, "to just wait a little bit and we would reopen." But most impatient were the women who could not afford to purchase pills at private sources and who did not want an IUD. They suffered.

Madame Hollant sums up the response: "We simply emphasized other parts of the work." The breastfeeding . . . the nutrition . . . the immunization. . . . Education and the radio program continued addressing other health issues as well.

Recalls Sue Klein on the scene during it all: "He took, I think, a very politically cautious approach of saying, 'Well, if that's what the ministry wants that's what we'll do.'" She continues: "He said that if they want to stop it, we'll have to stop it because apparently something has happened and we have to give it time to clear up, and eventually if we bide our time, the program will be reawakened. . . .' I think he was definitely upset, but he took what he felt was the only view to take and survive it—that is to wait."

For months Bordes had been planning to leave Haiti for a two-month training course in comprehensive health planning at Johns Hopkins, courtesy of a PAHO fellowship. He felt he needed the information for what he hoped to do in the "triangle." Three weeks following the decree, he left, not exactly happy, but philosophical: "This is the kind of thing that will have to wait for the bridge to come before it can be crossed."

For his part Dr. Laraque was unsuccessfully trying to get some members of the informal family planning committee to meet with an authorized representative of the health department, but nobody would touch it. "No action is being taken by the committee," he complained to his research counterparts in the United States. "Everyone seems to comfort themselves with a wait-and-see attitude." He was not sleeping so well anymore, very alarmed at the "disastrous consequences" on the ban for the large group of people practicing family planning, "the most severe setback" to the family planning movement ever.

It was during a morning planning course April 22, 1971, that a Ghanaian student gave Bordes the news. François Duvalier was dead after fourteen years of rule, succeeded by his son, Jean Claude, nineteen.

Earlier in the month Bordes had predicted to some American friends, while enjoying a leisurely beach day, that Jean Claude Duvalier would assume power on the 22nd of April. The number 22 was François Duvalier's favorite, an example of his oneness with the underworld of his culture, something he understood and used so well—some say believed himself. His Duvalieriste "revolution" began the 22nd of the month . . . many of his important state decisions were announced on the 22nd . . . the dedication of the new Port-au-Prince airport on the 22nd . . . always the 22nd. The possibility exists that his death was not to be revealed until the 22nd. A physician, Ary Bordes may have known the president was very ill, terminally so, when he left for Johns Hopkins; or maybe he was just perceptive about the ways of his president. The news was not a very big surprise.

He watched the events in Port-au-Prince on the six o'clock evening news in the university's television room—the funeral preparations; scenes about the presidential palace; the eerie quiet of the capital's streets, deserted in fear, pregnant with nobody-knew-what, but appearing expectant of the worst; the commentators wondering what might happen now; the U.S. State Department warning about intervention should violence begin; film clips of U.S. gunboats in the Port-au-Prince harbor.

Confounding expert predictions for years—books full of them— nothing happened. The transition was orderly, with no substantial threat ever made to the government, internally or externally. Thousands of emigrés in the Caribbean, North America, and West Africa lacked a central organization and were wracked with dissension and rivalry. Five unsuccessful invasion attempts had been made during the years of Duvalier's regime, never once arousing the Haitian peasants to rally and topple the government. The invaders had been captured and killed or imprisoned in Fort Dimanche—something worse than death, although death came, generally within a few months. The Haitian exiles remembered their fate. It was obvious at home as well as abroad that the government and the armed forces remained in the control of the Duvalier family and their supporters despite the patriarch's passing. Like a Renaissance prince, Jean Claude would come to his maturity while president of Haiti, protected and advised by the economic power elite which always abhors change. Political power would remain in the family. Appointed President-for-Life, Haiti's ninth, by his father, Jean Claude Duvalier was endorsed in a so-called referendum—2,931,961 to one, with two abstentions.

With the change of presidents came another cabinet shuffle, including a new health minister, Dr. Alix Theard, a medical school classmate of Ary Bordes. In fact, if fighting ever brings people together, they were buddies. Theard was a sporty type, big and husky. Ary Bordes has had

WELCOME BACK

very few fistfights in his life—it is not his style; plus, he is small. Bordes and Theard were once on the point of blows when Theard took Bordes's size into consideration—"I appreciated that!" he says. As well as considerate, Theard was respected, competent, and bursting with initiative. He wanted a complete overhaul of the health department to increase its efficiency and deal with some testy issues: control of foreign assistance, tighter administration, a new planning unit—and a national family-planning program.

Immediately upon his return from Hopkins, Bordes was named to a committee charged with reviewing the basic law organizing the health department, including renewing family-planning activities, but under government regulation. The discussions were going full blast when Bordes joined in, the government having recognized the high priority needed for maternal-child health and family planning. During his absence the long-talked-about Children's Bureau had become a "Division of Family Hygiene." Bordes recalls exactly how: "I had just arrived and they were looking for a name and then the minister turned to me and said, 'Why don't we call it exactly as you call your center?' So that was my contribution."

Still, the area was highly sensitive and while Bordes was able to assure Laraque two weeks upon his return that family planning would resume "pretty soon," Laraque found it wiser to discontinue clinic sessions in two sections of the capital at the loss of follow-up of large numbers of his study patients. He was advised to be careful and to restrict his activities until the health department had clarified its position.

On July 29, 1971, at his eleventh Council of Ministers meeting, the new president okayed a strong position favorable to family planning integrated into maternal-child health. Shortly afterwards the Haitian Parliament approved the action and a nineteen-page revision of the Department of Public Health and Population was made into law August 26, 1971, with article twenty-six creating a Division of Family Hygiene. Article thirty-nine defined its responsibilities as "supervision and coordination of all activities, public and private, concerned with child health, including family planning, underway in the territory of the Republic."

Ary Bordes was selected to be chief of the new division. He did not want the job; he wanted to work in the rural area and if he must, have an advisory, but not executive, role in the emerging urban family-planning program. He had already done that. "But you have to!" pressured the new health minister. Theard absolutely insisted. Nobody else was so evidently qualified for the post and for the direction of a national maternal-child health and family planning program. Bordes reluctantly agreed after thinking it over and making a strong case for the development of a rural model for family planning extension.

He got both jobs—neither of them would be easy. He got the "Grand Chevalier" award, his government's highest recognition for health service—he would earn it.

[PART IV]

10

A TASTE OF HONEY

"I think that what Americans, or people who want to help, should not do is to come and do for us. They should find out who are the Haitians that can do the job—and help them do it. There are many jobs to be done, and Haitians ready for them. There are Haitians frustrated because they cannot do what they would like to do. They see a lot of people coming and doing instead of helping them to do. This to me is the attitude to take: know that in every country there are enough civically-minded people desirous to change the country and if you want to do something—find them; help them. Development is a national endeavor; only the nationals of a country will develop the country. If external development comes, it will be for the benefit of the external forces. The world is not idealistic and people do not give usually . . . very few people give for nothing. Usually it is give and take. But someone who is trying to give, should be trying to push toward self-development. It is more time-consuming, but more lasting."

"What is underdevelopment? Underdevelopment is a lack of administration and a lack of organization. Underdevelopment is not underdevelopment of the country, it is underdevelopment of the people and of the administration. This is the heart of it. And then underdevelopment is also created by all the surrounding forces . . . the big countries. Overdevelopment can only exist because there is underdevelopment of others, small countries in the third world. The causes of underdevelopment are primarily intrinsic, due to the country itself, and secondly, to other countries . . . so it's a very complex thing."—Ary Bordes

There had been this horrible pause in the poshly conservative office of the poker-faced representative of Cordelia Scaife May. It probably lasted only about two or three minutes in real time—still, a hell of a long time—but it seemed like light years for Ary Bordes, Sam Wishik, and Dick Steckel. They had come to call for money for the "triangle" project, the obvious follow-through of the three-year field laboratory funded by those nice little pieces of paper from General Motors and Coca-Cola. . . . About $325,000 would do very nicely this visit, thank you. It was June 1971, just about time for Bordes to return to Haiti after winding up his health planning studies at Johns Hopkins.

They explained what the "triangle" was about, the need to integrate health and education with economic development, to expand throughout the Cul-de-Sac Plain, to plan and test for the national family planning program about to climax. Willison listened. It all went very nicely, very politely, albeit noncommittally. That was expected, given the first time around. No problem.

Then Willison turned to Steckel: "You've been using our money for three years. How come I have never heard from you? And now you come back and want more money?!" Devastation . . . absolutely stunned empty time passing in the infinitude of existence . . . the anxiety of the human condition sprung loose between walls of mahogany paneling. Willison had never heard a word. Never gotten a single report. Had no idea of what had been done.

Steckel was dumbstruck. He had simply assumed that the donor organization was on the mailing list for the monthly reports that were circulating fast and furious around the foundation circuit like greyhounds at a dog track. They had heard nothing.

The funding had achieved what it had promised. The money had made possible the model being taken over by other international organizations about to expand in the capital and eventually to all of Haiti's cities. Ary Bordes had delivered the urban family planning methodology and now he was looking for the wherewithal for the rural model. The program had succeeded. But it had failed—as far as Willison was concerned. HE didn't know about it.

"You can just imagine what kind of situation it was," Bordes recalls, chilled all over again. He felt as if he had just been hit with a hand grenade, to be more accurate. "I KNEW I had sent reports every month . . . those minutes of stunned silence! NOBODY SAYING ANYTHING . . . IT WAS SO COLD!" He goes through agonies right there just remembering.

They argued. Okay, there had been a slip-up, each in turn admitted, unavoidable, of course. "Mea culpa, mea culpa, mea maxima culpa." There was a lot of flagellation, with deeply sincere regrets about the

A TASTE OF HONEY

goof, preparatory to the recurring conclusion. BUT. The project has come through!

No change in Willison's position. "If we do see our way clear, it won't be very much," was the way he concluded the talk. They chatted about other things, most civilly, clinging to some remnant of reality, but mostly feeling the absurdity, and began to make moves to depart. As Bordes was leaving the room, Willison seemed to warm a bit to him personally and asked how things were in Port-au-Prince. He mumbled something reasonable, he thinks.

"Steckel was absolutely devastated," Wishik recalls. "He just felt terrible about it! Because he realized what a horrible mistake had been made! Everything was in favor of the program. . . . If they had just been sending the right kind of periodic information about the accomplishment! And I said as we left, 'I would hardly think the donor should rate with everyone else on a common mailing list. He ought to be sort of special. You don't just send reports—you send special reports to him!' "

Steckel heard him but seemed incapable of even a whimper. It was a little too late for that kind of hindsight advice, clearly. He looked exceedingly pained . . . and appeared to be mute.

"I remember it was sort of like somebody had died," Sue Klein recalls their return. "They came back speechless. And it was the next day! There was all this soul-searching and wrenching . . . the grief had not subsided enough to even say 'What do we do next?' It was all this backlooking kind of thing. . . ."

Life goes on. About a month later, Bordes had recovered enough to act. He wrote to Willison, July 12, reestablishing some personal communication clinging to that "How are things in Port-au-Prince?" social lubricant. He told Willison of breaking developments in the national program and expressed his appreciation for services rendered. He still had hopes that maybe the slight thaw on the way out might mean something. It was a kind of this-is-what-is-really-happening-in-Port-au-Prince response, what he had remembered in the shower later, what he should have said on the way out.

To everyone observing his exterior, Bordes seemed undaunted. Very busy. Actually preoccupied at the moment with very immediate demands. The national program negotiations were taking a lot of his time and energy. Interiorly, he continued to ponder the "triangle" project and while he had developed a more precise idea of what needed to be done, he didn't have an opportunity to write it up. A little denial, maybe.

That summer there had been an outbreak of polio along the Dominican Republic border. A massive vaccination campaign had been organized by the health department, including the Cul-de-Sac Plain, to reach children three months to six years—5,000 of them. The radio program backed up the polio blitz. The soundtrucks blared away. Bordes was out in the plain organizing the immunization day after day, too involved even to take time to eat. From the end of July to mid-August over 6,600 children received their first oral dose of live polio vaccine and during September and October, their second. He used the opportunity to get better acquainted with the area and talked to the staff out in the field with him about building on what was being done now in the months ahead. He spoke of the "triangle" frequently, almost as if it were to come to pass as surely as a Haitian mosquito knows how to bite. He just went on about it, talking it up, planning more of the details, acting like it was already in the can.

By fall, the uncertainty began to take its toll. A rare thing for Ary Bordes, he started to complain. In an October 11 letter to Boston he referred to "this floating period in which we are presently living . . . not really a very pleasant one." The Ford Foundation had been approached with the "triangle" proposal and a John Trowbridge was the new hatchet man to be dealt with. Bordes had been asked to be chief of the division at this point, but his appointment was still not official. He had begun to think of other possibilities, other directions to pursue if the "triangle" did not come through, and even the worst possibility— ending the program. He wrote Steckel again the same dreary month: "This morning while sending you the financial report, came to my mind the unsympathetic idea of the end of our program. Unless one of these three alternatives comes up. . . .": the complete "triangle" project; a partial project with a five-mile radius of one of the points, Croix-des-Bouquets; or a health and family planning education study. He had submitted that to Ford too, a research proposal to explore the acceptance of family planning in mothers with one child versus mothers with several children. He wasn't terribly enthusiastic, however. It was a research project and what he wanted, of course, was an action program. But then, you don't always get what you want.

Steckel replied immediately. "This floating period is all right with me as long as we don't sink!" He had met that week with the Rockefeller Foundation, he reported. They were interested, at least politely, but he had no real way of knowing if they would help. The whole scenario distinctively tasted of that September through December 1968 period when the family planning field laboratory was going through its labor pains. That baby had come into the world, howling happy . . . this one had complications.

Bordes wrote Willison again in October when he was officially appointed chief of the new division of family hygiene, noting well that the very title derived from the project he had funded three years earlier.

"This position could not have been given to me without the experience I acquired during the past years of work . . ." he also made note, tellingly, obviously, hopefully. With the United Nations concentrating in the capital, "an effort in the Cul-de-Sac rural area would be most productive in paving the way for the extension of the family planning program throughout the country." He concluded, "May you keep helping us. Thank you." Not much else to be said.

Sue Klein had an idea. "It was fairly incestuous as these things tend to be," she recalls. That October 18 she had lunch with a buddy named Anthony Drexler, who had just gotten a new job as a program consultant for Family Planning International Assistance (FPIA), a new consulting outfit formed that July. Drexler was the ex-husband of another trainee at the Institute for the Study of Human Reproduction, headed by Wishik. The two women interns had been friendly, had mutual friends, one of whom even lived around the corner from Drexler's parents in New York City. All very tight, as they say. So "Tony" had a new job, about $4 million worth of U.S. Agency for International Development funding and ". . . now I have to find a whole bunch of projects to fund," he said to Sue with his mouth full of hamburger.

"Got the project for you, Tony!" replied Sue. "It will be one of your star programs." It was almost a joke. It had all started with a casual telephone conversation about what's new, not business at all. "I just told him that the best family planning program I knew of was in Haiti and in danger of going under for lack of funding," she recalls. It was that simple.

Sue Klein finished her hamburger, finished her talk with Tony, returned to the institute to write a memo to Sam Wishik, off globe-trotting at the time. It was dated October 20, 1971, titled "Funding possibility for Dr. Bordes's program in Haiti," and destined to become a very important piece of paper in Ary Bordes's life. Sue obtained a copy of the 1970 annual report on the program to send to Drexler, but couldn't find a copy of the proposal. She called Steckel in Boston. He and Wishik had already been in touch with Family Planning International Assistance earlier, he told her, taking her aback a bit. At that time they had not been interested, he said, his voice tone sounding most weary, almost hurt. Drexler was new to the job and maybe unaware of some limitations, he continued. But he had been extremely enthusiastic, she told Steckel, adding brightly, maybe policy had changed. She would proceed informally, they decided, and if there were indications of movement, she would put Drexler in touch with Steckel. Sue Klein did not feel as triumphant as she had when she dialed.

The program was scheduled to terminate December 31, 1971. In a last-ditch effort to raise funds, Steckel arranged to have Trowbridge from Ford, accompanied by a Dr. John Funari, flown to Haiti in November to talk with Bordes directly. Maybe the quiet charisma would help. The November 22 meeting did not go well, ending badly, in fact. They did not seem to want to discuss the proposal as Bordes had expected. That evening he pondered at home, long and heavily, and reached for some Haitian adaptability; the next morning, prepared to probe other directions, such as funding possibilities for the national program. When you have Ford moneybags in your office, you don't let them get off easily if there were any chance of getting some. Trowbridge seemed mildly more receptive, but chances were still not over 50 percent, he said, and flew off to Mexico City to hear somebody else's pitch.

Five weeks left. Bordes's thoughts turned once more to his loyal and committed staff, and the painful task of composing the proper way to announce their dismissal and the shutdown of the center. There was gloom and a we-shall-overcome false bravado all mixed up—and down. On an emergency basis, the Service Committee had dug deep for funds to continue operations until mid-February, extending the deadline another six weeks, giving the project every possibility of survival.

Bordes's determination was in gear. He wrote Steckel, who was getting discouraged. "We should realize it, we will realize it. We will have a positive answer from the foundations. . . . " Aroused, Steckel wrote Willison November 15, "The project is indeed the pattern for the national family planning program. Dr. Bordes has now been given key responsibility for coordination of family planning and basic health efforts in Haiti. This can only strengthen what exists and what we now would hope to do." He enclosed a quarterly report. He had learned about sending reports.

November 30, a meeting with Planned Parenthood/World Population at their request. No definite answer. Four weeks left to Christmas telephone time.

"Our program has reached the point of no return," Bordes wrote Boston December 9. "Whatever happens, it should continue, it will continue. The ties with the Unitarian Universalist Service Committee will not break soon. Friendship and cooperation will last, irrespective of the final link. With Christmas in the air, hope in the future prevails. . . . There remains Pittsburgh. Mr. Willison. Our Christmas gift."

The Croix-des-Bouquets clinic was at the launching pad, he wrote, and the countdown had started for a program with the health department. The division had finished its preliminary contacts with all those involved in family planning delivery. The United Nations project was moving toward the implementation stage. He was going to write a letter proposing a private voluntary family-planning association. "As you can see, Dick, activities are in full swing. I have read recently this word of a French general, the famous Foch, during the 1914-18 war: 'My center yields, my left is falling back. Excellent situation, I attack!' How do you like that?" The local situation was good; the atmosphere favorable; the answer due soon. He still hoped.

Steckel wrote to FPIA: "It is a matter of some urgency that action on funding be taken in January in order to preserve the continuity of the current activities." He offered another field trip for on-site inspection of the program to move things along as quickly as possible, or anything else they needed ... more information ... recommendations ... budget clarifications. ... anything!

Christmas 1971 ... no telephone call.

The telephone rang the early afternoon of December 27 with a belated Christmas present from Cordelia Scaife May, a certificate of 1,710 shares of common stock of Aluminum Company of America. Value: $75,453.75, to be used over a three-year period to support a Haitian family planning program under the direction of Dr. Ary Bordes. Not everything, but something. There would have to be modifications, but still promises to keep. 1971 had definitely had its ups and downs, or downs and ups.

"It ends wonderfully," Bordes wrote Boston. "We did overcome.... More valuable it is by coming then, when it became doubtful." It had been soooo close this time ... who would have thought it could have been any closer than that last time? "The meeting we had in Pittsburgh, for many reasons, is unforgettable," Bordes wrote Willison January 10 of the new year, 1972, sending his "warmest thanks." It looked like a very good year. Ford even had come through with the research program which was passed over to the Haitian Center for Social Science Research. Why study when you can act? Bordes reasoned.

There was this little matter of a missing $225,000 or so....

There was a lot of hustling going on in the States. The problem was pretty much family planning. It was too large an expenditure of funds for a limited population, International Planned Parenthood Federation had concluded with their rejection notice—actually a skewed perspective, since the package being sought was for so much more than family planning. All that basic health care, education, and economic development; what Bordes really wanted to be doing, all of it. The Population Council was not interested, either. Not enough family planning, they said. It looked like Family Planning International Assistance was the only chance. But that required the U.S.A.I.D.'s okay; always for family planning, apart from maternal-child health. So what would be the chances of getting basic health services, education, economic development? They attract people to family planning, argued Bordes's supporters. So what? A.I.D. money came from congressionally mandated Title 10 family planning funding, with very decided constraints. Family planning would have to be separated out . . . or at least on paper. It was getting urgent. Family planning money was to run out in mid-February. It would have to be rammed through the A.I.D. machinery for okay if the deadline were to be met—if the proposal were to be funded. Or maybe some of the many United Nations agencies might fund an integrated approach, or at least portions.

Lots of hustling.

Family Planning International Assistance accepted the invitation for a trip to Haiti. On the flight down, John Palmer Smith, the boss, told Harold Crow, the program consultant, to take the lead in the discussion and proposal evaluation. Crow had experience in program development, particularly in Latin America. A strikingly handsome man, Crow is part American Indian and looks it, prematurely gray, generally tanned from some trip, sooooo well-modulated of voice, impeccably tailored, and Rothschild smooth. When Harold Crow sits in the back of a taxi, it turns into a limousine, a style he has cultivated into a science to camouflage his climb up. If, as Freud said, it is all love and work, then the Crow profile goes—very ruthless with women, very professionally skilled. There were overlaps, and his calculation was positively seductive.

"I remember commenting to John on the flight that I thought it was important for us to get to know Dr. Bordes and, perhaps, evaluate the man prior to evaluating the project," he reveals. "Neither of us knew much about him, other than the fact we had had some good references." They arrived that January afternoon, a lovely time in Haiti, mild, sunny and crystalline clear, not quite sure if Bordes would be meeting them at the airport.

"Is any one of you John Palmer Smith?" They turned and saw a "lovely" man, Crow recalls, with white flowing hair, a dark face, rather short, and in a white medical coat. "Welcome to Haiti," the man said, and smiled.

"It was such a warm greeting," Crow recalls. "It was very hard not to like him from the immediate start." Even Hal Crow, Prince Hal, could be affected by the charm. They checked into their hotel and went downstairs shortly afterwards to get acquainted and taste the rum punch. They asked some questions about politics in Haiti under Papa Doc. Bordes declined to comment. They had been indiscreet and knew it. They told a few jokes. They had several rum punches.

"It became apparent very quickly that he was the kind of man we wanted to work with. That he was a man of integrity. That he knew a lot about his country and a great deal about the health field," Crow recalls his first impression. "I just got the feeling that he was in Haiti because he had a strong dedication to help his country, which is quite rare in developing countries." He had not bumped into that kind of solid patriotism too often, ". . . to find a man so well-prepared who wanted to stay . . . . Dr. Bordes had chosen to stay in Haiti and to do his best for his own country and his own people. I greatly admire him for that—and it was all apparent when we first met him."

Next morning they drove out along the bumpy road to Fond Parisien. It was to be market day, Bordes said. Crow was delighted with visions in his head of his Latin American experiences and a chance to get a real feel for the community, to touch the local color, taste the food, join the merriment, work, but have some fun. Smith was pleased as well, as was Miss Lee Hall of Planned Parenthood, accompanying them on the project exploration.

It was not what they expected. "We arrived in the town and Dr. Bordes said we were in the market. What I saw were maybe fifteen to twenty small huts. What they were selling were various kinds of products . . . really kind of frightening and shocking. Suddenly we immediately realized right as we stepped out of the car how difficult life was in this community. I don't recall seeing any green vegetables. . . ." Perhaps the greens were fed to the livestock, he thought to himself, noting the beetlike roots and dried beans for sale, the eggshells, rather than the eggs, pounded into powder and used in local dishes. Hal Crow is no stranger to the suffering of the underdeveloped world, and he was bowled over. There were some scraps of newspaper being sold to wrap up tobacco and other little items sold by local merchants during the week. It was starkly poor. "I recall Lee, a very lovely, sensitive person, walking away from the market area back to the car and beginning to cry. . . ."

This is where Ary Bordes had chosen to work. Crow noted that. He also noted that as they drove out to the village, Bordes knew where he was going, in contrast to many other government and high-ranking officials in capital cities in his experience, who, when they invited him out "to meet the people," very obviously did not know where the people lived, depending on the driver to get them there.

He also noted that Bordes needed no introductions, another good sign—he had spent a lot of time in this community.

"The people flocked around him. He knew them . . . their first names. He talked with many of the mothers who had been to some of his clinics in the past. One woman, I recall, who had two children, walked up to him with a great big smile and talked about her IUD and how very happy she was with it and how she had no problems. It had been in a couple of years and she wondered if it might be necessary to change it, would it dissolve. . . . He assured her. . . . Many other people came up to ask about some minor illness of their children or vaccination programs and other kinds of concerns. In each case he talked with the people in a very personal way, a familiar kind of way. I was very impressed with the way he handled the people," Crow sums up, "the way he worked with the villagers. The way they respected him." Bordes was passing the first test—what kind of man.

They visited the other two triangle points that same day, an exhausting venture. It was the same at each location. Bordes was known by the community, the leaders, the children—who sang the family planning song for the visitors. They really grabbed the FPIA heartstrings. "He'd already had a tremendous impact in this area, working with limited resources," Crow could see. "It became obvious he had to have some support to bring his work to greater heights." Crow was getting hooked. All the while, Bordes was describing the total community development program he had in mind, at its base, providing Haitians with the option to truly exercise family planning in its full meaning, doing what was best for the entire unit's well-being.

Next morning, they started to work, discussing the proposal at great length over the next couple of days. Crow noticed Bordes's approach— and he respected him for it. It had to be Haitian. "I made several suggestions for the program, some of which Dr. Bordes accepted and was very pleased with, and others he didn't feel were too good and would reject. He was willing to have the inputs, the suggestions, the technical advice from outsiders . . . but he wanted to adapt the ideas to the Haitian environment. He believed very strongly that if development were to occur, it must come from within and not from outside," a position in line with the Crow development philosophy. Crow helped write it all up, brought it back to New York, worked on it some more, submitted it to A.I.D. for funding.

Less than two weeks later, they had the okay. Crow's association with Bordes would continue throughout the "triangle" years and beyond. Bordes would watch his performances with amusement—"He thinks he's so great!"

Bordes had felt very confident when they left, an impression confirmed in a March meeting in New York with Steckel in which the "triangle" project was called "the biggest and the best we have." With a verbal okay to proceed from U.S.A.I.D. and a formal "yes" in writing expected by the end of March, it all seemed fine, although the formal agreement lingered around without the signatures for months. Bordes waited, his natural optimism intact, working at the Croix-des-Bouquets center, operational for twenty years, but never like this.

He was starting slowly . . . step by step . . . having many fights. The national program was signed in April and the FPIA contract finally signed and sent back to New York in May. There had been a little unfortunate shuffling around, more family planning emphasis. FPIA was trying its best to have a wider perspective than its family planning specialty, but still, there were limits. . . . Whatever the compromises and adaptations, the integrated approach had money in the bank, to build a model for the rural phase of the government's family planning program, now very secure, rady for expansion and intensification.

The "triangle" even got a presidential endorsement.

In his annual message in January of that year, President-for-Life Jean Claude Duvalier had focused national attention on the efforts about to begin at Croix-des-Bouquets. He was telling everybody, including the testy medical community, that it had his backing. The behind-the-scenes support building had paid treasure too golden for any bank to confine.

The president spoke in a nationally televised address, in his formal tails, flanked by his family, his once-nurse mother particularly imperious and haughty as she listened to her son, the camera playing prominently upon her, focusing on the previous Duvalier generation, giving the son time to become a more familiar face. Pudgy but maturing, the young president was making his first state-of-the-union address, intoning in a singsong but firm-voiced cadence, at some length, with a good portion of his speech accorded to health.

One of the first steps of his new government had been the evaluation of the medical-sanitary needs of the people and identification of the public health problems requiring priority action, he said, deadpan, in regal repose like a lion in a game park. He was about to provide dispersion of resources, he said, to parallel the necessary improvements in the existing structure. So . . . "I have decided to strengthen the medical-sanitary infrastructure," he stated, getting perfunctory hand-clapping from the audience of bureaucrats and military, strange look-alikes, that same deadpan expression, suit and body posture of their new leader, a cameo in a large cast.

"With the goal of previewing competent and motivated structures for the rural part of the country, my government plans to construct in the area of Croix-des-Bouquets a center for training in community medicine. With a well-regulated work plan, this institution will become a veritable laboratory to study in detail the different aspects of our medical-sanitary problems. Students of the School of Medicine will be able to be exposed in the beginning of their clinical studies and initiated into the practice of community medicine in a center not far from the capital. At the same time, personnel of other institutions of health in different parts of the country, regional leaders, through a rotation schedule, will also benefit from this institution, and all necessary training for their preparation...."

He went on. The program was to be carried out through the cooperation of a variety of government agencies "to develop programs aimed at the promotion of health and economic development of the masses of the people in a conscious and motivated effort. When the ways are prepared and found in this special place of work, they will have been prepared for the objective of close collaboration with the masses of the rural countryside, firmly founded for real advancement."

When he concluded his remarks, a military officer took the text from his hands. He stood for the national anthem, all dignity, and unsmilingly, left the room, followed slowly by his entourage. All had just heard the party line about many things, including the objectives of the new Croix-des-Bouquets clinic—community medicine, training of staff, creation of a model for development of the rural area. To know the possibilities, understand the difficulties, set the price, evaluate the efficiency. It was to be a reference point for all concerned or those who should be.

The timing was important. Discussions of a national health plan were underway, pushing the idea of decentralization with a system of district hospitals around the country and surrounding health centers. What would be the role and function of these centers? Nobody really knew yet. Any national health plan needed a try-out on a minor scale before large-scale extension. The Croix-des-Bouquets center, only a twenty-minute drive from the capital, might provide some answers as well as training for present and future "district" staff around the country. It had been thirty years since Haitian law made it obligatory for young doctors to devote their first years of practice to the rural area. Maybe the time also was ripe to redefine and review the role of rural residency and its special work conditions. The Croix-des-Bouquets center also had that potential. Then, the center might stimulate more interest in the medical school faculty as well as medical students in the problems of their community and how to involve themselves in their unique national milieu.

This was the place. Even the president said so. Only eight kilometers north of Port-au-Prince, Croix-des-Bouquets was well-connected to the capital by paved road and a crossroad for a number of other roads in varying degrees of disrepair. It was a semiurban sort of place, consequently, with all that transportation to the urban Mecca by colorful public buses and multi-passenger station wagons coming and going and bumping into each other all the way. The accident rate was horrendous, but braved. On one end was the dirt road leading out from the town, past the "flamboyant" trees, the hens and the chicks crossing the road, burdened pedestrians and hoeing farmers. Then came the life-size and white-enamel-faced crucified Christ in thorn-crowned blood, the Calvary scene of every Haitian town of any size, just to the rear of the yellow cement inspection post with the military ready to check every move and all papers—both strong indicators of town life. Then a Croix-des-Bouquets resident could be off, onward to the wonders of the capital. The trip was frequently, often desperately, made by Croix-des-Bouquets residents and escapees, as well as marketers. The proximity weathered the face of this peripheral town into a certain expression, given its grabbing distance to Haitian sophistication.

Croix-des-Bouquets was in close touch with Port-au-Prince on a number of lines, including its educational sensitivity—some newspaper readers, the only two secondary schools in the entire "triangle," and eleven primary schools, reaching nearly 1,000 children. Also, there was the health center, shaded by a huge manguier tree, all round and green; under its shelter the human relations toward patients lived straight out of a caste society; irritation compounded by no water and the minimum of equipment and drugs. The town also had some piped water provided by a hydraulic pump and a canal system, a sanitation problem of immense magnitude. People understood water for thirst and agriculture, but not its connection to pollution and disease. There were some houses with latrines, some electric lights along the dirt streets, one telephone and postal service to and from the capital, as well as six radios for every 100 townspeople. There was a mayor in charge, a peace tribunal, an army barracks, a tax-collection office, and many churches. The slaughterhouse was an abomination beyond belief. There was a little bit of cottage industry underway, but the main thrust of the economy of the town and its environs of about 30,000 farmers, was the usual—sugarcane, maize, beans, bananas ... with an abundance of good fruit trees, mangoes in particular.

In short, it was a strange blend of town and country. A very quiet place, still save for birds chiping in the many trees lush with velvety unripe fruit, roosters crowing. The usual passers-by and their balancing act, stopped to chat and were off barefoot in different directions with their arms swinging, an almost military intensity of movement. Men urinated along the sides of the roads. Schoolchildren in blue-checked shirts and khaki shorts, books under their arms or in little briefcases, made their way for a school day. Good-day greetings came soft and melodic. People gossiped and spit. Children screamed as their hair was combed in the front yard. Pigs wandered for the day. Madame Rosaire maintained the major hairdressing establishment in town down the street from the green and yellow and very large Catholic church.

The best-maintained building by far was the tax-collection office, across the street from the Haitian Institute for the Promotion of Coffee Exports, not in such great shape, in turn next door to the most frequently used of the three—the lottery counter. The mayor's headquarters was built in 1921 and featured the usual Duvalier family portraits; next door was the telegraph office and across the street, the military post. The water pump station made a racket and lightbulbs strung in front proclaimed the initials of the national planning agency, CONADEP. "The Nation Has Chosen Planning . . . Here Is the Logic of Development" was written along the building's side, a quote of President François Duvalier, but the hedge had overgrown the word "planning." The pumping station had just been built in 1970 and featured a life-sized statue of a calabash-bearing woman outside, the old method still most widely used. In its core Croix-des-Bouquets was a town with tin-roofed cement houses with strange little metal gables in front; houses arranged along almost blocklike streets, quickly yielding to cement houses with thatch roofs, then finally, mud and thatch huts, and banana groves. Another block away—open farmland with cornstalks glistening in the sunlight and the lavender mountains off in the distance.

On Fridays the place came alive with market life, some 4,000 to 5,000 people buying and selling from the capital and nearby regions—meat, livestock, foods, mats, textiles, everything. Every day could be heard the sounds of the iron cutters, for this was the home of this unique Haitian art form of metal sculpture, found by simply seeking the origin of the hit of sledge hammer on metal; the artist sitting on a rock as he plied his trade.

Croix-des-Bouquets was a strange place, of strange ingredients, creating a strange blend. There was to be a strange beginning. The clinic was small and in terrible shape physically, a few rooms and verandas, wooden, white with green trim and green benches, a tin roof and not much else.

Dr. Antonio Narcisse remembers it well. In September of 1971, when he came to Croix-des-Bouquets to begin his rural residency, "there wasn't much," he says flatly. The equipment? "There wasn't much . . . certain necessary apparatus was missing . . . no refrigerator . . . no transportation . . . no drugs. . . ." The administration? "There wasn't much . . . the administrator came three times a week and did not have strong enough control over the personnel." For Narcisse to take a position, as strong a position as this, the conditions had to be BAD!

Dr. Narcisse is a heavy-set, actually fat, man with a ready laugh and a ready anything-for-the-boss insecurity. The eyes behind his black-rimmed glasses often change expression, hard as marbles; vulnerable as a kitten; cruel as a bully. Without much provocation his arms wildly flay the air, overwhelmed, overcome, overwrought—for Dr. Narcisse does not have much resiliency to stress. He can change pattern with the wallpaper in the room; outrainbow any chameleon within the national boundaries; very accommodating face-to-face; behind-the-back dangerous.

He moves with the deliberateness of a chess game played by correspondence. He has always been dependent, like most members of Haiti's middle class, and he is a fearful person, politically hypersensitive, suspicious, and nervous about his position and well-being. On the other hand, his social position within the Haitian milieu has helped him to stay close to the peasantry. While he is highly authoritarian, sometimes very harsh, he also knows how to work with the people, to joke and to reach them. He says he liked rural medicine and wanted to work with the peasants when he was assigned to Croix-des-Bouquets, where he would live in a small but comfortable house with his bourgeois wife, two children, and one maid. Years later, when he was given an opportunity to get a master's degree in public health medicine in Israel, he would fly back after three weeks when one of his children developed diarrhea. He wanted to come home, where he felt safe.

In 1971 he was a young doctor, eager, and attempting to organize different clinical services. "I had a great deal of trouble because the staff was not accustomed to supervision or control. They came late and left very early," he says, the biggest of all difficulties. The community? "What struck me most were certain diseases—infant diarrhea, umbilical tetanus, respiratory infections, malnutrition—the biggest problems. Also, the lack of good sanitation. There were almost no latrines in certain areas of the town. And the way the people used the water! They didn't understand the need to boil water, and in the rainy season . . . !" He concludes: "After Dr. Bordes arrived, things changed a lot."

Reconstruction of the building itself was an impossibility with the available funding. No change there. The equipment, however, could be beefed up—at least to a minimum of a stethoscope, child scale, syringes, blood-pressure gauge, sterilization material . . . something. The same with the drugs. Aspirin, antibiotics, sulfa, antacid were assured, while others were provided more intermittently.

Then, there was the problem of the passive personnel. That was the hardest. Ary Bordes was about to have some of his highest-pitched screaming fights ever at the Croix-des-Bouquets clinic. The staff screamed in protest against their new director's demands—for attendance. Absenteeism is one of Haiti's biggest calamities in health and everything else. People will pick up their paycheck religiously, but they won't work. Bordes wanted work, more work, even work in the afternoons, out in the community, no less! A terrible blow to their status as special and above the mass.

In short, he had the money from the outside, but he didn't have the people power from the inside. There was patronage. Ary Bordes was not always able to pick his staff and appoint whom he wanted for what job, and he could not fire if they had the job, even though they were not doing the job. He had to live with them.

During his many visits throughout the "triangle" years Sam Wishik was to note this tragic flaw in the program. "The things Ary was trying to do were right. The weakness was that he did not have the people to do it. Everything he was doing, I believed to be right. He was sound—but try to get the Haitians to do it!" he sounds disgusted. "There was this gap between the professionals and the people which did not and does not exist with Dr. Bordes in the way he meets the people and works with them. But many of the professionals did not give a damn about the people. And they had the job . . . that attitude. . . ." Things had to be changed despite the resistance.

Bordes simply screamed louder. He was quite a sight exhibiting that suppressed pure Haitian emotionality in staff meetings and confrontations with the resident physician, head nurse, and five auxiliary nurses of the original crew. They had nothing to work with for years, and not so surprisingly, had done very little. Attitude change was underway, assisted shortly by a salary supplement. It was almost an emergency and had required that kind of countermeasure. Also, the people of the community were very dissatisfied. Somehow Bordes had to move quickly, improving the efficiency and human relations of the center, providing better services so the people would use the facility, realizing that times and a lot of other things had changed.

The old director was not exactly delighted about all of this, you might say. Technically, he and Bordes had equal authority, although theoretically, Bordes was the one in charge—the kind of situation which could pain like bursitis in a joint. The problem was not easily resolved, even by screams. The doctor on the scene simply was not oriented to social medicine and was not interested in any shift in his personality and/or medical practice to direct a "triangle" type of project, and he made it all—and repeatedly—loud and clear. He did not want to cooperate, frankly.

It took four years, four l-o-n-g years, to get a change in staff. It was a government facility with government personnel, and it had to be lived through. The situation was bad, and what Bordes really wanted to do was make a sharp karate-chopping motion. That was the feeling; the action taken, softer. The objectives were long-term and his better judgment restrained his impulses. Instead, he pushed the program as much

A TASTE OF HONEY

as possible, avoiding too much damage by demanding results too quickly. But on many a drive back from the Croix-des-Bouquets center, sometimes a daily trip, he would be virtually talking to himself. Most people talk to themselves. He had his reasons.

Bordes did his best with what he had to work with. He had no choice. He worked and worked and worked. . . .

A medical-social survey conducted that March by 130 students from the Auxiliary School of Nursing with the help of the bureau of statistics had put the Croix-des-Bouquets health situation in the full harshness of documented Haitian reality.

Laumaire Elias suffered from the edema of malnutrition, as did eighteen others found March 7; on the same day, tetanus of the newborn killed Myriam Sagesse, two weeks; Solon Nau, forty, and Andre Alexis, seventeen, also died. It was like that throughout the survey period, defining the problem: 222 cases of intestinal worms; 3 of tuberculosis; 112, skin infections; 66, heart disease; 327, repiratory infections; 40, diarrhea; 247, other kinds of problems. Voilà, the pathology to be dealt with. The previous year, fifty-four deaths had been officially recorded, fourteen within the first year of life and nine from the age of one to four years.

Whence it came? The slaughterhouse and the badly constructed and waste-filled water canal system, blatantly obvious health hazards, with repercussions on the entire community. Of the 2,961 inhabitants in 704 houses, only 95 had running water by pipe; the rest used the canals, public water fountains, or other contaminated sources. There was one water-flushed toilet in the entire town; 523 latrines of some kind in courtyards; 89 houses without any kind of waste disposal. The tiny houses were packed with people, from five to ten or more in 40 percent of them. There had been little immunization to protect them against disease. Only 109 people had received their first dose of typhoid vaccine; 245 people, their first dose of polio vaccine; only 173, their first dose against diphtheria, whooping cough, and typhoid; only 111, their first dose of tuberculosis immunization. Again, only the first round of the series of three shots. Progressively smaller numbers of people had received the total. It was hard not to get sick in Croix-des-Bouquets; people were most vulnerable to the contagion around them, malnutrition weakening their fight.

There was a lot of work to be done. The survey had shown a predominance of women, 1,650 over 1,311 men—with 1,200 of the people in the peak fertile 15-to-40 age group. Only 27 people practiced some form of family planning, but 181 said they had heard of it; 204 said they would want to participate in such a program if it were available to them.

Most cited "Radio Doctor" as their source. The program would not be starting cold. It was 1972 and they had gotten the word.

About forty-five minutes away in a northeasterly direction could be found the second angle—Thomazeau—along the same paved road that five miles outside of Croix-des-Bouquets turned into bumpy dirt and headed all the way north to Mirebalais in the Artibonite Valley. Symptomatically, the way to Thomazeau was always rocky and/or dusty and/or muddy, depending on the season. Consequently, the town was much more isolated than Croix-des-Bouquets.

Between the two towns stretched the splendid sights of Haiti . . . the sunlight . . . the sugar cane . . . the glistening waterholes . . . the sensual bathers . . . the densely populated rural life of this country. Beyond sprawled more density, more and more rurality, the true mountain people of Haiti. Some 1,000 to 1,500 of them routinely came into the center of town every Thursday for market, boosting the town's also-sprawling population of about 2,000 people, with another 33,000 estimated to be in the immediate vicinity. Moving out from the core, Thomazeau became more and more like Fond Parisien, almost identical, in fact, only on the other side of Lake Azuey, dry, arid, full of cactus and bayahondes, the same HASCO sugar railroad tracks, the same skinny wandering animals and chickens. Thomazeau also had been an area of prosperity in colonial times, of agriculture and small industry and good animal breeding, supporting some 30,000 people then, with a souvenir of its good old days: a big chimney of an indigo factory. This had once been the home of many Lebanese merchants, whose contemporary hold on the economic life of the capital is bitterly resented; a coffee stronghold of the wealthy Brandt family, probably the richest in the country, who a few decades back loaned the government millions of dollars to pave the capital, repaid by returns on the gasoline tax.

Now agriculture was devastated by drought and only 174 of the town's surrounding 857 carreaux of land were under cultivation. Market prices for goods were twice the Port-au-Prince figures from whence they came. There was no organized fishing on this side of the lake, either. Charcoal manufacturing was flourishing, the recurring sign of economic desperation.

Today's Thomazeau seemed unique only in the making of mats from vegetation in nearby marshland. It would always be the weakest of the three angles in the "triangle" project, its physical appearance very telltale; wide-open streets, randomly organized merchants and houses also widely apart; an ever-so quiet, dusty and sleepy town with scatterings of houses of various states and status, a little bit of veranda juxtaposed with mud and thatch, and the tiny, one-room Hotel de Ville. The biggest complex of buildings was the Catholic church and rectory of the

French missionary father. There was no electricity and no running water. There was a mayor; an army barracks; a court; some churches and three schools; one telephone and postal service with Croix-des-Bouquets and Port-au-Prince. But almost anyone could meander around the army barracks, and, incredibly, no khaki-clad soldiers ventured forth to demand on what business, or to ask for papers. Birth certificates were said to be often issued by the local magistrate, but not always entered in the town's register, the money not always declared.

It was an easygoing place, marked more by the clang of the blacksmith and the buzz of the small grain-threshing machine than by anything else. There were groups in Thomazeau, but that was the problem—there were too many of them. No group cohesion. Efforts would be made to draw them together, but never really successfully. It was all rather like the justice-of-the-peace office, the red-and-black Haitian flag blowing lackadaisically in the wind beneath its red support pole, the building's aqua doors, green shutters, and peach stucco wall—not much color coordination. "Her brother used to be the mayor and now he is in jail, so she lost her job," went one comment, typical of local politics. Thomazeau was more divided, more provincial, more institutionally scattered than Croix-des-Bouquets.

It had had a health clinic since 1946, a small house down a long driveway, in a corner of the town opposite the market and mainstream of town life, and next door to the French Catholic mission. The clinic had no water and nothing else. It had been without a resident physician for the past fifteen years, somebody getting his paycheck, but not on the job. An untrained auxiliary worker was there, sometimes, but the people did not have too much confidence in her medical prowess and did not come. Basically there were walls, a staircase, and two goats living in the dispensary. Nobody had cared to or could change the situation, it seemed.

While the preliminary medical-social survey of Thomazeau was sketchy, it did show a stable population, with a median age of thirty-one years. Of the 341 people surveyed, nearly three-fourths had no education at all; only five percent could speak some French, the sign of some status. There were even fewer newspaper readers here than in Croix-des-Bouquets. Of the 399 houses in the town itself, none had running water. There was only one water source for all the people. There were 183 latrines. From a sample of 190 Thomazeau residents, data showed that about 60 percent had not vaccinated any of their children under six years of age; 25 percent had vaccinated one child; 72 percent of those with children seven to fourteen years of age had not been provided with vaccination protection. In still another survey of 283 adults, 65 percent were not vaccinated. In still another survey of

392 mothers, the women were pretty evenly divided about the possibilities of their babies' getting tetanus of the newborn; only nine percent of them were vaccinated against that disaster. Interestingly, only three percent in still another survey of 338 people felt that it was their responsibility to take care of immunization. The vast majority said it was up to the health center.

Personal initiative was at the same very low ebb in Thomazeau as was basic health information. In the survey of the 392 mothers, 94 percent had weaned their babies very abruptly, they said, in order to avoid sickness; only 15 percent of them ever sought the advice of a doctor or a nurse in their lives; but over half claimed or complained about having been sick the previous week. They seemed to have very little information about nutrition. Eighty-one percent of the people studied did not know anything about family planning, although 71 percent said they did not want to have more children. Only two percent were using a method of contraception.

There was a lot of work to be done in Thomazeau, too, with its health program as viable as the mythical resident physician.

About thrity-five kilometers east of Croix-des-Bouquets, stood the third "triangle" point, approached along a bad road, gradually leaving behind Croix-des-Bouquets's fertile growth and grazing animals and white water fowls, past an occasional multi-colored cemetery and farmland, until the dryness and the cactus and the wasteland took over. All over. Rocks. Gutted land. Primitive plant growth. Past Ganthier, its scattering of 193 houses and 1,500 people, the site of the first mobile-clinic outreach a few years earlier. Now the land became very, very, very dry, with a gutsy patch of stunted corn, a pathetic attempt to eke out life from a desert; the beauty of Lake Azuey lay off to the left, but mostly there were the gulleys and hills of ugly aridity. Past the little cottages of City Rurale, a token attempt at a government housing project, miniature tract housing, all the same with little porches. Then, a right turn over a drainage ditch, the jeep leaping down and up, into the sheep grazing—almost starving, and finally, the village of Fond Parisien—already familiar.

Here it was rural all the way, without major buildings or streets, water or electricity, a mayor or city council. It was the poorest of the three points. But its 4,000 residents and 11,000 neighbors had been getting weekly medical attention since 1965. There was the little clinic; Dieumaitre Jacques and his community workers; the educational and economic efforts; some succeeding, some failing. There were the mobile clinics into the environs. The program had a beginning here.

Within the "triangle" boundaries were an estimated 154 square kilometers with an estimated 100,000 to 150,000 people, nobody really could tell more accurately, concentrated mostly around the towns, and particularly south of Croix-des-Bouquets. The conditions were pretty much as Fond Parisien in the beginning. Umbilical tetanus at birth. High morbidity and mortality among the estimated 15,000 preschoolers. The same infectious diseases, malnutrition, poverty. The same scarcity of water and nonexistent sanitation. The same six to seven percent literacy rate. The same transportation by foot or donkey along impossible or rare roads. About two radios for every 100 people. High birthrate. No knowledge of modern theories of illness. Not a single pharmacy where people could obtain drugs. Not a single hospital bed. Of the estimated 3,000 births a year, nine out of ten babies were delivered at home by traditional midwives, the lone exception venturing into a maternity ward in Port-au-Prince, the only source of medical care beyond the Croix-des-Bouquets clinic and the traditional healers. There were few ideas, scant stimulation. It was "the village" of Haiti in all its grace and sadness; beauty and desperation; courage and suffering.

It was about to change. In fact, change had already begun, even before international assistance had been finalized. The Mellon money had made the Croix-des-Bouquets center viable. "A most interesting little town where an impressive program could be carried out. . . . I have now a precise idea of what is being done, of what needs to be done," Bordes had written Boston back in August of the previous year.

Losing no time, first had come the surveys in March 1972. The supplementary salary had changed the atmosphere of the health center somewhat, which in turn had begun to change the image of the center, away from irregularity and inefficiency to more attention to the needs of the people, a place that really belonged to them, that existed to serve them. It would take time to gain their trust, but the effort had begun. The same March, the center started a first-aid course in cooperation with the Red Cross, and the very popular child health course pioneered in the capital. With the funding go-ahead in April, three doctors, a public health nurse, auxiliaries, and a sanitation inspector were hired and brought to Croix-des-Bouquets for training in the program's objectives. There was enthusiasm. They were to live in the communities they served—very important—backed up by Bordes's private center in Port-au-Prince as their administrative headquarters, with a field office at the Croix-des-Bouquets clinic.

There had had to be some adjustments in the plan. "It's too bad," Bordes had confessed in a letter to Sue Klein, thanking her for her enormous contribution, that contact with "Tony." About half of the money had to be directed to family planning; consequently the program of community health and economic development had to somehow be organized around family planning. In short, it had not been possible to persuade the funding agency that in order to provide family planning, they had to have more latrines. . . . But still there were great hopes, along with the pragmatics of necessary bending and yielding, for a broad and general development program, aimed at meeting many of the needs of the people.

The family planning line had always been improved quality of life over the long term—so said the technocrats around the world. Now here was an opportunity. Family size, nutrition, health, and economic status were obviously so interrelated and interdependent that family planning alone, or for that matter, any single one of them, could bring only very limited and short-term improvement. To meet the long-term objective of a better life, family planning had to be part of something bigger, and so it was to be—curative and preventive medicine, environmental sanitation, health education, and economic development. Even on a small scale, it was an ambitious undertaking, requiring creativity, commitment, and community involvement far beyond even the fantasies of Lyndon Johnson and his "War on Poverty."

The coordination was left to the Haitians. They did the mixing from several sources, Bordes stirring the brew. The Haitian government's Department of Public Health and Population was providing the clinics at two of three locations, the medical residents, a sanitation agent, some minimal materials and drugs; the Department of Agriculture and Natural Resources and Rural Development, an agronomist to organize agricultural improvements and an agricultural extension agent—in total, about $30,000 a year on the Haitian side. Another $90,000 worth came through the Unitarian Universalist Service Committee as the administrating agency, working with Bordes's private center, maintaining the Fond Parisien facility, the jeep and other items, educational materials, and a loan program for economic cooperatives. That money in turn came courtesy of the Mellon fortune, later supplemented by $14,000 from the Veatch Committee of the North Shore Unitarian Society on Long Island; another $14,000 from a small foundation, the Robert Sterling Clark Foundation. There was more: $31,000 would subsequently be kicked into the pot by the General Services Foundation of St. Paul, a small family foundation, hardly of the Mellon magnitude, but helpful, and would continue the work until phase-out, planned for May 1975, and government takeover of the rural model. It was designed to be a multi-supported, multi-faceted—action—program of three years' duration. Not a "research" project or a "pilot" project in those pristine senses of top efficiency without much change or replication, but adapted to the local situation and local resources, to obtain better results and better organization than currently available—something that could be extended.

Some basic agenda items had to be covered for the "triangle" to be a successful "action." Bordes hewed and sculpted. A model rural health clinic had to be organized. Everybody's job had to be defined for its precise role and optimal effectiveness. A method of work had to be established from the hours of the center's operations on through its actual activities of clinical medicine, maternal and child health and family planning, the control of communicable diseases, school health, gathering of data, health education, training of personnel, involvement of the people, exercise of community leadership, all the ins and outs of community medicine . . . to some efforts at quantifiable evaluation.

It was a big job, beginning at square one. The patient arrived at the clinic . . . so there had to have been some outreach. The patient had to be registered . . . so there had to be new forms. The patient waited . . . so there could be education. The patient had a problem . . . triage was the rule, an important innovation: treatment by a qualified person, but proceeding up the chain of expertise from auxiliary, to nurse, to physician—if necessary; on to the laboratory, the pharmacy, or whatever next step; everything explained along the way, so modern medicine would be demystified. After consultation, treatment, and advice, the patient left. The records had to be filled. If needed, there were to be follow-ups.

Specific clinics were developed for prenatal and postnatal care, for pediatric care, for general health care, for schoolchildren, for dental care, for family planning, for immunization. The prenatal clinics were organized so the women would systematically be vaccinated against tetanus. The pediatric clinic was more refined so the auxiliary nurse routinely saw most of the children with minor problems. Special attention was paid to determining the extent of malnutrition and diarrhea problems in the area, and to eradication of tetanus of the newborn—the great health hazards of Haiti. Everybody who set foot into the clinic heard about family planning and the various methods through individual counseling or in groups.

There was the question of coverage. How well was the center really doing if it saw 300 pregnant women a year? It might be a very good clinic if there were 350 pregnant women in the community. Suppose there were 900? Evaluation procedures were worked out to determine approximate targets. Objectives were set . . . the first year, 30 percent coverage of pregnant women; second year, 45 percent; and on. . . .

How to simplify the record-keeping? How to see that the records were kept—an index card, a rendezvous card, a clinical form for each patient. Where should the vaccination be done? What about educating the captive audience? How should it be done and who should do it? What was the best path for the patient from entrance to exit? What about fees? Should they charge? Health was the right of the people. Right. But most countries of the world charged something. They were not sure, which was not unusual, but they decided upon a twenty-cent fee, something adjusted to the level of the people and returned to the clinics in some kind of needed item, like a pressure cooker for sterilization—making sure to inform the people that their contributions were being returned to them in another form. Every single detail had to be worked out, conceptually, and then in day-to-day operation.

Next, the making sure it was done, the hardest part, the hollering part. There were regular staff meetings at Croix-des-Bouquets every Friday and training seminars, courtesy of the government and the Pan American Health Organization. Every afternoon the staff was supposed to go into the community home-visiting and educating people about the program of community medicine, relating all activities to family planning. Group meetings were organized according to a schedule. Coupons were distributed. The soundtruck was put to good use. Home visits were paid to pregnant and newly-delivered women with an eye out for malnourished children and follow-up visits for family planning clients. The schools got the message about health care, elementary physiology, and reproduction, the concept of the small family and population problems, using the available educational materials. There was the "Radio Doctor" broadcast daily and the "Health Class" on Saturdays.

By June that first year, a physician, nurse, and medical auxiliary were located in the small clinics of Thomazeau and Fond Parisien, using the same approaches developed at Croix-des-Bouquets. Neither had dental or laboratory facilities, their only differences.

In July another massive vaccination campaign was conducted throughout the "triangle" from the three clinics and with mobile teams going out every day. Everybody got into the act, including volunteer medical students and health course participants. In addition to polio, this time tetanus, diphtheria, whooping-cough, and tuberculosis shots were given to children and adults from thirty-four vaccination points throughout the plain. Huge numbers of people were vaccinated, 1,000 an hour— 67,000 shots were administered the first three weeks to over 37,000 people. Bordes did not like it. "It was a kind of scientific picnic," he complained, with too much concentration on numbers and not enough on educating the people on the significance of immunization, not enough record-keeping, follow-through, not enough attention to the people as people, his usual themes.

But the campaign had its value, particularly in that stage of the work. "It was a way to really meet the people while they waited in line or had their cards filled. We could talk with them and really get to know them," Madame Hollant says, recalling the experience warmly. "It gave

A TASTE OF HONEY

us, I think, some feeling about the people we were about to work with ... going out in the soundtruck for days before ... the group meetings ... visiting the "houngans" and leaders. ... We toured the entire Cul-de-Sac."

The same month of the vaccination campaign, July 7, to be precise, the health ministry announced, blessed, and signed an agreement with the Family Hygiene Center for "The Interdisciplinary Field Laboratory for Community Medicine and Family Planning" in the Cul-de-Sac ... the "triangle" to its friends and supporters.

11

THE PUNGENT TASTE OF RURAL MEDICINE

"We are producing a lot of physicians, now close to 150 a year. The point is—do we wish to have their training balanced in such a way that they can have a basic preparation and on that preparation build up enough clinical and community knowledge to be able to cope with the problems of the country? One of the big discussions we are always having here is should physicians be prepared as universal physicians able to practice everywhere in the world—because a doctor has no country and is supposed to be able to apply his science everywhere in the world. This is one part of it. Another part is, should we prepare physicians for our own country?

"Now there are partisans of both, but the main line of thinking has always been, at least in the medical school, to prepare physicians of the universal type. When you look at it, there is a certain preparation that physicians everywhere should have; and then there are some special problems to each country that the physician of that country must know more about than another. As usual the truth is in between. We should give basic knowledge to our physicians, but they should be prepared to work in the country itself and on its particular medical problems so they will be able to cope with them.

"On the other hand, besides the knowledge a physician has, there is the attitude a physician has, the will to serve either his own private interests as a Haitian or to serve the community during his career. Interests of people vary. There are people who have more scientific minds and there are physicians who are interested in social medicine and the people. After the required period of serving the people that

Haitian government and law requires, each one can follow his own philosophy of life and own wishes. Those who are interested in science and teaching can go into that branch; those who want to just make money can go into private practice and make money; but those who are interested in social medicine must have basic financial support.

"We have not been able to develop a good attitude among our young physicians to want to serve the people. That is why I think we need to develop in our physicians a knowledge of the problems of the country and an attitude preparing them to serve the country, while continuing with their own medical careers. And until that change, we will have a lack of physicians in the rural area. When the change is made, we will have a number of physicians, not large, but still enough to serve the needs of the people. I think the School of Medicine is interested in trying to make that change.

"If you have three hundred physicians scattered throughout the country in the rural area they can do a lot. Mostly, if they become organizers and try to extend this kind of community medicine. We feel it is much better to use the physician as an organizer at the level of his knowledge and have the nurse and auxiliary personnel see the bulk of the patients who have known diseases. Well-trained nurses can do a lot about treating common diseases, really, as well as the physician.

"Suppose there is a child with malnutrition. The auxiliary can see it very easily and give advice and treatment as well as the physician . . . the same with skin diseases, eye diseases. . . . And if the physician helps her, her skills can increase, sharpen, and she can be in a better position to determine who to send to the doctor and who to treat herself. A well-trained nurse and an auxiliary nurse can give the same results in the rural area. The auxiliary nurse will work to her fullest capacity and apply all her knowledge. She will work at her top. The nurse can also work very much at her top while seeing patients. The physician is the one working at the bottom of his knowledge because he has only his eyes, his ears, and his hands while he has been trained to work with a lot of apparatus and laboratory equipment. The physician in the rural area cannot do the laboratory research he needs, then examine the patient, take the X-rays, and all the rest, then review in his mind quickly all the different pathologies it could be and come up with a diagnosis by putting together all the different patterns he knows, weighing the facts and eliminating this one and concluding that one. He is lacking all the means to be used to the fullest of his capacity.

"This is why the physician in the rural area should work in a hospital, or if there is no hospital, then work very much as an organizer with the paramedical personnel under his authority working to their fullest capacity. Then, he can use his knowledge to the fullest in a few cases, *or maybe in a mobile clinic, leaving the center or hospital where the patients have already been picked out and chosen by the nurse or the auxiliary. He cannot do much more for them."—Ary Bordes*

The people came. On January 5, 1973, a ten-year-old boy huddled in pain on the Thomazeau clinic porch, wincing in terror at any suggestion of touch toward his right arm. His face was down, hidden close to his shirt under his little straw hat, the puffiness still visible despite his hunched-up shoulders, defensive and protective, his left hand gingerly holding his upper right arm. His mother squatted in exhaustion next to him, her face an exclamation point of pathos, looking up at the doctor, eyes silently pleading for help, collapsed arms resting on her kneecaps, so very utterly spent. They had walked four hours over the mountains to come to the clinic, she said.

An examination of the boy indicated a compound bone fracture. He had been hurt on the Feast of the Assumption of Our Lady into Heaven, the woman said. August 15—five months earlier. Treatment began with a SCREAM of pain!

Bordes used the case as a teaching lesson. "We cannot wait for the sick to come . . . this is what will happen." He sounded upset, angry, and sad by this prolonged and unnecessary human suffering. Ary Bordes always felt for his people, and this eloquent testimony to the essentialness of his work affected him, even after all these years. "We will see them five months after the start of their difficulty! We must structure our medical care here in two ways, first, the clinics to see the patients, and second, go to the patients with community workers.

"Get a list of all the sick people and their homes," he instructed the staff, all business now, emotion past, "and find out which ones come to us and which ones don't. Otherwise, a lot of sick people will stay in their houses and die without medical care . . . that's why educational and community medicine is the way to do medicine here, not just clinical medicine." He sounded calm, but ever so firm. This is what he wanted.

Inside, a serious-faced father held his sad-faced three-year-old son, with the weight of a seven-month-old baby, the too-familiar red hair, swollen feet, utter listlessness, and isolation within self of classic kwashiorkor. Bordes asked the father, "What is wrong with the child?"

"I don't know," the man replied almost in a mumble, speaking ever so softly, twisting his torso in a faint rocking movement of paternal comfort for the child he held. "He is just sick. They told me it is lack of food."

The father was instructed to give the child beans, milk, and meat. "I will find the meat," he said, without a shadow of doubt in his tone, despite his poverty. If this is what must be done to save his son—was the quality of his determination. But his comment lacked vitality somehow. There was a deadness in this man, a resignation while going through the motions, doing what he would somehow have to be able to do. He supposed he would, as he always had. The father had some of the listlessness of his sick child, perhaps irrevocably damaged himself by his life of infinite and unrelieved struggle—now this burden.

He was given powdered milk and told to mix and cook it well with cereal; if it were not done properly, with potable water, it would cause diarrhea. "It is the bad water that will go away first," bearded Dr. Jean-Robert Leonidas told the father, following along with the folk theory of disease that worms caused malnutrition edema, maybe exacerbated by a little too much teasing. With treatment, the child first would lose the swelling, alarming the parents generally with the apparent weight loss. It was crucial to the child's life that the feeding schedule continue and he be returned to the clinic for follow-up. So the resident physician mixed modern and folk theories together to get the child back to him for further treatment. Leonidas concentrated on teaching the father what he should do now to help the child, not teaching him the actual causes of the problem. With the child's recovery, time, and education, it would change.

Bordes heartily approved. It was a very functional, practical approach: behavior change first, then attitude change. "These are the types of things I want you to put in writing," he said with obvious enthusiasm, "so the other doctors can benefit from your experience. Here you not only have to help the people with your community work, but you must also share your experience, the way you deal with people so the program can benefit from your stay here and you can be beneficial to other doctors," he continued, pushing for more recording of observations and experiences. Good work excited him. "You are the one in the field," he added.

"I don't have enough time to write this up outside of my work here," Leonidas complained, an edge of exasperation with this man's many demands in his voice tone. Doing things right only seemed to add to his work load; and if he did things wrong . . . that was even worse with this Dr. Ary Bordes. It had been a lot easier going to medical school, Leonidas recalled with nostalgia at those bygone days in the capital, not in the middle of nowhere as in this hick town of Thomazeau. He had enough problems without these inspections. . . .

"No," said Bordes with that characteristic firmness back in his tone. "If you desire to, you will find the time. There are a lot of things I do outside of my work. It is not a question of time—it is a question of enthusiasm." There was a note of finality here, and Leonidas recognized it. He had been through this before, many times before, with Ary Bordes. There was no point now in a reply, that he knew all too well from previous experience.

Next in line waited an elderly looking mother with a marasmic baby in arms. The child was a study of wrinkled skin and tiny bones, with no subcutaneous or fat tissue, due to lack of calories. Both wore the physical costumes of premature old age, the child from malnutrition, the mother from a tough life. In ironic juxtaposition, in the background, on the wall, hung a large poster of a virtually bouncing, healthy, happy black baby, arms reaching forward in glee, a big smile of recognition for all to see. It was not a Haitian baby—it was a Zambian baby.

The poster came from the National Food and Nutrition Commission of Lusaka, Zambia, by way of a nutrition project sponsored by the Service Committee. Another Zambian poster in the clinic featured three babies on a scale in the three main nutrition states: the marasmic child on the left, with staring eyes, distended stomach, like a World War II camp victim; in the middle, the same gleeful baby; the skin-diseased and sad-eyed kwarshiorkor child on the right. The posters would be some of the best and most useful educational materials provided the "triangle" clinics through the years of experimentation with different techniques and tools. They compared and showed what a healthy baby looked like, so the people could recognize the difference. Surrounded with malnourished and sick children, the Haitians knew disease, not health. It was that bad. Health had to be advertised.

Celestin Rablaim, two-years-and-two-months, respiratory infection, second-stage malnutrition. "Why is the record not filed?" Bordes asked, taking note of the consultation procedures.

"I have run out of pediatric forms," replied Leonidas. That was all Bordes needed to hear, poked in one of many, it seemed, administrative tender spots. He was off and nonstop-running about record keeping . . . its importance to the project's success . . . proper evaluation. . . . "The project has many tasks to accomplish," he carried on and on and on, "including the development of a statistical system that can be used nationally. There must be a form for the prenatal patient, for the pediatric patient, for the general patients. . . . The forms must be used!" Bordes chastised.

Some of the standard forms of the health department were in use in the project, while new ones were being tried, using a chronological data system, developed with assistance from the department's statistical unit. Bordes was said to be a fanatic about wanting the statistical manual of the health department applied in the "triangle" project—the rendezvous card, the index cards . . . moving a little bit into prenatal and maternal-child health, pediatric and family planning recording. The records were piling up in the Thomazeau clinic, and he did not like that—at all.

"You must be interested in the records and very careful of the records," he said, sounding downright angry now. "What you do and what you file must be done the same day. Otherwise . . . how are you going to find them when you need them!?" he demanded.

"If I have to fill in records for twenty patients, I will be spending most of my time with the records, not the patients," fired back one irritated auxiliary nurse. This was too much!

Maybe some of the data could be eliminated, it is a little unnecessary, he thought to himself, while sticking to his stated position with the staff. Maybe what he was asking was too complicated, he mused further, resolving to give the matter more thought. Statistics would always be a problem in the "triangle," although the attempt would be made, albeit reluctantly at times, in contrast to many other health institutions in Haiti. Statistics would be a continuing weakness of the program despite Bordes's coaching and coaxing. Records were dry stuff.

Family planning could be more fun. In the Croix-des-Bouquets center now, Bordes teased and propagandized the four rows of pregnant women patiently waiting for prenatal care out on the clinic porch under the shade tree. They turned silent as he approached. He gently pointed a finger, asking, "How many children?" of one, and then another.

"I needed two, but I had to have four," one woman replied.

"And you?" he asked another, proceeding here and there, charming and laughing with delight, getting giggles in return.

"Four."

"And you?"

"Two."

"And you?"

"I asked God to give me four, but he gave me seven," complained her companion on the right.

"How many babies did Father God make?" Bordes asked.

"One," they replied, in obedient unison, like schoolchildren, sweet and gentle.

"Then, the good God did not make many?" he added, warming up and moving in for the kill.

"No!" their laughing reply—"just Jesus."

"Who gives the example of family planning first?" he asked, really delighted now.

"Father God!" they replied to his question. They cannot give any argument against that, he mumbled to himself as he moved away. "You're just following God's example," he flung back for emphasis to everyone's smiling face, pleased by all the attention from the important white-haired doctor. Here was Ary Bordes at his most relaxed, enjoying and working with the peasantry, full of fun, active, animated, in sharp contrast to the serious, almost preoccupied look he wore in the capital, rarely laughing, silent, self-contained, inexpressive, severe. It closed over him as he imploded into his fortress on the jeep ride back toward Port-au-Prince.

That was party time, outside with the pregnant women; now came the clinic hangover, inside with the staff. "Nobody here should have a fixed job," Bordes said sternly. Stone silence. Cold. "I don't want to hear anybody saying, 'Well, I am just here for that kind of job and I am not interested. . . .' All employees should have a team spirit," he said, sounding like a football coach at half-time, his team losing and his salary based on games won. "Everybody must participate in all aspects of the program. Whatever is needed—you should be able to do it, although that is not your particular work." For once, no arguments.

Another subject brought up for discussion: people did not want to hear about family planning at all. Dr. Narcisse reported the reason for the staff's discouragement and not-very good attitude Bordes had picked up on and would not tolerate. They could not even begin a discussion, he continued. The people just walked away uninterested . . . or worse, got angry. Narcisse went on at some length about all their difficulties until Bordes had had enough, interrupting . . . he had heard the problem and did not want any more of these laments. He had a suggestion.

"Don't begin any individual, family, or group discussions with family planning," he said, "but instead assess the people's priority needs and then work gradually into family planning messages. First, meet their main concerns," he counseled. As an added incentive, the clinic charge of twenty cents had been dropped for family planning services because it was obvious the people would pay for medical care but did not consider family planning—preventive treatment—in the same category.

Getting more mellow, Bordes added, "Nothing to worry about." He assured the staff that "the usual history of family planning is about the same as vaccination. It takes time to obtain the full three shots in the immunization series and it will simply take more time for this."

"It took fifty years from Margaret Sanger until now in the United States," he continued supportively, "and the suit of a ten-year-old does not fit a fifty-year-old."

Data showed that only about one of the eighteen people exposed to family planning came to the clinic for services. "You have to seed before you harvest," Bordes would repeat through the "triangle" years over and over again. First must come trust from the people, never easy, given their many unfortunate experiences. They must feel they are respected and understood, he would comment, having learned the lesson the hard way in the capital with the curve of IUD insertion—then withdrawal. It was clear from the urban model that convincing people did not really work. In a figurative sense the IUD had to be both in a woman's head and in her uterus.

"The real results will come in the years ahead," he summed up, assuringly, and was off to Fond Parisien for a monthly inspection. The family planning figures had not been encouraging here, either, and he wondered why.

Bounced along the road, Bordes finally arrived and moved among the villagers easily, clearly respected as special but somehow bonded, recognized, and familiar, the gap bridged by years of very evident concern, creating a now unshakeable rapport. He spied a group and ventured over, the people moving around him as he approached, receptive to his visit, welcoming. "How many children do you have?" he asked one man, just returned from a nearby market and wearing two straw hats simultaneously, the old and the new.

"I have asked three women to marry me but they all said no," was his sad-voiced reply, embarrassed. Bordes roared with laughter.

"I have five children and my wife is young," said another man, so very wrinkled and leathery of face, like a piece of embossed horse saddle. "I would like to stop. What can I do?" Bordes told him.

"Would it be better to send my wife or me?" inquired another. "You know, men like to run around," said the man, with a grimace, clearly concerned at the thought of any sexual inhibitions. Bordes roared with more laughter. "I don't do anything at home," the man elaborated, encouraged by the doctor's good humor. "I do it on the outside so I don't have to worry about pregnancy," he explained, backing away from any thought of a trip to the clinic.

"But it costs $2," said another, incredulous at the waste of money.

It was a new idea, and some were ready for it and some were not. The best prospects were the young. While he would have preferred another response, Ary Bordes was not expecting much different and was not dissatisfied with the present progress, just building on it.

"I want to have two children," said one woman, joining the group, curious, answering Bordes's question. "I want to be able to take care of them. Now I have just one and I would like to find a way not to have more children...."

"Oh, these women," grumbled a man nearby, overhearing her comment. "When you come back from the garden and you are tired and she is always after you...."

"Listen to him," she retorted, disgusted. "He talks like this and he doesn't even have a wife!"

The battle of the sexes would wage on, Haitian-peasant style, as Bordes edged away, mischievously pleased by all the uproar he had caused and off to the clinic to speak with Dr. Phyat Dessources about more emphasis on family planning.

They would quarrel, Dessources furiously resisting Bordes's criticism, aggressively presenting his defense: a bachelor, young, someone who could not go easily into the village and talk about sexuality and family planning without creating a scandal. "You have white hair and a prestigious position, that's how you can do it," Dessources shot back, hostile, his eyes flashing, almost hating, over a minor critique. The staff watched the confrontation. Silent. Embarrassed. "Maybe you are spending too much time reading and not enough time with the people," Bordes would conclude the debate finally—insisting on getting the last word.

The team approach was not working right now, and Bordes had to play the disciplinarian despite his work philosophy. His position was— the "triangle" staff should be motivated and enjoy their work—period. And his job was to make them feel they were doing something worthwhile; provide them with what they needed to do their job as much as he could; keep their enthusiasm up. While he did not enjoy the police work underway, sometimes he had to make what he called "observations. . . ."

There were the usual problems here as well as anywhere else in Haiti— not enough tools to heal, low salary, isolation. Bordes understood and did his best to relieve the hardships. The staff had a clinic, a program, his supervision—all designed to relieve their frustrations—and they had his support. Staff meetings were Friday-afternoon happenings at Croix-des-Bouquets, and all doctors were to come into the capital to the center, once or twice monthly, to report on their situations, sharing problems and observations, getting as much assistance as possible.

Most of all—to Ary Bordes in particular—they were following a plan, a thoroughly organized endeavor and one of the most exciting events in public health medicine underway in Haiti. He wanted everyone to feel a part of it; to involve themselves and the people in their areas; to work together; to develop precisely and rationally this phase of public health—and he refused to be demoralized by any little one thing that was going wrong, even Dr. Dessources. Always Ary Bordes was a visionary, looking at the totality—and it was coming along, despite some uniquely Haitian considerations for the community medicine program to deal with, many of them discovered and typed up—by kerosene lantern while batting malaria-carrying mosquitoes—by a young anthropologist named Gerald F. Murray, doing his doctoral research in a

Haitian village near Thomazeau. Something of a protégé of Sam Wishik's, Murray would speak of Wishik as his intellectual father, the man who helped him get the grants he needed to go all the way educationally.

Murray was a marvelous blend of enthusiasm and neurosis, somebody full of buttons, so an accidental brush inevitably activated rage, glee, passion, argumentation, argumentation, argumentation.... "There's been a little tension" was one of his recurring themes when he talked about anyone. Murray had a tendency to hide out from people—his thesis advisor, Sam Wishik, the U.S. Government. All of whom liked him because of his obvious charm and talent, however, they easily became opponents in his view. He had dropped out of college, gone into the Peace Corps in the Dominican Republic, where he met Maria D. Alvarez, an educational psychologist, whom he would marry just before he was about to head off to Haiti.

The couple would rarely surface during their plunge into rural Haiti, but occasionally Ary Bordes would be presented with some formidable piece of work, like their 225-page paper on "Childbearing, Sickness and Healing in a Haitian Village." It had the kinds of facts Bordes was looking for to understand better the traditional folk system which he seemed to be studying more and more, almost clandestinely. He pointed the Murrays in that direction but didn't seem to want anybody else to know what he was up to. Haitian folk medicine was taboo in modern medical circles of Port-au-Prince, and he had enough problems with a community-medicine program already. For her part, Madame Hollant was courting and making good connections with the Fond Parisien "houngans" to assist with the immunization program without Bordes's knowing much about it. Each saw and pursued the possibilities separately, keeping very quiet about what they were doing.

Meanwhile, the Murrays were operating as professionally trained objective observers and learning more about Haiti than most Haitians ever could, during their eighteen months of observations in a Haitian village during 1972-73. Murray, for instance, discovered that the name "doctor" did not necessarily carry the usual quota of prestige. For years it had been applied to roving and mostly untrained laymen who came from time to time to administer inoculations and pass out potions and ointments, selling "consultations." The villagers actually called such medical practitioners "charlatans."

Then, there was another breakdown of doctors into "doktè privé"— private doctors—and "doktè léta"—doctors at one of the capital's hospitals. The people preferred the private doctors, it seemed to Murray, because they got more individual attention, an examination from head to toe, while in the hospital, it was often a wait for hours and hours with nobody explaining when they would be seen, or simply a few words written on a piece of paper they could not read, and a "next." The people like a lot of attention, Murray reported to Bordes.

There is a certain reluctance to go to hospitals or any institutionalized health care facility, Murray reported, as a direct result of accounts of poor human relations experiences, passed from family to friend to neighbor; yet, there also appears to be some recognition that very serious illness has to be treated in a hospital because of the larger facilities—and if one "big doctor" did not know what was wrong, another might, he added. These attitudes had implications for the rural clinics being established in the "triangle," from the first, concerned about proper human relations.

Murray also found that the two young doctors at the Thomazeau clinic were suspect and not considered up to par—for just being there. Dr. Leonidas's beard lowered his prestige even further. "No great doctor would come to Thomazeau," Murray was told—they always stayed in Port-au-Prince. And while some villagers believed that, yes, good doctors could come to Thomazeau . . . if they were really good doctors they would not be walking around the countryside visiting the people as these young doctors were doing; instead, they would be in their offices and have the nurses and other workers out with the people. So much for appreciation of community outreach: just not proper high-status behavior, which was some indication of the low state of self-esteem among the Haitian peasantry. The people in his village did not go to the Thomazeau clinic, Murray noticed, except for minor illnesses cured with aspirin or an injection, saving their major problems for a trip to Port-au-Prince, where solid medical care—with status—could be found.

It was a problem, and would continue to be a problem. Health care was being brought to the people, but they dismissed it as inferior for its presence in their milieu. And there was always the local "houngan" and his healing, a constant problem.

Something interesting was happening here. Murray found that just as in Fond Parisien, where one of the "houngans" had come to accept the difference between natural and supernatural illness, so it was in his study village. After the voodoo diagnosis and treatment had been administered, the patient was advised by the "houngan" to go to the medical doctor. The "houngan" had taken care of the needs of the spirits, performed his rites, and collected his fees; now it was time for physical needs to be ministered to, the usual peasant flexibility. In short, the reasoning went, if the spirit had attacked and caused sickness, now the spirit was appeased and would desist; the poisons, however, had to be removed by modern medicine. If the clinic treatment came first and the poisons were removed, then the "houngan" came next so that the spirit would not strike again. It made a lot of sense.

Murray's recommendation was that the program's medical personnel be tolerant and interested in the folk rituals, but make no direct contact with the "houngans" to formalize a relationship which might only increase the latters' prestige as healers. It would not hurt to hire some clinic personnel involved in ritual healing, either, he added, because of the personal initiative and status associated with that position.

Murray also developed some very strong feelings about family planning potential in the vast rural area of Haiti—basically, he was pessimistic about the chances of success. The people demonstrate only the vaguest awareness of contraception, he reported, and children are always spoken of as products of God's will, which makes them pretty inevitable. Also, he believed economics made the small family being propagandized by the center totally impractical until the children had a higher chance of surviving to maturity, particularly newborns. He so told Bordes, citing the instance of one funeral he attended where both the mother and the grandmother lamented the death of the child because, "she knew how to sweep, to carry water from the river, to wash clothes, to buy in the market, to do errands."

Another observing scientist, Dr. Berggren, had some insights into family planning acceptance based on her work with rural peasants in the Artibonite Valley around the Schweitzer Hospital. In her opinion the single factor that played the largest role in resistance to family planning was the instability of the peasant's conjugal relationship. After five years of services at the hospital, never more than 10 percent of the women of peak reproductive age would be acceptors. While many expressed a what-can-I-do attitude about childbearing, studies showed that at any one time 30 percent of the heads of households in the valley would be women with no man present. So one-third of the women who had experienced a conjugal relationship at any one point were not sexually involved in a stable union, and consequently, had no need for family planning. Then there were the younger women who still had only one or two children and wanted a larger family. In short, the actual target group was far smaller than the reproductive age group indicated.

Despite the cultural complexities, the program grew. By the end of the first year, 9,500 patients had visited the three clinics for medical care, the vast majority babies and schoolchildren. Their problems? Respiratory infections, diarrhea, malnutrition, skin diseases, and intestinal worms. For adults? Respiratory infection, also number one, followed by tuberculosis, digestive problems, venereal and skin diseases.

About 30 percent of the estimated number of children five years of age and under had been to the clinics, not including those who came for immunization and who received home care. Over 500 pregnant women had sought out prenatal care, about 17 percent of the approximately 3,000 pregnant women in the area. And ninety-five patients had come for family planning in the two months of its provision that first year, a component not implemented until November.

It was the same trend seen for years in the capital—first came the children; then, pregnant women; then, family planning, in vastly descending order or priority.

The spread of the figures was interesting, too. By far the most successful clinic was Croix-des-Bouquets, reaching about 6,600 people; Thomazeau, second, with nearly 2,000; Fond Parisien, third, with about 1,000 patients. The spread made sense given the population densities and the familiarity with modern medicine. The Croix-des-Bouquets clinic had been operating, albeit crippled, for twenty years; there had not been a doctor in Thomazeau for fourteen years; Fond Parisien had never had a resident doctor. The sick did not flock to the unfamiliar, as anthropologist Murray had noticed, and confidence had to be built up in the centers and their staffs, as well as in modern medical care, by sick people becoming well and babies not dying. The traditional folk practices had a long head start and the centers had to work at building up community rapport.

The following year they did, with ten so-called "community agents," hired, trained, and assigned to each center following the methodology of work pioneered by Dieumatre Jacques. Each operated in a well-defined work zone within a five-mile radius of their clinic headquarters.

Also, for more outreach, more satellite clinics served by mobile teams were organized to bring services, including family planning, to the people in the outlying areas: four in Croix-des-Bouquet; a third mobile-clinic site added to Fond Parisien's two existing points; four in Thomazeau the next year. But the staff had a hell of a time examining some of their female patients with glaring-eyed husbands watching their every move. As they moved farther out from the towns, they encountered more and more hassles, less and less sophistication.

Still, over 12,500 patients were served in 1973 with these new approaches—a 32 percent increase in patient load over the first year. It all had to be written up, of course.

The emerging methodology was crammed into 156 pages of a new manual, gray this time, with the same compulsiveness of detail as its yellow-colored predecessor. It was titled, "An Interdisciplinary Laboratory for Community Medicine and Family Planning" and seemed to cover every possibility and nuance of the work underway, right down to what furniture the medical resident should have in his house, sanitation details of his environment, even his entertainment, to set a good example for the community without setting himself apart. . . . Very similar to the yellow manual developed in 1969 around the urban model then emerging, the new gray rural-model manual would find its way into the hands of most doctors, with Ary Bordes's constant push for more awareness of community medicine now taking an integrated approach. Two hundred copies of the methodology were distributed.

The manual particularly concerned three young doctors who sat down and helped write it after a year on the job, the resident physicians in the three triangle points who were out there every day developing what was put on paper into some kind of reality for the thousands of people of the "triangle." They did the best they could.

Dr. André Eustache had completed his obligatory residence in October of 1971 at the Croix-des-Bouquets clinic and transferred to Thomazeau to continue the work, turning down an opportunity for a residency in obstetrics and gynecology at the general hospital in the capital. His brother, also a doctor, had not spoken to Eustache for months afterwards, furious with his decision to go into public health. Grandson of a leaf doctor and son of a small businessman, a shoemaker, Eustache's father had struggled brutally to educate his children and pushed them all into medicine as the only way to have independence in Haiti. "My father saw this all his life, this spectacle of people fighting for jobs in a system which they were so dependent upon, stooping to this and that, doing things, competing with each other, and he didn't want his children to be like that."

Eustache suffers from a partial face paralysis, which only shows when he smiles, so he doesn't very often. His voice tone is morose and subdued, kind of tired; his perspective, wide-ranging, with a keen sense of cause and effect. He evaluates well but never categorically, for that would be too simple, and Eustache finds life very complex. He is a modest man, honest, unpretentious, and kind.

Married and the father of a son and daughter, both of whom rarely smile like their father, his wife would visit him in Thomazeau from time to time, preparing huge meals and using up a week's supply of prepared food in one evening. He was young and lonely there, but worked easily with the people, to whom he felt close.

His first hurdle, he says, was overcoming the prejudice of being there, that why-in-the-world-are-you-in-Thomazeau-if-you-are-any-good opinion anthropologist Murray had documented. Eustache did not wear glasses—another bad sign. He tried not to give prescriptions for expensive medicine if he could avoid it—not a good sign, either. His injections did not seem to hurt a lot—bad. A good injection gave you an overwhelming reaction, hopefully made you a little sick, and then you knew you were getting something for your money, went the prevailing opinion. A patient with a cut still had to have a stethoscope examination, Eustache discovered, even if it were on his knee. He did what helped, regardless of how ridiculous.

Eustache felt beleaguered at first, insecure about his new administrative responsibilities, left there all alone with maybe six or eight visits a year by Bordes. It was tough having a staff to supervise for the first time in his career, running a clinic, seeing that all the services were provided, organizing, evaluating.

When he first arrived he went out with the community agents and auxiliaries to home visit in the afternoons and help educate the people. But he quickly realized how much more efficient it would be to plan and help supervise the staff to maximum use. He divided the work at the clinic level, using the triage concept, delegating responsibility, actually concluding there was too much staff for the job of the clinic. One auxiliary really did nothing but clerical work, finished it all in the morning, and had little to do in the afternoon.

In his community organizing he studied the pattern of the agents and systematized their tasks, eliminating too much improvising, getting them to plan ahead and hold regular meetings, helping them with note-taking and reports, organizing their areas, developing new approaches to respond to common arguments against family planning, giving priority to certain services, evaluating their contribution every month.

He says he tried not to work too hard because otherwise nobody would want to work with him. The Protestant ethic does not flourish in tropical Haiti, although evangelism does and "excess-of-zeal" reputation could ruin his rapport. He brought his stamp collection to the clinic.

His biggest frustration? Not enough drugs and not enough variety. He just did not have what he needed to work with. There was a lot of vaccine and plenty of family planning methods, but the curative pharmaceuticals were lacking and desperately needed, particularly antirespiratory infection medication. Except for aspirin, he ran out of everything very quickly, and with his $10 monthly allowance for incidentals he bought ingredients and mixed up some of the formulas he had learned in medical school to expand his limited drug supply.

There was no laboratory, no x-ray machine, no referral system. He was operating like an auxiliary nurse; he lost a lot of patients as a result of these limitations, to his immense frustration. There was nothing he could do about it except learn to live with this needless suffering and death.

Eustache wrestled alone with gastroenteritis and malnutrition and respiratory infections. Intestinal parasites were very widespread but he could not do the laboratory analyses to isolate the offender and he did not have the proper medication, anyway. In the surrounding areas umbilical tetanus spores germinated freely.

He ventured out to some of the mobile-clinic sites and small medical outposts established in the environs, one day catching a community agent with some paramedical skills charging for an injection—he suspended her for two months and blocked her salary for the violation. He made the eight-to-ten-hour walk out to Grand Bois, where people had not had a doctor's services in twenty to twenty-five years. Eustache came to understand why. He made four trips, a horse or donkey carrying the medications and materials, and finally the doctor wearing a new pair of mountain-climbing boots. The boots were too tight, he discovered, ever so painfully, almost crying on the return trip. He removed them and put his shoes back on. Anything was better than this. He put the boots on the donkey's back just as the animal fell over dead. It was rugged, mountain terrain, indeed. Eustache made the journey to support the marvelous energies of one of the best community agents of the project, Erima Poigno, a woman with ten children who spent three weeks out of every month in Grand Bois. When Eustache later was transferred to the division headquarters in the capital, in October of 1974, promoted to head the section for health education, the deputy of Grand Bois fiercely protested the transfer to the minister of health. He must not leave Thomazeau, the deputy said, irate. He was needed in Grand Bois, and nobody else would ever want to make the trip. Probably true.

That kind of obstacle—the mountains—Eustache was willing and able to take on. Others were insurmountable.

The economics. "No matter how much education you give the people, they will always say, 'Okay, doctor, that's fine, that's fine. But can you help us to better our financial situation so we can put into practice everything you are saying?'"

The politics. The community council is becoming an institution of local government in Haiti, and so it was in Thomazeau. The former magistrate had formed a council; the current magistrate had his own council; the aspiring magistrate was developing a committee to form a council. Eustache could not possibly work with all three, because they could not work with each other. He attended a lot of community meetings, but held back because of the in-fighting, since any position he took might endear him with one group, inevitably at the expense of rapport with four others.

He was able to work with schools for vaccination and recruiting students for the child health classes. The Catholic priests next door refused to cooperate with the program because of its family planning component, but the twenty Protestant churches did. Eustache announced vaccination campaigns on Sundays.

The bureaucracy. The worst part of the job, he says, getting support from the central office of the health department. They just could not understand his priorities, what he had to deal with every day, what he needed and why he asked. They turned down a desperate request for $15 worth of antiworm medicine. Too expensive. Can't have it. "All you people in administration see in front of you is an accounting sheet," Eustache raged, knowing the long-term benefit for the people in Thomazeau. He was living with them. There they were. Full of worms. What could he do? Petty bureaucrats, he mumbled, instead of screaming, as he felt. Eustache prescribed what medicine he had available very carefully, knowing how many people needed it and did not have the money to buy it.

Or he would be packed and ready to go out on a mobile clinic, knowing people were out there waiting, depending on him. No jeep, the people's confidence shaken, and the program jeopardized. In his heart Eustache watched some administrator running around Port-au-Prince in a jeep on some silly errand, fuming at the bad consequences for his work.

Still, there were rewards. "You do a work and you actually see results," he said, a very simple and sincere declaration, like the man.

In his twenty-eight months at the Thomazeau clinic Eustache noticed an increasing interest in family planning and its acceptance, although he believed the IUD and vaginal methods unsuited to Haiti . . . too much physical interference with the sacredness of sex for the peasantry. And he said so. The pill, he thought, would be more effective and appropriate, but it too had its drawbacks, requiring a certain amount of forethought and regularity, considerable detriments to its use by large numbers of people.

And yet, there was an increase in family planning. Eustache wasn't sure why—whether education or simply better service; but, yes, it was happening to some extent, to his surprise, given the odds. He sounded melancholy and kept looking out over the mountains, wrinkling off into the distance through the open back door of the clinic.

Dessources had another view, the poor thatch-roofed huts of Fond Parisien, and while he had many of the same experiences as his "triangle" colleague Eustache, his perspective was different—it was all class struggle.

Fond Parisien's situation was the fault of the village elite, he maintained adamantly, without a hue of hesitation, his certitude almost papal. It was the responsibility of the so-called "negative leaders," the "privileged" who opposed the "enlightenment" of the rest, he continued, in a tone of contained fury, probably costing a few layers of stomach lining at the minimum. In the microcosm of this little Haitian village, Dessources saw the haves and the have-nots at each others' throats; the rich versus the poor. But the "elite" of Fond Parisien had to contend with him.

Recommended for the program by Dr. Laroche at the medical school, in his way Dessources was as remarkable a man in his achievements as was Ary Bordes . . . a peasant who had become a physician. The price had been high and his black, attractively featured face was sullen, full of anger, and yes, hate, from his struggle. He had had to slug his way through, a war really, and it had tracked him into the fight. Dessources was always fighting, feisty, defensive, disagreeable. Asked a question, he shot one right back. Privately, he confided he wished he were an auto mechanic . . . it would have been easier that way.

Dessources fought Ary Bordes, a Mulatto who had not had his hard times, although he did not know of Ary Bordes's own hard times. It was not so much Ary Bordes who bothered him, actually, but the class he represented.

There were times when Dessources's aggressiveness got to Bordes and he became decidedly irritated at this young physician's brashness and disrespect for a supervisor—and a superior, for Ary Bordes is authoritarian, too. He watched Dessources's face for signs of mellowing, that face so full of suffering and closed to life. He must learn to fight for the class of people he champions, Bordes thought, to see how he can change things and improve things . . . he is too much against . . . he has a lot of work to do with himself, Bordes speculated.

When Dessources arrived in June 1972, "there was almost nothing." The dispensary was empty, but shortly he was provided with the usual minimum of essential materials and drugs: an examining table, a wooden closet, baby scale, adult scale, table, two chairs, a little gas-run refrigerator, water basin, two file cabinets, a gas stove for boiling water—and posters from Zambia. Given the national situation, the resources were "pretty good." His problems were the same as in Croix-des-Bouquets and Thomazeau. He did what he could but the odds were bad, the suffering great, and it ate at Dessources because these were his very own people in a more intimate way than for Ary Bordes. It was in a village very much like this one outside of Jacmel that he had grown to boyhood; Bordes's hometown, too, but theirs were very different destinies indeed.

The people were uneducated, and at the same time they were seeing him, they were seeing the "houngan" nearby. He knew it but was smart enough not to fight the "houngans" of Fond Parisien. He worked for collaboration; sometimes it existed and sometimes there was friction, but he tried a little compromise for a change, a little negotiation, a faint juggling of modern and folk beliefs, avoiding a confrontation on this front, at least. He worked as best he could with all the leaders, the rapport laboriously built up over the years by Dieumaitre Jacques.

But while he worked, Dessources inside tended to the pessimistic. The illiteracy, the malnutrition, the lack of roads, electricity, irrigation—"all are obstacles that stop you from going anywhere," and at their base a certain mind set, the fundamental obstacle, he believed. "We have to take time to not only change the country physically," he maintained always, "but reeducate the masses and the elite. Often we think of the education of the masses; we forget the elite also must be educated because they are not ready." There was hostility to progress, institutionalized. "Fond Parisien is an element of the whole country, not an isolated area," he would often comment about this village where he lived. "For Fond Parisien to really move, the whole country has to move because if Fond Parisien moves—these other forces will come and overwhelm the spirit of Fond Parisien." And in this village he did not see the human and material resources for real development, for the triumph of real change—"habit and understanding." In time he noticed change here and there, but he was always prudent about it, not putting too much stock in what was in his opinion so fragile a thing and subject to overweening opposition. He acknowledged it, that was as far as he went.

But he often spoke out loud and clear, sometimes too loud and less clear, to those "technicians who live in Port-au-Prince." With them he was not as prudent.

"To understand the problem you must have the PRIVILEGE of living in the rural area," he would say. "You must know that the rural people have their own laws, which are not the same as those of the urban area. YOU with your education in the city do not understand the RULES of the peasantry," the obvious implication being that he did, very well. "Your methodology must be adapted to the concrete reality of the Haitian people," he would carry on, adding an almost threatening command, yet almost pleading and pathetic: "Don't infuse MY reality with YOUR theories from *another* reality! I am living with the illiteracy, the malnutrition, the absence of roads, no electricity, no irrigation, and the mentality that must be educated," he would say, pugnaciously, and be off to Galette Chambons to assist with the organization of a sewing group for young women, rather than come into the capital for a staff meeting as had been requested. He went off to work in what he called "the simultaneous tragedy and comedy of life," a classical existentialist with more than a sprinkling of peasant fatalism in his soul. "An existentialist must always have a project," he would say, shrugging some more. "It is not idealism that brought me to Fond Parisien . . . hard . . . difficult. Frankly, to work here you have to have courage and the call. . . ."

Basically he was having an easier time than Eustache, who was more isolated and beleaguered. While Fond Parisien was the poorest point, it had been the focus of a lot of activity since the nutrition rehabilitation days in the early 1960s. Still, he had no laboratory or X-ray machine; he had to be a generalist, not a specialist. He did have a jeep every Wednesday come with a consulting gynecologist for IUD insertion, a rotating service among the "triangle" points. On its return trip he could pack inside very ill patients for hospitalization in Port-au-Prince, the most difficult cases, often convulsions in pregnant women. For that reason not as many of his patients died while he watched helplessly—frustration he was spared, unlike Eustache in Thomazeau.

"Rural medicine has its logic," he would say philosophically and most insightfully. Conditions were different, and practice necessarily must be different as well. He too surveyed the scene from his position on the clinic porch, pensive like Eustache.

At the end of his residency Dessources was replaced, not by another physician, but by a head nurse, not so frustrated by the limitations of resources making impossible the use of a doctor's skills. Madame Marie Jose Moreau Julien, a large-boned, vivacious, cheery woman, also in contrast to her predecessor, had three years of clinical experience in Thomazeau before her transfer. She would be assisted by two auxiliary nurses. Miss Vierginie Justin, an aggressive, sparkly-eyed young woman, full of ability and thwarted ambition, who wanted to become a trained midwife but did not have an "uncle"—a patron—in the bureaucracy to ease her rise higher. And Miss Rosemarie Pierre Louisaux, quiet, pensive, suspicious and heavier, someone Ary Bordes, who rarely joked, called, "that one who looks like a potato." They would carry on well. The clinic record continued to improve with their provision of services, excellent human relations, and obvious talent. They would live together like sorority sisters in a modest hut, doing up each other's hair in rollers, paying their maid $6 a month to clean and cook, and escaping to the capital on weekends. They had courage, too, like Dessources and Eustache . . . and others.

Meanwhile, Dr. Narcisse was throwing up his hands in despair and screaming at the auxiliary nurses, overwhelmed by the crowd of patients surrounding him at every turn. . . . The schoolboy emergency in the examining room, the usual child who had fallen over from hunger in his classroom after a long walk to school without breakfast. The others waiting patiently for him, a lot of them. . . .

The Croix-des-Bouquets clinic was thriving. There was a sad-faced old woman, her pink patient card held carefully in her hand, crying gently in obvious pain, a clean white handkerchief reaching up to her tearing eyes every so often. Next, a woman in black mourning clothes with her schoolchild daughter in green uniform, dazed and leaning her head against her mother's shoulders. Next, a very malnourished child with the staring eyes of the hungry and thighs the size of her legs, connected by protruding knobby knees. The whites of those arresting eyes, yellow with illness. A maternal arm reached around her shoulder. Next, a man in total collapse, head wrapped in a towel—the sign of sickness—resting in the lap of his daughter. The veins in his forehead protruded in pain, eyes closed, seeking comfort within himself. . . .

As the program succeeded, the clinics as well as Dr. Narcisse felt the squeeze—the lack of drugs, shortage of personnel, the pressures of providing curative medicine compounded by a growing recognition of preventive medicine—immunization, health education, and family planning.

By the end of the second year of operation, about 40 percent of the children in the "triangle" had begun their immunization series. Prenatal care alone had jumped from the first year's figure of 17 percent of the estimated target group, to 30 percent. There were 1,678 new family-planning acceptors, and family planning services were being offered every day rather than assigned to any specific clinic schedule. Over $2,800 was contributed that year by the people's fees.

By the end of the third year, the patient load at the clinics appeared to have stabilized, probably due to the lack of drugs and limits of human relations rapport. But more than half of the pregnant women in the area had been seen in the prenatal clinics, 1,710 women. The number of new family planning patients had grown to 2,845—most interestingly, more men than women. The previous year, the women represented 60 percent of new acceptors, but by the end of 1974, they were only 27 percent of the total. There was a reason. . . .

During the third and final "triangle" year, 15,000 patients were seen in the three clinics. Eight out of every ten pregnant women in Fond Parisien were seeking prenatal care. There were nearly 1,000 new family-planning acceptors and over 2,000 new male acceptors.

Those were the numbers. Bordes did not play the numbers game. Hal Crow pressed, urging him to get more people to practice contraception, concerned most about the family planning aspects of the program. After all, a lot of the money was coming from Family Planning International Assistance. But Bordes could not be enticed into the game.

"Family planning was a major concern of Ary's, yet it was not his major concern," says Crow, as he recalls the days of those short-term goals, the target for one year, two years, visions of percentages of contraception users. Numbers.

Then Crow began to make some adjustments. "I think we achieved our objective in a roundabout way," is the attitude he holds in retrospect, having located something called the long-term view. Crow was learning about Haiti and about Haitian time. He lowered his targets, deciding that his objectives were unrealistic given the milieu. The targets would be achieved in the future, he began to think, a la Ary Bordes . . . since so much of the action was directed at young people who would be the adults of Haiti tomorrow.

"We did fall below those kinds of objectives that were quantifiable," he acknowledges. Yet, he never felt the project was not measuring up to expectation, those warm, wonderful expectations of his first Haitian trip, full of good will and good impressions. "I think it was so very obvious to anyone who came in from the outside that this program was making some significant contributions to the life-style, to the kinds of educational activity . . . just the awareness and concern about life."

He did occasionally lapse into North American numbering, however, urging Bordes to go faster, not able to hang on to his Haitian patience once in Manhattan, his outsider's view of the situation coming back like a mirage in the desert. Milk, honey, water, dates, IUDs, pills. . . ."I remember he looked at me once and smiled and then said, 'One thing that I have learned after many years of working in the field is that development is a slow process!'" He was like a guru—gentle with understanding, patient with experience. The Socratic method—knowledge must come from the learner, not the teacher.

Crow did learn. He comments, "Indeed, it is a slow process. It is true we do often make mistakes by pushing things to a conclusion much more rapidly than we need to. And then, the program falls apart after an outside technician or advisor leaves." He recognized the legitimacy of Bordes's position, the merits of the slow pace, the need to train large numbers of people and involve them with responsibilities so there would come—continuity. And he restrained his American efficiency, confident the program was going along as best as possible under very difficult circumstances.

To this day Crow refuses to comment critically or negatively about Ary Bordes. He just doesn't feel that way. Crow believed FPIA was getting its money's worth in the "triangle" and was full of admiration, very proud of his association, as was Alice Sheridan years before—"I was very, very pleased to be a part of it in some limited way," he comments. He believed, although he knew there were weaknesses.

There were weaknesses. Essential to the health program's success was improvement in sanitation, far more acute a problem here than in the city, and most essential to any breakthroughs in diarrhea and other infectious-disease control. There would be no substantial change over the years. The water stayed the same, as did the latrines. They tried... failed.

The solution to the water problem in Croix-des-Bouquets was simply piped water—beyond the means of the project, which was heavily weighted in its contractual funding to family planning. The people of Fond Parisien were talking about potable water by 1974 but nothing ever came of it. They were even talking about it in Thomazeau. Nothing.

Virtually the same with latrines. They tried a latrine-construction project in cooperation with the sanitary-engineering section of the health department, and trained a man to make the cement slabs and locally manufactured filters. They were just beginning to have some success in Croix-des-Bouquets—fifty-one contracts signed at $1 down and 50 cents a month until the $6 charge had been paid off. The sanitary officer emigrated to Canada. That was the end of that. In Thomazeau there never was a good sanitary inspector. No contracts at all. In Fond Parisien the latrines would increase in time, but they would be the old style, unsanitary pit type. A mason was trained, but the people did not have the $6. Economics.

To develop more community involvement and rapport with the program, from its very earliest days health committees were started at each "triangle" point with local people—the magistrate, the military commander, the deputy... fourteen others. They didn't work, either. Meetings were held in a little house near the Catholic church in Croix-des-Bouquets, with Bordes attempting to rally support, to get the leaders involved in community medicine—informing, motivating the people they were in a position to influence... many meetings were held over many months, for a couple of years. There was a president, a treasurer, three counselors, the fourteen members. Virtually no work was done. Talk. No work.

The same in Thomazeau. The religious, civil, military authorities met, even the Catholic priest, but the members of the town's top were too divided by internecine warfare to cooperate together, although, again, there was a lot of talk.

Fond Parisien had its paper committee in one of Dieumaitre's big black Mephisthophelean ledgers, a compilation of his lists. They never got much done, either. The thirty members would meet every Tuesday afternoon, but gradually dissolved with the pressure of farming duties, until finally, only a few faithful met monthly, without much result.

Initiative seemed to be missing, although the problems were obvious enough, just from the five subcommittee titles—distribution of food for the pregnant women, for the malnourished children under four, potable water, health education, latrine-building. . . . The people needed to be trained to handle meetings, do a little planning, raise funds, learn the techniques of motivating other people, as well as themselves. Nobody on the staff seemed to have the know-how or the time, although the auxiliary nurses had that potential. It was never capitalized upon, a weakness of the organization which showed up without being overcome.

The same with human relations, another major debilitating factor, a huge anchor on forward movement. "I will come to the clinic and be hollered at when I am sick," complained one furious woman who stormed out of the Croix-des-Bouquets clinic with Madame Hollant chasing after her to find out her problem—"but I will not be hollered at for family planning!"

Human sensitivity to others. The recognition that every human being is a special case was not a strength of the Haitian social system—consequently, a weakness of a program staffed by Haitians with all the typical prejudices and insecurities. Proper courtesy to people you are working here to help would be the theme song heard incessantly, daily, angrily. It is their center—not yours. But status, authoritarianism, and fear are sizable human hurdles to jump, given the small egos of the race and the heights of human pettiness. A Haitian felt taller when stepping on someone lower, not a unique trait.

There would be more luck with the drugs than with the humans. Croix-des-Bouquets had always had a pharmacy, but not the other two points. Drugs had first come from a share of the very limited $3,000 the center budgeted for that purpose. Slowly the idea actualized of a local community pharmacy for Fond Parisien. Its evolution began in 1974, from basic medications at first provided by the program, with 10 percent of the sales put in the bank. In eight months the pharmacy was self-sufficient, in more time supported by a revolving fund of $400 to $500 annually—the consultation contribution of the people, an accumulation of the twenty-cents fee rotating back, full circle.

It was hardly your corner Rexall. The sign read "Pharmacy Communi" —on the second line, the rest, "ty": not enough planning—"of Fond Parisien." It was a very small, one-room cement building with a tin roof and shuttered doors, across the way from the little clinic, and maintained five days a week, since its inception, by Madame Bonard Polynice, a former community agent, cousin of Dieumaitre's, like a lot of project people. Inside on crude wooden shelves painted burgundy and a table covered over with pressed-down tin Pepsi-Cola can metal could be found a variety of simple medications, many samples or surplus items. Painkillers, tranquilizers, penicillin, vitamins of all kinds, nutrition supplements for the malnourished, Band-Aids, antihemorrhoid medicine, coughdrops. . . . It was a minipharmacy, but adequate for the needs of the people.

Bordes loved it. The pharmacy was something he was extremely proud of because it assured continuity and self-sufficiency—his obsessions. It was THE formula he was attempting to carry to completion in every aspect of the "triangle" project. Now whatever happened in Port-au-Prince or with the international organizations would not affect the drug supply of the village.

One month before the "triangle" experiment concluded and was taken over by the government, the drug-shortage problem in Thomazeau would find the same solution through the efforts of Eustache's successor, Dr. Michael Leandre, the model replicated within its own ranks.

Perhaps Madame Monpoint put the total health package best: "You can see it in the church," she said of her Croix-des-Bouquets base since 1973. "Every afternoon it was once full of funerals, particularly baby funerals, and maybe five or six adults. The church is closed in the afternoons now."

12

UNITED WE STAND

"This is a very arid country, and what we are going to do in these very dry areas where the people barely have something to eat! Are we going to tell them to eat meat, eggs, and drink milk? I think in a place like this unless you bring in agricultural development your program will not have much success.

"That's why I think more and more we should try to have the understanding to see if we can't all work together. I don't want the doctor to be an agronomist, but if he works somewhere he should try to see that an agronomist is there to help him, a literacy man to help him; and know that he can do his best, but he cannot do his best by himself. He needs all these people to come and give him a hand and everyone working together . . . I don't think we can continue by doing separate programs.

"We are specialists in health, agriculture, literacy—but the peasant sees his small community as a whole and he does not come and ask us to develop one piece by one piece. He asks us to come and help him in his total life. So we have to bring our thinking to the level of the poor peasant and the rural masses who need a composite type of development. This is the specialist thinking that has to change. This is the way I look at it now."—Ary Bordes

Bordes was always off in a beanfield someplace, coaxing.

"Your future depends on uniting your efforts," he would say, his arms thrusting upward, index finger characteristically pointing up all the way, as far as he could go, urging unity out of the brilliant Haitian sunlight, incredibly clear but deadly still.

So it seemed with the village's economic development. The issue was obvious enough ... there was no movement.

"You must be your own developers," he would say, another time, another beanfield, white hair mussed by the prevailing winds of Fond Parisien, taking away the precious topsoil as he spoke. Nothing done about it that time either.

"The water will only come if you will to do it," he would respond to complaints about irrigation. "You must be the ones to do it," he would continue, warming up, shouting above the complaints and protests, ignoring the folded arms of passive aggression, the blank sometimes sullen expressions under farmers' hats, faces patinaed with the harshness of Haitian peasant life, hardened, hurt, beaten, tired, gentle, respectful of this doctor's carryings on.

"It is not money and machinery that will make the water come down. It is you, with technical help on the side. If you don't want to give your manpower—it won't happen. It is your will power that will do it."

No visible willpower, although the manpower showed tough enough on the muscled bodies bare to the waist, thin-framed but strong.

And on it would go through the years from 1965 ... Bordes encouraging, cajoling, charming, advocating, exhorting, provoking, demanding, hoping, believing, reasoning, enticing.

"It is our responsibility. It is our country. Nobody can do it for us. We must save ourselves! Nobody else is going to save us."

Nothing. Still ... he persisted ... another year ... another group of farmers ... another field. "You must take development in your own hands ... it is us who must make the progress ... we must unite. ..."

They tried to get together. Three, four real efforts in those early years. All failures. While it was known that progress was being made in the village through the health program, nothing really showed. Fewer people were dying, of course, and that was very important progress which the people were well aware of; but a medical program could not really develop the village, make that evident and invigorating change in conditions for the better. Bordes had a dream of improving the standard of living of the people ... the fishing dream ... the block-making dream ... the bread-making dream. Nothing seemed to come of it, even after all those years in all those beanfields.

A church had been built with community assistance from funds provided by the Mennonites working in the area. That was it. The babies cried, the pigs squealed, the donkeys brayed, the cocks crowed on as usual. Everything was as usual.

Somebody was thinking. Somebody began to have some feelings of initiative, some response to all those years of apparently fruitless but persistent stimulation. His name was Lemé Jacques, a most unusual man, immediately visible in his appearance. For one thing, he was physically much larger and more robust than the usual peasant, his body a fullback proportion, broad-shouldered, wide-torsoed with particularly strong arms and large wide hands. Also he wore a beard, a short, black growth, unique among his peers and contributing to his apartness from other men. He grew it because he read in the Bible that all the leaders in those days had beards, he says, and since his grew naturally, he did not cut it. He was also one of the most educated men in Fond Parisien, the holder of a primary-school certificate awarded him in 1960, so he could read and he could write well.

In 1957 while he was a schoolboy, Lemé along with other boys in the village had been a member of an organization called the 4-Cs—like a Midwestern 4-H Club—representing "corp" (body), "cerveau" (mind), "coeur" (heart), and "cooperation" (the same in many languages). The boys had learned agriculture—growing tomatoes, cabbages, eggplant, peanuts, corn—together. It had been very successful, and Lemé in particular had distinguished himself by winning four diplomas for his farming prowess. In fact, he had been named president of the group and took his responsibilities very seriously, pushing others to act.

In 1971 Lemé remembered those diplomas and the cooperation that had made them possible. He began to meditate and to plan. He had an idea. He wanted to organize a cooperative, a voluntary organization of farmers working together to improve their productivity, just as they had done as children.

Lemé was now twenty-eight years old, married at twenty-one to a village girl of fifteen, the father of four children with another on the way. He had married well; his father-in-law was very comfortable by village standards, and the family since 1965 had lived in a relatively middle-class peasant house with fancy cut-out wooden trim, furniture from the capital, lots of glasses, and even curtains. There was a nice porch in front and Lemé's farm animals wandered nearby. Lemé had a wristwatch and a ballpoint pen. He wore socks and shoes and clean clothes with considerable dignity. His oldest child, a daughter, Mary Myrlene, attended the village school. But there was also Bertha, four; Jean Claude, three; Simone, fourteen months; and soon another, since his wife had expelled the IUD from the clinic twice. His bad luck, he supposed.

Lemé was doing his best for these children he had fathered. They were immunized at the clinic; they wore shoes; but he wanted more for them, particularly more education. His parents had done their best for him, the third of eight children, but they could not afford more schooling and now it looked as if he would not be able to provide more schooling for his children, either. It upset him, for Lemé was a caring and gentle father. His children would run to greet him, cuddling around his tall legs, as he caressed the tops of their heads affectionately while Madame Jacques for her part ran off to the "kitchen" to prepare his dinner now that he had returned from the fields. He would be willing to work at something else to provide them with more, even to live in Port-au-Prince; but there was nothing else for him to do but farm in Fond Parisien.

Like many in this village Lemé was a tenant farmer working another's land, which he rented. He was never able to save money and really stock up produce and move forward, despite his backbreaking hours under the hot sun, digging away with his hoe six days a week with rest on Sunday. It didn't seem to matter what he did because he never got anywhere. He needed to do something to improve his prospects, he decided. He thought about how a lot.

Then he talked with some other young men who were his age and a little younger and also had the same problems, the same fights over water rights to irrigate their fields, the same incurable sicknesses in the plantings, the same inertia, above all else.

It took only three days for him to organize the first meeting. The meetings continued, the visits to other houses, the talks at one house after another. More discussions. More meetings. They studied the question together. It was difficult to get people to agree, he discovered. Two of the original group dropped out, discouraged. Not Lemé. He hung in there. He was the president of the group, after all. Gradually the group began to grow and routinely hold weekly meetings. There was always something new coming up for discussion, but there was one main recurring theme. How could they increase the productivity of their land? They all had such small, dry holdings. They needed more land; they needed more water.

In time, twenty-nine young men joined the group, and three older men. One of the original drop-outs changed his mind and was trying to come back . . . he was accepted. Lemé began talking about the cooperative virtually all the time, Madame Jacques noticed. He spent much of his energy trying to keep a spirit of cooperation alive in the membership, maintaining contact with them, holding the initiative together. He seemed able to do it somehow, in his soft-spoken way, for there was in Lemé a great strength of personality without dominance or intimidation or overpowering of others. He did not impose his view; he listened always are carefully to the others, drawing them out; when he spoke, they in turn seemed to pay attention. He had command in his voice alone, rarely gesturing or becoming animated, that royal lack of necessity. Presence seemed enough. There was something in Lemé, deep in him, a confidence that he was special, and it gave him an innate assurance about himself without swagger or the arrogance that distances others, who sensed his power of personality and responded to it and respected him for it. He was quiet, self-contained, and a loner, but he was liked.

The group called themselves the Cooperative of Bois-de-Mieux, their neighborhood in Fond Parisien. Their formal organization, January 12, 1972, signified the beginning of this village's economic resurrection—and more.

Enter agronomist Marcel Depestre, someone recommended to Bordes as a good choice to head the economic component of the "triangle" project. Bordes called Depestre to the center, talked with him about his hopes for Fond Parisien and the entire "triangle," for that matter—and the need. Depestre remembered. Twenty-five years earlier as an agronomy student he had been in Fond Parisien and he knew the desperation. He recalled how at the time he was particularly impressed by the limitations, the constraints, the obstacles in this village. Overwhelming. The land parcels so small. The rains so erratic. The harvests often ruined. More and more the land eroding and losing fertility. The many years of drought. The prevailing winds. Bordes in turn was impressed with Depestre's sensitivity, technical knowledge, experience, and zest of personality, just right for the work he had in mind. Depestre accepted the assignment. He did not need to be pushed.

A short, stocky man with a wide smile and pleasant, friendly, easy-going manner, somehow sloppy-looking in a suit and tie, Depestre looks as if he belongs in open-collared khaki work clothes out in the field in the hot sun with the peasants. Somehow he is a little like Santa Claus out of costume and season, not as portly, perhaps, although heavy around the middle, but full of jovial, generous, in-the-spirit, good will, and brotherhood of man. He also is smart and skilled, a careful listener and an excellent speaker, all of which helped his career advance along very nicely. His technical expertise is superior, transcended solely by his enthusiasm for his specialty. Depestre loves his work as much as Ary Bordes loves his, and, similarly, often keeps his wife waiting, a long wait, as he completes some assignment. In 1972 he was assistant director of the national Agricultural Extension Service, long past his days in khaki. He had done that for thirteen years in the Jacmel area, and now was an administrator. But . . . he liked a challenge. Back into khakis.

"Fond Parisien was considered a closed area where nothing could be done because the conditions were so difficult," he recalls. "We were told we couldn't possibly succeed. I wanted to see what could be tried. ... The area was extremely poor," he admits, "really poor! It was supposed to be hopeless and had been abandoned. Except for Dr. Bordes, everybody thought Fond Parisien was simply beyond being helped."

He began to work part-time, three days a week summoning forth all his insatiable energies and superb rapport with the peasantry, assisted by a capacity for flights of rousing eloquence. Tomatoes could be poetry when described by Depestre, whose encouragement, assistance and undaunted as well as knowledgeable support also were of hyperbolic quality. But when Depestre first arrived the people wanted him or the center or the department of agriculture or somebody ... to give them a hand-out, give them development. "Men, women, children, each season, were above all waiting for us to give them something, food, everything!" he says, chewing on the idea because it was his number-one difficulty. Instead Depestre unequivocally reiterated time after time their personal responsibility. Fond Parisien had been reduced to childhood by years of assistance from international organizations providing a custodial type of care and commensurate decline in individual responsibility, on par with a mental patient with twenty-five years of institutionalization under loose-fitting hospital pajamas. So near to Port-au-Prince, Fond Parisien had attracted everybody's attention, particularly the compassion of various religious groups, who were doing this and that from time to time in a completely dispersed and disorganized manner—17 different ones were functioning in the village. The missionaries came in for one, two or three years, accomplished something, and left, abandoning the people to themselves once more, falling back into a situation even more difficult than originally. It was a common phenomenon, dangerous, and had hurt Fond Parisien.

"We all know that development can only take place through local initiative," Depestre says as flatly as he told the peasants they had to develop their village. And the charity had "damaged somewhat local initiative and created a climate which killed the national spirit, the human strength and dignity of the people," he continued. "You know, the peasant is very intelligent," he looks wily just talking about it, "and he easily arranges to receive what we are willing to give him. There were some peasants," he laughs heartily, "who were Mennonites, Adventists, Evangelicals—all three together—because that was the best arrangement!"

So. "We didn't begin by changing the attitude of the peasants," Depestre explains, "but by changing the attitude of the givers of aid. This was really a most difficult thing," he adds, without going into the details of their resistance, their sense of superiority, their ... it got

UNITED WE STAND

messy at times. That was the first thing, passing the new word on how development was to proceed in Fond Parisien from now on.

Then there was the sheer desperation, the isolation, the desolation, the competition, the internal division—"and we couldn't continue to have that, either," he says, beginning to get more powerful and graceful, "for the base of development must be human. This is the fundamental factor. The vertical axis of development is above all—man!"

So he told the villagers over and over and over.... He told everybody. An intensive training effort was undertaken at Damien, the headquarters of the department of agriculture, for extension agents assigned to work in the village. They were trained anyway, but more theoretical and practical as well as on-site education was fed the personnel who would be handling this most difficult of all tasks, the alleged impossible. What was development, really? What was proper coordination? What was the work to be done? What was the government's policy? What was popular participation? What was the importance of this integrated approach with health and education? Depestre constantly repeated, "The essential factor is man!"

"The peasant must play the essential role in what concerns him most. His own self-interest must dictate his involvement in the development of his country," Depestre hammered away. "With this assumption of responsibility, assisted by intervention and coordination, time and money, development will happen. And if it can happen in Fond Parisien, it can happen anywhere in Haiti!"

The technicians were aroused by the challenge, too.

The search for community leadership came simultaneously with the training of the personnel at the site. Everybody had an eye out, inventorying available human resources through contacts with the center's staff, Dieumaitre Jacques—"who was very knowledgeable about those in authority," the pastors, the teachers.... The agricultural agents in particular investigated the villagers who had participated in past development work, such as the youth groups like the 4-C clubs, and the former domestic training corps for young girls. Now they had grown up and maybe retained a little of what they had learned. It was here that Lemé Jacques was rediscovered and nurtured along.

Also, group meetings were held to let the people know they were there and ready to help. Notice was taken here of those who seemed the most capable—the activists, the decision-makers, the people who could rise to the surface—the leadership material to be connected with the technical assistance with the potential for transmitting the information to others.

Now working with the natural leaders they had ferreted out from among the many villagers of Fond Parisien, the agricultural agents began to form very small groups of ten and thirteen people, meeting regularly each week for about six months. They conducted educational sessions, exclusively devoted to the rationale for the new cooperative rather than to the traditional, individual way of doing things. They spent weeks discussing the importance of assessing facts, of arriving at a group decision, and the wisdom, above all, of planning in advance. It was an acutal class, like a Chinese commune session. A certificate went to each member who completed the training. Throughout this early phase, cultural norms were carefully respected. Fond Parisien had many geographic sectors, for instance, with some distinction in their character and conditions; neighborhood identities were honored with a separate study group with a unique identity and special attention to particular problems. Bois-de-Mieux, Pengano, Gaillart . . . where the conditions were dry, maybe cattle grazing was a solution; where the water pumps were available, maybe tomatoes; where the. . . .

Depestre personally attended every single group meeting of the emerging cooperatives, orienting the members: "It is good to receive help," he would say, "but it is more important to have your own identity. The aid will not go on forever." There would be nods of agreement because that had been the history.

"You have to plan," he would always say. "You have to plan everything for every growing season. Everything. When you plant beans, you must know how much money will be spent for water, for seed and plants; what quantity to plant; what quality of the plants; what is a good price for the plants; what are the potential diseases; what are the insects; what kind of fertilizer and insecticides are best; how much should be invested in each phase of the operation; what time are you going to harvest; what are you going to do with the profits. You have to PLAN!"

The technicians collated the information; the people made their decisions. It began with Lemé Jacques and Bois-de-Mieux and the first thirty-two cooperative members, each paying $2 to join the group, and attending a meeting organized by Depestre, sprawling all over the clinic benches and porch railings. They wanted to plant tomatoes, they said, and each came with their estimated amount of land for a tomato planting. Then, they jointly determined—after a wide-ranging discussion with Depestre patiently waiting for their conclusion—how much, indeed, should be planted. Then, with a blackboard, Depestre calculated for all to see: the costs; the insects; the pumps; fertilizer; the quantity of water; where they could get the fuel. Everything was planned, down to the minutest detail—except for the vagaries of the weather, unpredictable.

It was only then that a delegation from the cooperative, composed of

President Lemé Jacques, accompanied by the coop's treasurer and secretary, took the "tap-tap" to Port-au-Prince and paid a call at Ary Bordes's center. They requested the necessary funds—a loan. Bordes questioned them thoroughly to test whether they really were prepared for the undertaking. They were prepared. The blackboard had informed them well. It was July 1972.

"I could see the people had the will to change," Bordes says, "but there was no change. Then ... suddenly ... in the middle of 1972 they seemed to wake up; they had reached a turning point. We had made some plans for them, but they came out with their own plans."

They didn't want fishing and they didn't want block-making, and they didn't want brick-making, and they didn't want ... they wanted to grow tomatoes. Period. That was their group decision. It was very evidently a "working" cooperative and Bordes was *delighted*, ready to rally support in the tomato fields this time. He put his own ideas aside without a moment's hesitation. They had the initiative now. It had finally happened, an effect of time, lots of spade work, the emergence of indigenous leadership.

Lemé signed the contract, a short-term loan—"It must be repaid," Bordes emphasized—of $422.50 to purchase tomato plants, 110,782 of them, rent the five-and-a-half acres of land for the tomato field, pay for the insecticide, the fertilizer, the crates for transporting the produce to Port-au-Prince for marketing. The contract was in turn signed by every member of the cooperative, all taking equal responsibility for repayment of the loan and agreeing to follow the recommendations of the technicians assigned to assist them in fighting insects and plant diseases, coordinating irrigation and assisting their organization. It was terrific!

Bordes wrote Boston: "I assure you spirits are high here. Our common endeavor is developing and taking on more and more of the shape that we have been dreaming about. In Fond Parisien the agricultural program has really changed the sight of the village. It is now largely covered with tomato plants....

"It is thrilling after seven years of work in the village, after that long sleeping period, to see definite signs of awakening. The initiative is changing hands. Propositions don't come from us anymore, but from the villagers themselves. Time and effort are bringing the desired results. The village is starting up on its road to recovery. The marriage of health and agriculture is producing fruit." Then, he added most prophetically, "The economic program definitely is going to help the family planning program and enhance its necessity."

The project was providing some of the means; the people, the labor; everyone cooperating together. The people individually cared for their plots but coordinated as a group for the purchase of seed and fertilizer. The center provided insecticide pumps to combat diseases which in the past had preyed upon the plants, a kind of preventive agricultural medicine, raising production. Also, they made the jeep available to cut down on transportation expenses for the technicians as well as to bring the produce to market in Port-au-Prince.

The department of agriculture had its technicians in the field, improving sometimes backward farming techniques—plants put too close together, choking each other; five or six, even ten seeds in one hole, a waste when three or four would suffice. Also, they made available certain fertilizers at low cost and carefully taught proper drying and storage techniques to cut down on waste.

With only a few demonstrations, the people readily adopted the new techniques. They seemed very open to learning once the methods had proved themselves. All kinds of educational approaches were being used to push the new ideas—home visits to individual farmers in trouble, demonstrations, group meetings, constant attendance at each and every cooperative meeting, little skits and theater pieces on proper agriculture, animal-raising and domestic economics, teaching as well as entertaining the people at gatherings on community feast days. The cooperative members of Bois-de-Mieux even were carted off to other cooperatives working with the department, developing a little bit of competition, which never hurt.

It was all precisely calculated and planned every Monday morning with a meeting between Depestre and Bordes, discussing the situation as it was developing and exchanging ideas on every detail and possibility—a constant process of review. It was a most respectful collaboration, each affirming the other's expertise in their respective disciplines and understanding the total objective—development. Bordes considered Depestre the "artisan of the agricultural program," the master craftsman to be supported like a good talent known to a Renaissance prince. While keenly interested in everything, he was careful never to try to be the agronomist; emphasizing how most advantageously to merge health and agriculture.

For his part, Depestre considered the weekly sessions "really magnificent" support. He had confidence that Bordes would back him up—"his regularity, his reliability, his punctuality, a certain firmness." The loans must be repaid. Money must never be given away. Even if the crop were lost, the money was due—all at once, not in little installments, unless there was a very good excuse. Depestre knew he had a strong ally. "The direction of the program was correct," he sums up.

The coordination paid off. The loan made by the Bois-de-Mieux cooperative was repaid before the due date, with the sale of tomatoes

UNITED WE STAND

totalling $3,042.30. Profits after expenses were $57.94 per coop member in an area with one of the lowest per capita yearly incomes in the country, and for that matter, in the world—$50.

The delegation returned to Port-au-Prince to repay the loan and had five percent of the profits, $49, put into savings. They obtained a $1,000 loan for a red-bean project.

The women had done well too, selling tomato paste made from the inferior and bruised produce. They sold $71.40 worth; made a profit of $28; started their own savings account at the center; asked and received a $336 loan for a rice-marketing project, to be repaid the following June.

The cooperative began to gain momentum. At their own initiative, exclusive of any support from the program, each coop member agreed to contribute $6 to purchase communally twelve goats for breeding purposes. The department of agriculture agreed to provide the cooperative with a bull to improve cattle-breeding among animals owned by the membership.

The next planting of the Bois-de-Mieux cooperative—protein-rich red beans—needed more water for success. The center agreed to contribute seven cents per gallon of gasoline to run the pump. It frequently broke down, alas, and there were many nights when Depestre would be up until all hours repairing the machinery with the local Mennonite pastor. For a while, it was a very bad spell—seven consecutive nights. On another occasion, Depestre spent a full day and a half without a break, desperately resurrecting the equipment, for the fields were at a critical juncture and water shortage could make or break the harvest. Such was his commitment, and the people saw it. For his part, Bordes continually pushed the nutritional potential of the bean crop and its mixture with cereal, preventing malnutrition in children.

It wasn't all smooth. There was some dissension among the membership, endangering the delicate group cohesion being fostered. Wandering farm animals of some members were grazing on the property of other members, and the quarrel had to be resolved quickly before a real rupture occurred. In addition to problem-solving, Depestre was busy introducing some new ideas, oxen as plow animals replacing the traditional hoe and man. A demonstration was arranged during the field preparation for the beans. Then, there always was that "What have you brought me?" mentality to be dealt with—actually a literal part of a Haitian greeting after an absence. With the beans beginning to grow in the field, about four inches high, still, Bordes was asked: "When will we have a program of food for work?"

"The beans are food. You will eat the beans," he replied firmly.

"And after the beans are finished?" the farmer persisted.

"Then you can plant corn, and eat the corn, and after the corn, you can plant rice and eat the rice," he replied.

There was to be no food provided for economic development—a strict policy at that time. They were to do the growing; otherwise, there would be the constant problem of food distribution, and if the food ever stopped, so would the work. Food was to be distributed only for health reasons, for pregnant women or lactating mothers or small children— not as an incentive for economic development. Bordes argued with the combative farmer while the others watched and listened. But Bordes was absolutely determined about this point.

"Progress rests on the courage of the people here," Depestre agreed, standing nearby.

That was obvious at a weekly meeting of the Bois-de-Mieux membership, imperfect, but present. Men and women, no longer meeting on the clinic porch, but now at the cooperative headquarters they had built, identified by a primitive little sign and the tattered Haitian colors on a crooked flagpole attached to the side of a rickety little yellow and green out-building. The people, in various postures of head-in-hand and arms folded, were arranged along the sides of the straw "tonnelle" above them, shielded from the sun. In front sat Lemé Jacques behind a little table with the ledgers and copy books of the coop's business, with three other officers around him. To the side sat Depestre and an agricultural-extension agent, Théoma Bellanton, who had worked for many years in the area, only in the recent past getting some visible rewards. They both sat quietly, but very intently, listening, sizing up every nuance, nothing in particular escaping Bellanton's big, staring, bulging eyes in a face that was a study in concentration. Bellanton seemed to capture the vibrations like walls in a recording studio, every so often registered by a small muscle flinching or a slight frown between his eyebrows. He controlled his obvious urge to participate.

At 10:50 A.M. the meeting began in silence, as people collected their thoughts once Lemé had called for order and opened the floor to discussion. "Robert's Rules of Order" were not officially known, but politeness, a Haitian habit, was in full sway, along with that capacity for total stillness, the absence of impatient stirrings or interruption.

There were a few mumbles. After a time, an old man rose, white-haired with a stubble of beard on a face marked by many years in the sunlight. There was a ruler in his yellow shirt pocket. He said the cooperative was "not going well. The pump is taking too long to deliver water. Why?" he demanded.

"There has been trouble getting the gasoline," Lemé explained quietly. Despite an inspection every month, the pump had had some more mechanical problems. "The members are not paying their dues," Lemé added, warning that the money was needed to repair the pump, paying for the parts. With three failures to pay dues, "a decision will have to be made" about whether these members could continue to participate in the Bois-de-Mieux cooperative. Depestre nodded agreement, expressing satisfaction with the firmness of the leadership. From the beginning it had been established that the group must pay dues and demand to know why any member did not attend a meeting. Three consecutively missed meetings were to be punished with a fine of forty centimes.

Another long silence. More thinking. Another member rose, young this time, with a scar on his cheek. He stared at the ground in thought and then began. He had planted beans as he was instructed, he said, but he had not been getting the necessary water for them. Another man, then a woman, also rose, voicing the same complaints.

Elisma Oscard, a nondescript-looking man except for his total lack of teeth, explained the problem. He directed the pump. "I had to change the order of irrigation after the pump broke down," he said, defending himself. "I did not change the plan."

Loud mumbles, a few inside jokes, sarcastic laughter. Another member rose and with a leer, commented, "People come to the pump director to ask for water, but not everyone is a bigshot and can come and ask and get it." His implication was clear to all—the pump director was being paid off by some and getting preferential treatment.

Lemé intervened. "Normally," he explained, "if a person thinks he is a bigshot, he thinks he can get things done that way and quickly—but we cannot do it that way," so they had all agreed, he said.

Lots of grumbling. The cooperative paid $1.28 for each hour of pump water, twenty-four hours a day. The gasoline price hike had wounded their finances deeply and now some of the people were saying they would not plant beans again. They did not want to participate.

In the far right corner there was talk of terror—a "sans pouel"—a secret society of malevolent people who performed ceremonies at night and often killed others with their black magic. One of the farmers was saying that when he went out around 1 A.M. two nights earlier, his time to open the dikes for the irrigation of his bean field, he had seen their characteristic blue light, the killing beam off in the distance of a "sans pouel."

There were squeaks and a few cries. He elaborated animatedly, encouraged. The people stayed quiet and listened, frightened at these revelations of dangers and how this farmer had fought his apprehensions the previous night, venturing forth with his hoe all alone in the pitch black roads of the village, into his garden. How his heart had pounded all the while and what courage it had required for him to do the irrigation.

"It was a Tuesday night," he continued, the tension registering on his face as he recollected that awful time for Tuesday and Saturday were the worst days for these regiments of bad spirits on the move. His listeners "aahhhh" and "oohhh" his commentary. His very time for irrigation, he added, was the very worst! Between 11 P.M. and 2 A.M., the peak hours for "sans pouel" destructiveness. They nodded. He could have been killed instantly by the blue light or just withered away, suddenly taken ill, gradually but surely to die.

Things were getting out of hand. Depestre rose, and things quieted down. "I don't like the tone of this talk. We should not fight or be defiant, but speak in a spirit of cooperation." Then he quickly changed the subject away from bigshots and peasant spirits to more practical matters, the bickering and fear probably not forgotten, but momentarily arrested. Next time there was to be a planting of corn on a communally operated field, a new twist and a new kind of corn of an experimental and high-yielding, low-water-intensity variety. "Is everyone agreed to pay for the irrigation of the corn?" he asked.

More mumbling. Only one person had agreed. The others said they had not seen the corn. "But it belongs to all the members," Depestre added. "After this meeting we must all go together and see the cornfield and make a decision together," he said, and sat down, watching some more.

This morning things were not going too well in the Bois-de-Mieux cooperative and this dissension and passivity had to be changed. He had other thoughts and musings as the business and the discussion continued. . . . Off in the distance was the lake with its protein-potential, as yet untapped, a continuing vexation, but maybe with some justification. He had once brought some fish home for testing himself, had become ill, as did his dog, who had munched on some remaining scraps. Further away . . . the rocky, deteriorating mountains, the meanest problem, the erosion the people struggled with as they attempted to turn the corner of their destiny, so arbitrarily dictated by nature. This nature that was pushing the cornfields and the palm tree right-faced in the wind. A cock crowed. A woman walked off, burdened with firewood, an enormous quantity on her head, but borne without a grimace or look of strain, the stoicism and endurance of Haiti passing in review while under the thatch emerged cooperative initiative, regardless of its weaknesses. Lemé was ending a statement, ". . . it is us that must do it."

Depestre's cue for a contribution. He rose again. "I have several things to talk about. First, we are already in the second period of the year and next week we should prepare a program for the year. We need to work on the fuel," he continued, giving details on the gasoline price rise to be expected, possibly an entire ten additional cents a gallon.

Also, Depestre spoke of measuring the bean planting in all the gardens before harvesting to see what the proportional share of the profits should be. "No one is to cut down their fields before the measuring next Wednesday," Lemé reiterated.

"We cannot have this done by one man," jumped up one cooperative member. He was seconded. A third rose to support him. A fourth.... There was suspicion. Depestre agreed to see that the measuring of the harvest be done by a few agents to eliminate any chance of graft, and so instructed Bellanton. Cooperative or no cooperative, it would take a lot more than that to eradicate envy and distrust among these Haitian peasants.

Then Depestre made another point, holding up a sample of a little gray bankbook for all to see. "We could have a little bank to put in and take out money," he said. "You have often asked to have a fund. Today you can put your money in the bank. And next week, if you need it, you can take it out again—it is your money."

The people listened carefully to this suggestion. Traditionally, land, even left unused, and farm animals, however skinny, were money in the bank. This was a break with the past, and going even further than the idea of the five percent savings kept with Dr. Bordes.

"There will be a receipt locked into the strongbox. Even your wives will be authorized to take the money." Hoots of laughter! Doubled-up bodies with derision!

Hiding his amusement at the reaction, Depestre carefully placed his clipboard on the table and with incredible deliberation put the cap back on his fountain pen. "The next time we meet we can talk about this program together some more," he said, sensing the tide of opposition. The wives must be kept away from the strongbox at all costs, was the obvious prevailing opinion. Gambling is a major domestic sore point in Haiti.

There was other business that morning. One bean field had developed a disease—eight out of ten plants were affected and the garden must be burned, Bellanton said, lest the sickness spread to the others. Wandering cows and a horse had been by the pump, dirtying the water which was used for drinking and breaking the basin, he continued. "This had to be controlled," he said, given its sanitation hazards.

But the people of the area were not helping to restrain their animals because it was not their fields that were being irrigated and they had no lands to lose, was the gist of several replies. "They do not care," one member complained bitterly. It was agreed that the now 40 members of the cooperative could apply a great deal of pressure to the offenders by going to the commandant. He would respond.

"No, no," a subgroup protested the suggestion in unison. "If we say we will all do it—then nobody will do it," summed up one.

Everybody roared with laughter in agreement. Depestre joined in. That was the way it worked generally. Everybody began to talk at once. There were shouts of anger and there was laughter. The final arrangement—a delegation was to inform the commandant.

Lemé wrapped the table for attention—and got it. "Before we leave, what is it that we have to do?" Lemé asked. They had to look at the experimental corn. They went off with Depestre.

It was noon, and they would meet again the following Wednesday.

Despite all the meetings, encouragement, the proper planning, the assistance—there was discouragement. The fields had been in very good shape, the water was coming, the plants were flourishing—then the drought. The absence of the expected rains and the mechanical failures of the pump hurt the beans, and by the spring of 1973 the food shortage in Fond Parisien was serious. It created a huge setback to the enthusiasm that had been so very fresh in the minds and hearts of the people, and consequently, so very fragile. "The sky of development is obscured," Depestre reported one Monday morning to Bordes, not discouraged, but a little down about it.

Then came that remarkable Haitian quality—vitality in the face of constant bludgeoning with adversity. The people got angry about what they had gained and what they were losing. It aroused their fight, that will to live in their souls. They rose up, speaking more and more among themselves about the need to work on an irrigation project from the Lastic River, nine miles away, that river which had once channeled prosperity through Fond Parisien.

That was in March. April: the drought persisted and so did the response to the drought, the will to live growing stronger. By May, Bordes spent a very special evening of his life in Fond Parisien. It was May 3, 1973, to be exact. He stayed until past 9 P.M. in Fond Parisien, talking with the cooperative members and accompanying them on the long trek to the Lastic River source, urging on their growing motivation to reconstruct the irrigation system. By June, the center had agreed to provide tools for the work; Church World Service, to supply engineering help and food for work since the people would have to be away from their own fields if they were out by the Lastic, digging.

"If the water is brought to the village, it would be tremendous," Bordes summed up in a letter to Boston. By November, any lagging enthusiasm had been revived by a very, very successful tomato harvest once again, and $700 of the original $1,000 overdue bean loan was repaid, the rest to come the following March along with the new loan of $1,300. It was the proof that the people would respond positively given adequate guidance and resources.

A very adult sense of responsibility was growing up from the childhood dependency that had characterized the village, noticeable in the calculation and use of the profits from the tomato harvest, for example. A funny phenomenon.

From the first, the people had agreed to evaluate their yield in the presence of each other, just to keep things honest. But still, a gain of 200 gourdes—$40—was calculated at 40 gourdes—$10. Depestre knew it, but he let it pass, waiting figuratively for the kids to stop filching nickels from his suit coat in the closet. Little by little, with each harvest, the truth progressively emerged—first 100 gourdes, then 150 gourdes, and after a while. . . . "We were close enough to the truth"—the 200 gourdes' worth. Depestre laughs, remembering the machinations. "Confidence was more and more established, and even though we were not told 200. . . . Still, it was very close." He laughs some more.

What was to be done with the profits? A major issue. There was a thriving lottery—to be avoided. There was a chance to take on a new wife—and have more children. There was a chance to buy farm animals— and have some money in the bank of sorts. The people were taught how to save their money, to buy goats and cattle with that year's earnings. So, should bad times come, they could sell the animals, repay the loan, and never go into debt. Some money was also put into a more formal savings account at the center, first 10 gourdes, 15 gourdes . . . and it would grow into the thousands in time. Then, Depestre was working still on that little gray bankbook. It was all noted.

On balance the Bois-de-Mieux cooperative was doing exceedingly well, and the people watching in the background started to move. It was obvious this was a much better way to operate than to depend on outside assistance or work alone. "The people have recognized that they have to work together and with deliberateness," Depestre reported back to Bordes. Following the first successful tomato project, four other cooperatives had organized themselves by the end of 1972, in their respective neighborhoods, following the same crop choices as Bois-de-Mieux.

So on Tuesdays Depestre must be in Pengano with the thirty-nine members there, who met from 10 A.M. to noon. The next meeting was very important, a discussion of milk distribution for the entire village since that neighborhood was a good area for cow-grazing. The same day, at 1:30 P.M., he attended the meeting of the Gaillart cooperative of thirty members. Here the land was dry and the emphasis on cattle-grazing. . . .

By the end of 1973, the original Bois-de-Mieux cooperative had realized a magnificent $200–$250 gain; twelve cooperatives were functioning in Fond Parisien, a total of 363 people—282 men and 81 women.

Engaging that many villagers in the development of their community, given its conditions and history and in a mere fourteen-month period, was some achievement. There were about 1,500 people in the entire population of Fond Parisien who could be considered in the most active age category, and now over 350 of them were working for their own interests and for Fond Parisien. So Bordes had dreamed from the very beginning, some day to reach 300 to 400 villagers. "Then, things will really change here," he had said long ago. "Then maybe by the year 2000 this community won't be like this anymore. They will move forward. I know they won't be rich," he had said to the skeptical, "but I think they won't be poor, either. They won't be hungry. They will eat. They won't be affluent, but they will have satisfied their basic needs."

It started to look like that. A number of projects were underway, backed by $4,221 in loans—beans, sorghum, and rice selling; cattle and goat improvement; turkey-raising; fruit-tree planting; tomato and vegetable growing, with tomato paste on the side; needlework by some young girls; and that continuing talk about organizing irrigation from the Lastic River. Each project had been initiated by a cooperative working within the "triangle" project with the program's techniques available to help the membership realize their desires. But always the initiative rested with the people themselves. Although it was harder that way, the chances of permanent initiative were better and education and motivation continued in every cooperative meeting.

The tomato- and vegetable-growing had been by far the most successful undertaking. The 209 villagers involved made a profit of $13,522. The original cooperative of Bois-de-Mieux by the end of 1974 had an average profit of $130 per member; again, in an area with a $50 per year per capita income. They easily managed to repay fully that failed-beans debt. All the other projects had gone well, too. Depestre particularly was pleased when the young girls organized to sew layettes for babies, so instead of going outside, the girls arranged to make the baby clothes inside, keeping Fond Parisien self-sufficient in that item, the money circulating at home from pregnant customers. "Another striking example that the program is going well!" he reported one Monday morning, very excited about initiative in so young an age group, the first breakthrough with the next generation.

The bull had been a disappointment, however. "Inefficient animal," went the report. No progeny and no consequent genetic improvement for the cattle of Fond Parisien. Oh, well . . . you can't have everything.

UNITED WE STAND

With the growing spirit of cooperation and responsibility, so came self-confidence. The villagers agreed to contribute five percent of each loan repayment to build up a revolving fund once the Unitarian Universalist Service Committee withdrew as planned in the spring of 1975, a year and a half down the pike, but an eventuality to be prepared for. The $8,000 the Service Committee originally had contributed, however, was to remain behind.

The villagers understood now about planning ahead. The community seemed to be overcoming that egocentricity which the *News of Fond Parisien* in its final edition had scolded them about. Group decision-making, while never easy, was happening. There was planning before action. There was hope for something more, replacing the passivity and acceptance of what was. By the end of 1974 there were thirteen cooperatives with 464 members—364 men and 100 women—101 new coop members.

Now increasingly Depestre concentrated his efforts to gain greater coordination among them. The peasants themselves favored more cooperation, for they recognized now, two years since the experiment had begun, their dependence upon each other. A federation was formed, beginning with a group meeting in the health clinic of all the cooperative presidents, all the secretaries, all the treasurers. "Fond Parisien is very small," Depestre told them, "and a house divided against itself cannot stand," he added. The Bible was always an effective reference point, he had discovered early in his career. There was agreement, as he had anticipated.

An even larger meeting was convened, bringing all the cooperative members together, an enormous group, including many of the curious not yet attached to a coop, but considering. "Real economic and social development can only take place with the agreement of all the people together," Despestre addressed the gathering in his inimitable style, including more biblical quotation and more oratory and more agreement. "Only with a large structure can we find the assistance and the necessary cooperation. . . ."

And he went on. "Instead of the international groups and the religious groups giving you four sacks of rice or other things, you must group yourself together, really organize yourselves, to bring the water back to Fond Parisien." This is what the federation was all about—the Lastic River irrigation project—bringing Fond Parisien back to its former prosperity and the days when it was a food source for the capital, rather than a subject of Port-au-Prince dole.

"Now Fond Parisien can receive all or nothing. You must have the human will. . . . The possibilities of Fond Parisien are immense—but there has to be water! Water for all the acres of Fond Parisien!" He was really excited now, and the people listened intently . . . responsively. He grabbed his audience and was squeezing out their hopes and faith in their future and their children's future, their constant concern. "With water, at any moment there can be corn, beans, vegetables, fruit trees like papaya, greens for feeding the animals!" It all sounded great to his listeners.

Depestre had begun to perspire a little. "The fattening of the pigs now is very inhibited because there is no food to give them. The chickens are in competition with the humans to eat the grains! But if you have the grain for the chickens, you can eat the chickens and have a good yield of chicks as well!! The production of milk also would very certainly rise!"

Depestre was getting passionate. The words shot out of him, bursts of possibilities, little explosions of enthusiasm. His voice tone rose even higher, but held firm. "You could have more cattle, goats, sheep. You could have a multiplication of these animals and a large quantity of their products because you already know the techniques now. You have the training! The motivation! Some of the resources! But you could do more! Much more! There are people in the Cul-de-Sac Plain producing five times more than you."

That really aroused the audience. They groaned loudly at the revelations. Depestre was a skillful organizer, and now he almost seemed to be venturing into the realm of fantasy, speaking of the chances of a surplus of water, once the irrigation project was underway, and even electricity to refrigerate some of the produce. It was mind-boggling!

He started his summation: "The development of Fond Parisien is possible with water. The transformation of agriculture is possible with water. It could be marvelous!" He was just about ready to talk about the possibilities of the lake—his dog notwithstanding—and of mineral exploration, even oil! But now was the time to keep both feet on the ground and be realistic, inventory the available resources, sustain the motivation that was there.

Depestre used the Fond Parisien example everywhere in the "triangle." The largest loans ever would be made for a pig-fattening and sales project in Croix-des-Bouquets—$3,000; it was the most successful of all the projects, always with excellent to fair results, for the pigs were not as susceptible to the vagaries of the weather as was farming. Depestre faithfully supported the group every Sunday morning at their 7 to 8:30 A.M. meeting. In time, there would be three cooperatives in this "triangle" point, another keeping Depestre hanging around for their Sunday 3 P.M. meeting, and bring him back the same time on Thursdays. In Thomazeau it was Sunday mornings at 10:30 for a vegetable project underway outside of town, and shakily. It would always be so.

UNITED WE STAND

By the end of 1974 the revolving fund of loans had grown from $8,000 to $10,180; the people's profits, $5,731, not counting the produce which they retained for their own nutritional purposes. About 4,000 papaya trees had been planted in Fond Parisien, with fruit sales estimated at a minimum of $1,000. The goat-raising of the previous year had increased the genetically improving goat population of Fond Parisien to 111; the so-called "inefficient" bull had managed to produce four progeny—two males and two females. With the news of the Croix-des-Bouquets pig project's success, Fond Parisien decided to try it, too—completely on its own, with its own community funding. They did the same with a small peanut project.

The women were moving, too, particularly the women of Ganthier, the first mobile-clinic site years before. On their own initiative they had begun a cooperative, the only group maintained exclusively by women, although a real try had been made in Fond Parisien, a much larger village, without any success. Depestre was on the scene every Monday at 3 P.M. to maintain the spirit, with agent Bellaton untiringly helping and Bordes occasionally visiting to stir up more enthusiasm. Depestre, however, was the real hero. "He is our father," commented President Ordanie Pierre, a woman who oozed wisdom as well as aggression, with some of the Lemé Jacques quality in her. She was all shiny-eyed and appreciative of Depestre's support.

In 1975 many women involved in the cooperatives of Fond Parisien reinvested their profits in sorghum, and in time they would have a savings account of $2,135 at the center in Port-au-Prince. The Gaillart cooperative had planted palma christi bushes for oil-making that year. The bull and goats were continuing their reproductive ways.

As the Service Committee phased out its funding of the "triangle" economic component in the spring of 1975, the loans continued because of the revolving fund that had been supplemented the previous year with another $211.05 contribution by the cooperatives. Eighteen loans were made that final project year, totaling $22,700 from the original $8,000 from Boston. All the loans were repaid. Bordes was ecstatic about the program's success. "Every time I talk with people and tell them about the cooperatives—they just feel it is unbelievable!" Only $5 were outstanding from the thousands which had been loaned out through the "triangle" years.

Bordes wrote Boston just a few days short of termination of the project: "I was in Fond Parisien this week and it made me feel so glad to see the tremendous changes in the mind and spirit and responsible behavior of the cooperative groups. With the big help they have obtained through the Service Committee program, these men will soon make the material progress they need. Their lives will be different as they already understand the prominent role they themselves have to play."

There was more. Before year's end 125 village volunteers trekked out to the Lastic River twice monthly to begin preliminary work on "bringing the water down." In mid-December of 1975 the department of agriculture had begun studies surveying where the canals might go. The village was a place of firm-jawed determination. But what of the other "triangle" points?

Sure, pigs were fattening and goats growing in Croix-des-Bouquets, and some vegetables were growing outside of the mainstream of semi-urban Thomazeau, but this was hardly of the magnitude of Fond Parisien's activity despite employment of the very same methods. It was a flaw in the work which showed up without being overcome, and Bordes thought about it a lot. What was wrong? Why had the program been so strong in one point and weak in the two others, very much so in Thomazeau? It had implications for any replication, serious ones. Bordes and Depestre discussed the situation on many occasions, and both pretty much recognized what had gone wrong: the lack of what Depestre called "Fond Parisien's peasant purity."

Thomazeau, for instance, had a big central church, schools, a weekly market day; it also had more autonomy, more confidence, and more division, what Depestre called "certain divergence of opinion. Leaders who were not really interested in economic activity and who had influence over the people, interfering with group motivation." Eustache had had the same problems with local politics, and the Thomazeau clinic had never been able to establish itself as the focal point of community organization that the Fond Parisien clinic had become, its porch a veritable conference room and town-hall complex.

Simply, there was not the local leadership, and consequently, there was not the harnessing of community participation in development, the participation that could make or break a project. "To work in a village there must be a cohesive force," Bordes concluded after all his analysis. "In Fond Parisien, Dieumaitre was the cohesive force because he was a man of the community, well known, respected, with contacts everywhere. He represented the program which was bringing help to the village, so there was this very good link between the community and the program. But in Thomazeau and Croix-des-Bouquets we never had that leader taking charge of the program.

"It is very difficult to organize people from a health point of view," he continued. "This is one of the lessons we have learned. In order to have success you must organize people, and to organize people, you must go along the lines that will permit them to change their lot. In most places in Haiti, this would be with agriculture."

It must be written up, all of it, what worked and what did not, Bordes

UNITED WE STAND

said. Depestre hesitated. Would it be useful? It would be a lot of work, that was certain. Bordes told his standard write-it-up story, the chemistry teacher in medical school who had said, "Every serious work must finish in a book."

A 108-page green manual was published, detailing every phase of the achievement of the alleged impossible in Fond Parisien and the entire "triangle" economic case in point from defining the problem, the program philosophy, on through training of personnel, description of the particular conditions to be overcome, identification of projects, and a detailed analysis of every one of the projects and their results. . . . One hundred and five copies of the manual were distributed widely in Haitian government circles, with another edition of 105 requested one month later, because of the response.

For his part Depestre was doing some propagandizing beyond the labor of the manual. "This is what we have achieved here," he would say, getting the word out in seminars and meetings with other Department-of-Agriculture authorities and technicians in other disciplines, "because . . . we have considered the essential fundamental factor—man!" That was his recurring theme; Fond Parisien was his prize. He used it to motivate other agricultural-extension workers to the enormous possibilities of their work when properly approached.

"If in Fond Parisien, a village so poor, we could have these results. . . . Here is the example to be copied all over the Republic," Depestre told them. Wholeheartedly, he would continue, "We have learned that when we have the peasant's participation and when he takes responsibility and there is coordination and time and money and technical assistance—even the impossible can be done."

Something else was becoming a theme—the concept of integrated development, working with health and education for more action in agriculture. What Depestre called "more beneficial action."

You might say the action had been . . . very beneficial. That family planning trend of male participation transcending female, a two-to-one ratio, began through the agricultural cooperatives, particularly striking to Bordes when he recalled that just a few years earlier condoms could not even be given away.

No mention had ever been made of family planning in the beginning of the cooperatives' evolution. But once the people began to gain something, once they had a little more money in hand, then Depestre went back to the blackboard and diagrammed land holdings and why it was most important now not to have more children.

"Suppose you die and you have four children," he explained, dividing up the block he had sketched into four shares. "This is what it will look like for them!" One one-fourth to each. . . .

A very simple illustration, but effective, and it attracted a lot of attention, reiterated by other agricultural agents at every coop meeting and every chance. "It is the way to hold onto your gains," they repeated, "a fundamental necessity" for your development and your children's future; that future which had been an inspiration to Lemé Jacques as he caressed the heads of his children.

Condoms were distributed at every coop meeting. With the more aggressive pushing of this method of family planning came the male breakthrough. Finally. For his part, Bordes had always been convinced that the condom was a good method—the male phase of family planning, necessary and a helpful facilitator for the female phase. For once a man began to use a condom, he was contraception-minded and that meant his wife could more easily be too, particularly in male-dominated societies.

The figures indicated the same. In February 1973, there were 236 cooperative members—178 men and 68 women. None of the men were practicing contraception; 23 of their wives were and eight of the women coop members. By December of the year after those diagrams on the blackboard, the membership had grown to 363—282 men and 81 women; 61 of the men were using condoms; 32 of their wives practiced family planning, as well as 11 of the women coop members. The results were exhilarating to the program: an increase in family planning practice of 28 percent—20 percent of the men from zero and 11 percent of their wives; 13 percent of the women members.

It was a strong indicator that agricultural organization could assist family planning—and Haiti was an agricultural society. By the following year the figures were even more impressive, beyond the indicator stage—40 percent of all cooperative members were practicing family planning—42 percent of the men and 24 percent of the women. The percentage held steady, and by the end of 1975 the division of family hygiene was organizing a special seminar for agronomists to use agricultural projects as the basis for family planning acceptance nationally.

No place else in the Western Hemisphere has there been such a case as in the "triangle" project, Boston reported back. Their inquiries had indicated only Kenya and India had had such success with the use of condoms, and only after expensive and extensive marketing and advertising campaigns.

13

THE LOCAL CONNECTION

"I was going from Croix-des-Bouquets to Fond Parisien every week and seeing each trip, that until we arrived at the village, there was no health care. So the idea was that we had to give medical care to that area. We had to extend. And from the "triangle" we had to extend even further, to the entire country.

"My thinking is always ahead of my present; I am very interested in planning—I have to have a goal. And I really like that line of psychology—psychocybernetics—which says you must have an objective that you are trying to reach. And my main objective is to arrive at good health organization countrywide. This has always been in the back of my mind since I came back here and wanted to do public health and be helpful to the Haitian population . . . and I have been aiming at national coverage since the first health center was created to find out what were the health problems and what were the solutions. It started out as a center and ten years later it was a division with national coverage.

"I think there must have been something going on in the back of my mind, in my subconscious thinking. The actions taken were the results of that work being done over those years."

"There are two ways to look at an experimental program: one is to see how you can have maximum efficiency—the best way to arrive at the greatest results; the second, less efficiency but applicability all over the country. Most experimental programs follow the first approach. Get a model, the best model, the best results—but not applicable na-

tionally. We didn't pick that. I am not looking for the best efficiency. I am looking for a program that can be applied all over the country, the fastest way with a certain degree of efficiency and improved efficiency on what we have now. In an experimental program you can have a more dedicated staff, better organization, a smaller area served, and lose sight of the proper objective, which is expansion at the national level. The goal is improved efficiency with wide availability."—
Ary Bordes

A clear plastic phallus was being waved in the air of the Croix-des-Bouquets clinic by community agent Madame Louis Juste, young and vivacious with mischievous eyes, her earrings swinging vigorously along with her speech on family-planning methods.

It was another day at the clinic, with the usual family planning introduction for the rows of patients awaiting their turn for medical care for a variety of reasons, including a very evidently ill old woman who put her head in her hands, struggling to maintain her seated position, varicose veins like road maps in her legs from her many pregnancies. All listened silently—no choice—as the community agent explained about condoms, stretching one about eighteen inches to demonstrate the elasticity of the rubber.

"I will take one hundred!" hollered out one man, breaking the silence, collapsing the entire clinic and Madame Juste.

Family-planning education had its humor during its evolution through the years of the "triangle" methodology. Everything was being tried and tested, with the particular goal of reaching all age groups, vital to the program's success and to any future national maternal and child health and family planning program. Not even inoculations were supposed to be administered without an explanation, for health-with-education was carved in stone somewhere in Ary Bordes's work philosophy.

Once a week Madame Juste and all the community agents in the "triangle" spent the day at their headquarters clinic, talking with patients like these, easing their anxieties, creating a comfortable atmosphere, performing a few administrative tasks like registration, but mostly the little acts of public relations that could make or break a program's success. The original community agent, Dieumaitre Jacques, had demonstrated that.

Meanwhile, community agent Revalin Cham was busy out in the field, conducting a group discussion he had organized. There was a certain style about Cham, a kind of itinerant Ivy Leaguer of the rural area—clean cut, strong and healthy, an open smile, smart and sure, neat mustache. He looked as if he had it easier than those surrounding

THE LOCAL CONNECTION

him, standing out in his clean shirt and pressed trousers, a little dusty now about the cuffs and lower legs. Most characteristic was his alertness of mind and deliberation of speech.

"It's the good Lord who gives children! It is for him to decide!" shouted one pink-bandanaed woman in the group discussion, her eyes narrowed in hostility.

"Madame, it is not the Good Lord who sleeps with you," replied Cham, with a certain professional patience, getting hoots of laughter and approval for his quick wit, and slow, effective delivery.

The woman looked crestfallen momentarily, then she smiled, too. Haitians like to joke . . . it was a good argument.

Then he was off, his cuffs to become even dustier as the day progressed, venturing into the outlying areas of Croix-des-Bouquets four days of the week, mornings, and afternoons, carrying a little plastic briefcase designed by Madame Hollant with all the project's booklets, samples of the family-planning methods, coupons, his registers. The briefcase was Hal Crow's idea; the registers came from Dieumaitre's compulsion to list.

Cham had a household register to ensure that all families received a visit for information about the program and for special households in particular situations which should receive a re-visit; a postpartum register for all pregnant women in his territory, with their probable delivery dates so he could follow them along, urging prenatal care, check out the postpartum situation, and push for family planning; the family-planning register for all family planning clients, to make sure they continued with the method.

It was all very much a la Dieumaitre, right down to the propaganda at the cockfights and in the marketplace, smooth relations with the "houngans" and other natural leaders, short public speeches whenever the situation presented itself, but mostly, the basic tool—home visiting and group meetings out there in the villages, in the dust and the sun and the suffering; sometimes in the rain and the mosquitoes.

In 1974, 1,385 home visits were made in Fond Parisien and 169 large afternoon group meetings organized by community agents assisted by the soundtruck blaring out messages and music, rounding up 6,133 people who heard the word, many receiving pink rendezvous cards for services at the clinic; in Croix-des-Bouquets, 4,255 home visits, 94 group meetings, with 2,772 participants; in Thomazeau, 1,425 home visits, 161 group meetings, and 4,066 people.

The use of the community agent, following the Dieumaitre model, was the single most important way of getting people to seek out clinic services and family planning; to inform, motivate, educate, recruit, and follow up potential patients; to achieve a maximization of community medicine in the Cul-de-Sac Plain. An auxiliary nurse might get the same answer as a community agent—not the same results:

"Do you agree with family planning?"
"Yes, I agree with family planning."
"Are you going to come to the clinic?"
"Yes, I am going to come to the clinic."
"Will you use family planning?"
"Yes, I will use family planning."
Nothing.

It would happen over and over again, polite noncompliance. Family planning was hard to make tangible and understandable. It was not like a vitamin-B shot. Somebody from the community had to be committed to the program and have the rapport to make it desirable; otherwise, yes, they would do whatever you say. Haitian politeness, a throwback perhaps to the student-teacher relationship or the cultural authoritarianism which the medical and paramedical staff could not overcome despite their good human relations—when they existed. A case in point. Nobody's fault—but a failure:

Doctor to patient: "Why don't you come and do planning?"
"No," replied the woman receiving care for an intestinal problem, "I don't think so."
Doctor: "How many children do you have?"
Patient: "Two."
Doctor: "Do you want more?"
Patient: "No."
Doctor: "Then why don't you do planning?"
Patient: "No, I don't think so."
Doctor to nurse: "Difficult case."

Later the woman, leaning over the railing of the Croix-des-Bouquets clinic, spoke with Madame Juste: "Don't you think the pill is better than the IUD?" It was a very simple misunderstanding because for so long the IUD had been the only really widely available method of contraception, and synonymous with family planning generally. Madame Juste clarified; the woman was very ready to "do family planning." She would not have made such a comment to someone with the status of a doctor, only someone like a neighbor, someone of her own social level—like Madame Juste, who knew how to demonstrate the value of the service and promote it in the community, her community as well.

The community agent's job had been nicely tidied up with concepts like priority groups, targeted messages, the registers, more precise duties, schedules and reporting . . . after a year-and-a-half of investigation by an American graduate student intern from Johns Hopkins. Of course, Dieumaitre Jacques was watched in fascination—"There were things I felt and knew conceptually, but he put them into practice!" comments Norine C. Jewell, impressed. It was her challenging task to systematize the community agent's job and develop a training program, based on the "triangle" experience, for the emerging national program.

Pert, light-hearted and laughing—on the surface; underneath, hypersensitive, deep, committed; the talent was evident in all layers and she would present Ary Bordes with a good training manual. "Norine has been very influential," he later would say of this small, delicately-boned, "girlish" woman of thirty, whom he worked to death for three years and who would be that rare phenomenon in his experience—"the perfect consultant." She would do other training manuals, write up graduate school applications for doctors she liked, press for a promotion system at the division of family hygiene—and fall in daughterly love with Ary Bordes, a surrogate father.

The national takeover was moving along, spreading out, with Bordes constantly juggling his two hats, directing the "triangle" and simultaneously, the division. In January of 1973 he had written Boston of his return from the Northeastern health district, "where I presented to a large seminar of teachers all of our booklets related to family planning and the concept of the small family. It was an enriching experience which further enhanced the value of our laboratory in the Cul-de-Sac." That was the way it was going, like a bicycle-built-for-two: first, it had been the physician and the "houngan"; now, it was the "triangle" and the national program peddling along in unison, gradually gaining speed.

That October he reported back to the Service Committee on another seminar, this time organized for the press, to inform them of developments in the population issue and the family planning effort—"a big push for the national program," he wrote again. Always the national program . . . extension.

Meanwhile, from the very beginning months of the "triangle," Dr. Narcisse had been busy teaching the child health course to reach young women, fifteen to twenty-five years of age, patterned after the most successful Port-au-Prince model. The first year about 150 young women at the three "triangle" points took the course, passed their examination, received their certificate; 180 the following year; 232 the third year. They developed a habit of hanging around the clinics where they had spent their afternoons, even after the course had been completed, for this was where their new status was—their education. They were put to good use as volunteers and general helpers and propagandizers, just as the neighborhood workers from the early days in the urban model.

Narcisse taught the theoretical aspects of the course and Madame Monpoint the practical, twice a week, October through May. The students came from all over and were almost fiercely interested: "In general, Haitians like to accumulate diplomas and certificates," says Narcisse, philosophical about the response at his "triangle" point, remembering in particular one student who had emigrated to Canada and sent her father to the clinic to find her certificate and mail it to her.

The radio program was absolutely skyrocketing, along with Madame Souvenir's reputation. When she visited the Cayes radio station on her first trip into the provinces, she was assailed by a huge crowd, screaming and pushing and cheering. "Fannie! Where is Ti Dio?" In the sound-truck touring the town, she was applauded like the President of the Republic, chased some more by a flood of people shouting her radio name; when they drove past the market, all the women agreed to go off to the clinic, some following the truck. Hardly your basic-model wilting flower, she got more than a little nervous by the size and enthusiasm of the attention.

"Radio Doctor's" daily broadcasts and twice-weekly presentations on family planning were the single main source of information on family planning for the entire Haitian population, studies showed. The program's popularity in the "triangle" zone was precisely available in a 1973 survey of 1,330 radio owners, one for every fifteen to twenty-three families, a 50 percent increase in radio ownership over a similar study done in 1969. Almost every single radio owner contacted knew of "Radio Doctor."

On Saturdays the program "Health Class" was broadcast. During the first "triangle" year the bicycle contest had brought in 10,865 written responses from 62 localities, more than doubling the second year to 22,226 responses from 171 localities, and sliding a bit the third year to 15,478 responses, but extending to 194 localities nationally. By the end of the "triangle" years, more provincial contestants vied for the bicycle than in the capital, absolutely inundating the center with replies to the five health questions. In time, the procedure had to be changed to a more local tabulation from the toll of the mounting mail-bags, arriving like CARE food packages, and their impact on the center's secretary.

Same with the school health song. Originally conducted by Dieumaitre Jacques, now the baton had been passed to someone very different. Philippe Alies had thirty years of educational experience in the rural area, school inspecting, supervising curricula, teaching health, checking buildings.... It had all made him very nervous, apparently. He was on the defensive all the time, all the way, like somebody who had been beaten up every day for years. It had stopped now, but he was expecting a resumption momentarily. Recommended for the job of school-health director by Depestre, he was old-faced, white-haired, yellow-toothed, with that "do unto others as they have done unto you" mentality.

He was severe. Armed with copies of Madame Hollant's booklets on the concept of the small family, "When We Grow Up," and the population problem, "By the Year 2000," and the manual of the child-health course, he ventured into the schools of the "triangle" beginning in July of 1972, a presence most assuredly noticed for a number of reasons.

Eugene Paul had been teaching for sixteen years when Alies paid his first call to his little three-room schoolhouse in Croix-des-Bouquets, a few wooden benches, two blackboards and some pictures of the presidential family, a few maps on the whitewashed walls, topped with a tin roof. "There is very little to work with," he told Alies in total resignation, itemizing his lacks, " . . . no water, no toilets, no recreation . . . only half the 300 students can afford to buy books." The students sat there silently staring in their blue-checked uniforms with their teacher occasionally rising to sternly admonish one or another, shoo this one away, snarl at that one. He straightened up proudly with each act of authority.

Alies nodded in understanding of the situation and the style and began his job. He was practical. The children learned in their schoolbooks to wash their hands before eating, but did not wash their hands before eating lunch at school. He noticed this and was aroused. When Monsieur Alies arrived at a school and saw children with dirty hands—he sent them to "wash your hands!" If he noticed a child could not hear well, he GRABBED him and put him in a seat closer to the teacher. The same with sight problems—MOVE closer to the blackboard! A sad child—extra servings at lunch—can't you see the child is starving! Above all his objective was to each the children how to avoid sickness and develop better health habits, to push for immunization, propagandize the clinics and their use, the importance of insecticides to control mosquitoes, the dangers of contagious disease, the essentialness of potable water. Water really got him going. WASH! he would say. Wash yourself! Wash your clothes! Wash your house! Wash everything! WASH!

LISTEN! Listen to the program "Health Class" every Saturday on the radio. A lot of the children apparently thought they had better if any one of the two per 100 radios were in their vicinity lest Monsieur Alies hear otherwise. Only about one percent of the "triangle" children participated in the contest when he started working in the program; a year later, 20 percent did; the following year, 28 percent.

"We must change the Haitian mentality," Alies would rage. "Don't you see the consequences and impact on the population? The children don't go to school . . . they stay at home! The children are hungry . . . almost nude! They are sick and die for lack of medicine! If the parents have five carreaux of land and two children, each will receive only two-and-a-half carreaux! If it is insufficient to feed the children, there will be even more problems!!!"

He could be very persuasive in his authoritarian way and schoolmaster Paul for one heard every single word in his ever-so-soft-spoken manner—when not speaking with a student. He nodded in quiet agreement, his brown eyes, sad; his hairline, receding; his mustache, drooping; his spirits, as buoyant as the shining navy blue gabardine suit, dripping off his fragile frame. The impression was he would have to be reinforced with iron and covered with urethane plastic coating to contradict Alies.

By the second year on the job Alies had reached 147 schoolchildren and 30 teachers and distributed 730 little educational booklets. By the end of 1974, he had reached 3,375 children, had 29 percent of the teachers practicing family planning, and distributed nearly 19,000 booklets. The family planning song had been taped and played every hour he was in a classroom. That fall he visited ten towns nationally, contacting school principals about the radio program "Health Class" and the contest, the expanding national school health and family planning program. Really moving, he reached 198 school principals in each district with a personal call and another 1,204 by mail. By the conclusion of the "triangle" years, he had distributed the booklets to all the remaining schools in the Cul-de-Sac Plain. From October 1974 to April 1975, 12,513 schoolchildren had learned the family planning song. Alies had done his job. Alas, in time he would have to stay out of Ganthier, having gotten into a little trouble with a love affair, quite a disruptive factor to the educational program, given his status as a teacher and his contact with the children.

Finally in May 1975, Alies moved on to Thomazeau where another eleven schools full of children needed the health word. The going would be rough, and he would encounter the same terrain problems in reaching the population concentrations in the outlying areas that had hampered the medical personnel. In school health too, Thomazeau would be the weakest. Yet, 1,296 Thomazeau children would learn the song.

Children liked to sing—that was known. More precise testing, however, was needed to determine the effectiveness of the educational materials. It would happen in 1974 and prove to be both encouraging and discouraging, but important to the emerging national family planning program aimed at that age group.

The study was done by Madame Hollant in ten villages, including the main "triangle" points in May and June. Of the sample of 70 girls and

101 boys chosen from 141 different schools, most had received the booklets, they said—the first step. "When I Grow Up" had been read by 85 children surveyed and not read by only 11; 64 of the readers said that the message of the book was to have two children. It worked. Very important as well, 96 of the children surveyed knew the song— only six did not.

"By the Year 2000," the booklet on the population issue did not fare as well. While 63 of the children still had the booklet and only nine did not, a mere 19 respondents could tell the interviewer it was about the Haitian population problem; a small family—close; as many said they did not know. The results were a little shaky. Teaching the dangers of overpopulation to children was difficult, and before the book would become part of any national program it would be revised by Madame Hollant, away from a "balancing act" and statistics to a more personal approach, a dialogue between two children, Nicole and John. She got the idea during the survey, when one child spontaneously would often ask another's help to read the text.

The "syllabi" using the calabash concept also were widely distributed to adults in the "triangle" in 1972 and 1973, over 1,000 copies, and well over 2,500 by 1974. Despite the discouraging results first gained in Fond Parisien, every way still had its tryout in the rural laboratory of the Cul-de-Sac Plain, but again, the data would not be impressive, and in time the calabash would be thrown out. In a study in 1973 of eighty-seven homes, about half had received the booklets, but only eight were still around, a mere three copies in relatively good condition. They were not valued. Six had been given away and seventeen "lost."

Madame Hollant was beginning to have very, very, VERY serious reservations about the use of printed materials in a rural, illiterate milieu and she went back to Bordes. "To tell you the truth," she said, study results in hand, "I am not a believer in this type of material; I cannot say it is totally useless. . . ." But Bordes believed in print, that it had its place, although, yes, he agreed, it was a limited place. The "syllabi" would become part of the national program—all three amalgamated together: the baby, the pregnant women, and family planning, becoming the "Syllabus of the Haitian Family." Not for mass distribution to the people this time, but as a reference book for teachers, community agents, clinic staff, child-health-course students. . . . That would become the pattern—selective and appropriate use by personnel in the field.

Also, the line sketches of the originals would be dropped in favor of photographs—with the reason becoming more and more obvious through the intervening years along with the magnitude of the problem of visual illiteracy. The sequence went—line drawings, incomplete photographs, complete photographs. The posters had a lot to do with it.

People had difficulty reading—but certainly they could see! The assignment: posters preaching the five basic health concepts of breast-feeding, immunization of the baby and the pregnant mother, child spacing, and family planning. Sounds simple enough, as it always did until it was tried.

For instance, it took Madame Hollant a month to get the baby for the breastfeeding poster. Each day she drove out to the Croix-des-Bouquets center looking for a likely candidate at the pediatric clinic. Finally she found three, which was not easy, given the state of baby health; but their mothers refused to permit them to be photographed despite all her cajoling, pleading, charming.... They were frightened and fearful because of the voodoo beliefs that harm could come to their child through the recorded image.

The child-spacing and family planning posters did not work at all, although a lot of discussion went into their production. The concepts proved too abstract and difficult to illustrate and the hoped-for results escaped. The child is asking the mother for food, begging the mother for food, starving, went the feedback, "exactly the message I did not want to show!" says Madame Hollant in frustration. "The whole idea was that with family planning and child spacing there would be more food!"

It was the same with the big strapping photograph of community agent Cham, in his trimmed mustached and similar shirt; Creole caption reading, "All smart men should do planning." The message didn't really come across just looking at the picture and the people could not read. "The people thought I was making propaganda for Cham like the government does for Jean Claude!"

Each month from their production onward, the posters, about 2,500 to 3,000 of them—pastel-colored, standard-size, 8½-by-11 inches—on the five subjects, inundated the people at every possible turn. Meetings were held with all the "triangle" personnel to make sure everyone understood the messages to be communicated and could explain them, where to put them, who should have them. The community agents were given a quota of unloading 200 each month. Over 35,000 posters were distributed on vaccinating babies; 25,000 on vaccination of the pregnant women ... unsuccessfully mostly.

How does Madame Hollant know? "When you have posters on the wall and a lot of people don't even look at them, well, that's a sign," she notes with disappointment, given all the frustration and the time and the need. "They didn't even seem to attract people's attention!

Then, when we gave the posters and explained to them how they could put them on the wall and decorate their houses, and then, when we went into the houses and—no posters!" Another bad sign. The worst, however, was a walk through the streets of Croix-des-Bouquets or Fond Parisien. "I could see them all crushed up like somebody had just thrown one away." Or if they were used, it was more often for the precious paper, to wrap the sugar or the cornmeal.

Hal Crow was stunned by all the difficulties, the lack of translation of image in people's minds, particularly when he heard about the nursing mother, a torso shot. "The lower torso was not showing and the people in the village, when they were asked what they saw, said it made them feel very sad because the mother had no legs. This is how primitive the people were in the area when it came to reading the message that was being conveyed, or we hoped to be conveying into their lives. . . . It took so much time!" he wonders at it still, "to make sure we weren't making some serious mistake in some of these simple pamphlets, brochures, and booklets. . . ."

Madame Hollant kept learning, and, later, very much influenced by the successful Zambian posters, the batch of posters slated for the national program would be wall-poster size, not flyers—a big 16-by-20 inches, for one thing. Also, they never would be mass distributed to an illiterate population, but designed as support material in educational sessions, used to influence and teach people personally and directly for it was clear that pictures had to be explained to people. Also, Madame Hollant tried to stay out of the production stage since people did not know her and did not trust her. In the years ahead she would give Dr. Narcisse and the community agents a list of what she needed. She had learned her place, given her status and apartness.

Ary Bordes was busy with a poster too, full of tilting shapes and freewheeling fantasies. This one would succeed in finding its way onto the walls of hut after hut in rural Haiti, in time becoming the most widely known single piece of Haitian art in the country.

It was called "The Human Tide" and was the work of one of the country's top three primitivists, Préfète Duffaut. He characteristically painted out his imaginary visions and the exuberance he found in the hills and harbor of his native Jacmel, the crooked colored streets, the sailboats—all completely covered, dripping, packed with falling-off, crunched little human figures. Hundreds and hundreds of them, not even relieved by the overloaded boats in the harbor; people literally hanging onto each other in chains suspended from peninsulas of fantasyland, circles of substance, burdened bridges. In a way, it was grim.

The original three-by-five-foot oil-on-canvas was donated to the center, a gift valued at many thousands of dollars. The occasion? World Population Year, 1974, so designated by the United Nations and certainly an occasion not to go unnoticed by a family-planning project.

It was Hal Crow's idea. "Why don't we have a poster of Haitian art for population year?" Crow asked.

"Well, okay, let's try to do it," Bordes replied. It hung in the back of his mind for awhile, growing in enthusiasm in his nationalistic imagination. Why not?! Why not find a way to put Haitian art in the service of the Haitian people, their health and their development.

He went to one of the well-known moderns and explained what he wanted. There they sat, two famous members of the second generation of Haitian art, schooled and sophisticated. A painting on the population explosion? They looked at each other knowingly and explained painstakingly and more than a little condescendingly to this public-health physician about—the problem. "They sat me down and said that an artist cannot do a painting like that on command and some other very theoretical things about the function of art and things like that," Bordes recalls, unimpressed by their aesthetic philosophy. "And I said, 'Well, that's all right.'"

Undaunted as usual, he went to Duffaut's gallery, a man he did not know, but a native Jacmelian, also. Duffaut was less theoretical; his son was in medical school in Canada, as well; he was supportive of doctors and medicine these days, proud of his boy. He agreed.

The painting began March 15 and was completed by April 18. Like all his work, "The Human Tide," came from a dream—as well as the suggestion of Ary Bordes via Hal Crow. It was mystical and supernatural, topped by a trio of angels carrying the banner of the people and trumpeting for Haiti's resurrection and an end to the crowding on his spiraling imaginary island, so full of color and too full of life, to the point of the bizarre. The gift received widespread radio, newspaper, and television coverage.

Meanwhile, Madame Monpoint was like a pep girl before the big game, in a red wool suit, laughing and cheering on with her amazing energy, enthusiasm, and earthiness, and with her arms gesturing animatedly, surrounded by two benches—of midwives. The old faces of Haiti, lined with experience and serene with survival, the gaze secure with high social position in peasant society. Their wrinkled hands very clean for class, the midwives wore white headscarfs with tufts of white hair escaping, white sacklike dresses, and their shoes.

If there were fewer baby funerals in Croix-des-Bouquets's church in the afternoons, it had a lot to do with what was happening here.

"A midwife may not be a doctor or a nurse," Madame Monpoint was saying to the silent and attentive, serious-faced group—a peaceful group, just sitting there in absolute stillness, like the white crows on a tree limb in a breezeless afternoon, soaking up the day, this day in their life. Perhaps, it was just old age, most assuredly they felt wiser now since they had been taught about umbilical tetanus.

Madame Monpoint was gaining strength, her Creole coming machine-gun rapid fire, her voice tone rising and lowering dramatically. "A midwife is an agent of change in the community—her community." It was a recognition of the prestige of the group and they loved it, basking in her words. "This is a very serious thing we are involved in," Madame Monpoint continued, bringing the class into the total program of community medicine. "We are not just there to cut umbilical cords! We are there to talk with the women about changing their ways!" Very dramatic stuff, like a "For God and Country" parade, "We are here for family planning, for health, sanitation...."

Madame Monpoint had been at this job since 1973 after having identified about 150 midwives in the "triangle" with the help of the community agents. Forty of the midwives had been interviewed to learn of their methods—revealing the very worst, none of them had any real knowledge. The training was urgent. All the traditional folk methods leading to tetanus of the newborn were being practiced in the Cul-de-Sac Plain.

She began, developing a sixteen-lesson course, meeting once a week, covering a long list of subjects from the role of the midwife in a program of community medicine, on through a gamut of general health principles, to a very detailed procedure re-creating the entire birth sequence, almost a process of conditioning to change midwife habits at this critical moment.

It had taken a lot of Madame Monpoint's time to get them into the class, lots of persuasion and gentle touches to knee and thigh during many home visits and conversations—affectionate, close, laughing, dismissing their lies, courting. The thought of the class frightened them. They feared arrest, that they were doing something illegal suddenly, after all these years. If often took three or four visits—once they had been gently led to the clinic—before they felt secure in the physical confines of the building, apparently ready to spring out the door any instant.

One very powerful midwife, Madame E. Antoine Dieudonne of Croix-des-Bouquets, hesitated for two years before she set foot in the clinic. She delivered about fifty babies a year, getting paid $2, not the standard 40 cents, and Madame Monpoint had worked and worked and worked to get her into the program. She would visit, she would visit, she would visit. The midwife would promise, she would promise. Finally, it would happen. Madame Dieudonne sat on the left-hand bench, third midwife down.

By 1974 Madame Monpoint was commuting among the three "triangle" points to conduct the course she had developed. By the end of the first year, 27 of the 43 midwives of Croix-des-Bouquets had been trained; 24 of the 41 of Fond Parisien; and 22 of the 71 in Thomazeau, that persistently weak link. In addition, six midwives from Ganthier and five from Bas Boen, mobile-clinic sites, had received the training, a total of 84 of the 150 midwives of the "triangle," over half. Twenty-nine successfully passed their final examination, receiving their prized certificates, which they placed in little plastic bags and showed their clients, an excuse to boost their fees. The nongraduates would try again. Forty-two more midwives would be trained in 1975.

The data showed the midwives had been somewhat integrated into the total program of community medicine, another major objective, and were cooperating: twenty-nine women had been referred to the clinics for prenatal care; forty-two women and seven men, for family planning.

Madame Monpoint was at that stage now, distributing coupon books for family planning referral. "I know you know a lot," she said, as she continued to hand out the coupons. "You are very powerful people. We just want to make you more strong!" They giggled and purred with pleasure at the compliment.

A midwife rose, clapping her hands for attention. The class was getting more vivacious now, relaxed and less constrained. "If I see a woman with children, one after another, that she cannot educate and care for, I tell her she must take a rest." Wonderful approach, went Madame Monpoint's congratulations. The midwife leaned back in her chair, her legs extending out, like a poised corporation officer, contentedly powerful. All she needed to complete the picture was a desk in front, completely free of paper and reports . . . just there to think.

Another rose, a big woman, awkward and large-boned: "There is a big sickness in the land," she said, her eyes bulging forward, about to announce the horrible something that would sting the soul of every tourist not yet immunized against the scourge. "It is called," she paused lengthily—". . . malnutrition!" Madame Monpoint collapsed in laughter, shushing her gently, convulsed.

A quarter of an hour later she was swirling an IUD before the group, explaining that it was not planning, trying to cut down on that constant confusion. "Planning is a democracy, deciding when you want to have a child"—was her point.

"It is a rest," agreed a midwife off to the far left. Her name was Miracle, and she delivered just about the peak number of infants each year. Her family planning technique, she revealed to the group in a hushed voice, betraying her great confidence, was to talk with a family about just everything, she said, anything you can think of. Then, she continued her whispering, you say you must go visit next door, that you have to leave and talk about planning. Then, she continued, they insist you remain and explain it to them, in every detail. Madame Monpoint liked it.

Another midwife rose, standing erectly and explained about pill-taking, demonstrating through her missing front teeth. It was excellent and everybody broke into applause, Madame Monpoint particularly impressed by her use of the phrase "sexual contact."

Now it was the foam method, and with a plastic model of the female anatomy and a foam inserter she showed the proper use of the method. "It is even better when the husband puts it in," said one inspired wise-cracker, breaking everybody up, some clapping their hands high in the air to show their appreciation. "Yes, he'll know the direction," came the reply from her right. More claps. A few screams.

"If you have relations during the day are you supposed to use it?" inquired another. "It is the same thing you are doing, day or night," Madame Monpoint said, clearly enjoying her work. The class was fun. It would get funnier as she tried to get the midwives to talk about condoms.

Phase-out of the "triangle" was approaching with 1975. That February Bordes reported to the Service Committee his plans for the smooth transfer of the Thomazeau and Croix-des-Bouquets clinics into the expanding national program. Narcisse, the project physician at Croix-des-Bouquets, had been given the post of assistant director of that center, among other responsibilities—the teaching of medical students, Bordes added, obviously delighted at the long sought turn of events. Over the next months the national program would expand into Cap Haitian and Cayes, and Bordes was hoping to cover Haiti's ten main towns progressively. "There is plenty of work ahead," he concluded, always delighted with the prospect.

Meanwhile, Madame Hollant was into film-making in Haiti's rural area, without electricity and with a $1,350 budget. For his part Crow loved the idea, but did not think it possible to make a ten-minute film in color with sound for that amount of money. He had a great deal of respect for Madame Hollant—"a very talented worker ... very fine painter ... her great skill and dedication. ..." There were limits. The standard minimum for one minute of film is $300.

It was called "Modern Time is Different from the Old Time," very obviously a Haitian first—the first film about family planning and one of the very few films produced in Creole, another significant implication, nationally noted. It is very still when evening comes in the rural area of Haiti, only the sound of crickets and the voodoo drums; something marvelous was about to be added to the repertoire.

Raphael Stine, the producer, worked for the little money available and did just about everything—camerawork, set design, special effects, script rewrite, as well as all the technical production . . . what he was supposed to be doing. "It was very nice of him to do all that work for so little money," Madame Hollant comments in monumental understatement. The whole thing excited Stine enormously, the immense potential he saw in a Creole film as a social-cultural force in Haiti. The film was so very Haitian—its conception, realization, language. "Not one doubt existed in my heart," he later wrote in a newspaper article about his experience, "that this film will attain its objective."

The film was to present four basic messages to the viewers: 1) vaccination and nutrition for the pregnant woman; 2) preparation for childbirth; 3) care of the baby; 4) family planning.

The script would take two months of work and go into four drafts as the ideas were tossed around, the sequence of scenes debated, the plan of viewing time reconsidered. Madame Hollant completed the first draft, then looked at it again. "I can't read it," she said to herself, "what the hell is this? What's happened?" She passed it on to Dr. Bordes.

"I am sorry," he said, "but I cannot read it."

She wrote another script. She couldn't read this one, either; neither could Bordes. She thought she could write Creole, but apparently that was not the case. She took a Creole course; she tried another script; then, a final draft. People could read it.

The scenario occupied her greatly: the mother could come to the prenatal clinic of Croix-des-Bouquets for vaccination; then, she could go home and properly prepare for her baby's delivery; then, she could talk with her husband in the backyard of their house about family planning once the new baby was born; then, go back to the clinic for family planning; even meet a friend on the street on the way back . . . country scenes, clinic scenes, village scenes. "I knew approximately what I wanted," she says.

It took two weeks to find the house and the cast, with Madame Hollant meeting the community agents of Croix-des-Bouquets and explaining: "I want a baby. I want a lady. I want a house with a bed. I want a normal, typical lady of Croix-des-Bouquets, very clean, that's all, no necklaces and no gold watch."

They couldn't find a couple who could carry the parts. Sometimes the wife was good and the husband wasn't, or the reverse. Sometimes one partner was just too dark-skinned for the technical limitations of the production. Sometimes one or both could not act or would not show. The courageous partner could not take the part with another, without getting into trouble. They were playing the role of a couple and they had to be a couple for it would be very disturbing for a Haitian peasant to see his wife on film with another husband.

It was disturbing. The female lead would be the only nonlocal member of the cast. Marie Carmelle Blaise, in her mid-twenties, came from Port-au-Prince each day of the filming, a volunteer without pay, also very generous of her. She had done some advertising work for Stine and projected a natural feeling, unsophisticated and authentic to the milieu, just right.

There would be baby problems, script problems, transportation problems, power problems, lighting problems, camera problems, and emotional-support problems.

"What drove me really crazy was when the mother of the baby said she didn't want her baby in the film anymore! I don't know how many scenes we had shot with that baby!!" In the mother's mind the film was a series of pictures and she had second thoughts, fearful of voodoo abuses of her baby's picture. She complained that the father did not want the child to be filmed . . . the child had a fever . . . Madame Hollant did not try to persuade her. Should the child become sick for some reason, the entire program of community medicine in Croix-des Bouquets would be jeopardized. "Maybe nothing would happen, but I didn't want to take a chance." The whole thing had to be reshot with a new baby.

The script problem. Many members of the cast did not know how to read, so the script had to be put on tape and played over and over and over so they could learn their lines. It took a lot of time. With the slip of one word the entire scene had to be reshot . . . because of the camera problem. It was an old camera, not equipped with a recorder, and when mounting time came, the sound track would have to be synchronized with the visual image. Madame Hollant tried to limit the scenes to three takes . . . because of the budget. Finally, in desperation at the waste of film and time, she began changing the camera angle so the viewer could not really see the lip movement all that well. She never really knew for sure what was happening from day to day . . . because of the developing, to be done in New York all at once. But she carried on as usual . . . gracefully. There wasn't much choice, really.

The filming started the thirtieth of July and concluded on August 8, very l-o-n-g days . . . because of the lighting problem, Haiti's glorious summer sunlight. In bright sun the people's dark skins were masks without detail, the harsh shadows completely overpowering their features. The days also were long . . . because of the transportation problem. The jeep would leave Port-au-Prince at 6 A.M., deposit Madame Hollant and Stine, and be off for other duties, like mobile clinics. They would set up for early-morning and diffused-light shooting, beginning by 7 A.M. up to around 9 A.M.; then Madame Hollant would talk with the cast, have them repeat their lines, rehearse their scenes, and a big Nana would come and cook lunch; it would start all over again around 4 P.M. in the outdoor-scene shooting, again in that muted afternoon light. The indoor scenes using the clinic's electricity would go on for hours, until nine and 10 o'clock at night, because they couldn't work until all the patients had left. The set would have to be reorganized each day, the spotlights replaced, the cast put in the mood. "It took hours!" she recalls the trauma. "Rehearsals, tapes, then three shootings. So we really would run through something sometimes eight or ten times an evening, and if we started at six, we wouldn't finish until 10:30!"

Then, she would go home, where her three daughters would take one look at her in complete disgust and lack of interest in what their dusty, tired mother was out there killing herself trying to do. "Oh, no! Not another day in the Plain de Cul-de-Sac. You must be crazy!" one inevitably would say. They would never see the film, resenting their mother's exhaustion, absence from them all day, arrival home tired and hungry, rushing for a bath and a coffee, taking some time to chat with them, something to eat and then—bed. It all began again very early the following morning in the sun and the dust and the heat and the fatigue and the problems and the insecurity.

"I have no idea what we have," Madame Hollant said when she sent the footage for film developing and mounting of the sound track and splicing. It was a little tough on the New York laboratory, given they did not understand Creole. That's why Stine went to New York. The $1,350 budget included his round-trip air fare. Only two scenes would require reshooting—miraculously.

Two years later, when she made her second film "Health Is Wealthy", again funded by FPIA, again with the help of Raphael Stine, she would have learned a few shortcuts. For one thing there would be no script. "I want you to say you are going to the center for family planning. Put it in your own words." There would be nothing to learn and nothing to rehearse and it would go much faster. Next time, she would capture the sunlight of Haiti for her purposes, imaginatively getting around the lack of electricity. Stine suggested a mirror for shooting scenes inside houses. Impossible! Each day's jeep ride would shatter it to smithereens ... a little expensive. She improvised, using large five-by-three foot pieces of cardboard covered with aluminum foil and held, bent slightly, by one of the many children who crowded around to watch each day's shooting. It was better than a spotlight, created no harsh shadows, and cheaper. "Health Is Wealth," would be a technically improved production, presenting fewer concepts and, consequently, better understood. The premiere of "Modern Time Is Different from the Old Time" was a major event. Invitations were sent to the leading personages of Croix-des-Bouquets, the cast, their families, the extras. A very, very high protocol situation; the men wore ties; everyone, proper and tense. The chief of section was there; the mayor was there; the magistrate was there . . . everybody was there, but the army. The president's ranch was nearby and he was there; nobody was supposed to gather together in a large group in his vicinity for security reasons. With eighty people trying to gather for the premiere there was great confusion.

Eventually, there was great applause. One critic from the department of tourism, however, found the film "too primitive and simplistic, very disappointing, too low-level intellectually." Madame Hollant did not bother to reply: "What's the point of convincing that man from the Department of Tourism about an educational film for the rural area!"

The projections began in thirty villages, twice weekly from that July through December, at sites chosen carefully within the "triangle" area, exposed to vaccination and community medicine, accessible by road, with fairly good population concentrations. Rivière would push the accelerator of his "jet" and Monsieur Alies into the vicinity and they would drive around like crazy, bumping over ditches and ruts, bouncing and leaping into the air, Alies's insides juggling as well as the microphone to the sound system overhead as he urged residents of the village they were encircling to "Come to the cinema . . . a wonderful cinema . . . an interesting cinema . . . in color . . . with young girls and children . . . little houses . . . FREE!" The children would run and laugh and chase the jeep, peripheral residents coming out for a closer look at the commotion; the recorded music would play on and another announcement began again, "Come to the cinema . . ."

They would come, assisted by the community agent in the area, some volunteer assistants, all washed and spruced up for the occasion. Rivière worked quickly in the gathering dusk to get the portable electric generator going, and set up the screen and projector, in the middle of nowhere in the darkening Haitian night. Monsieur Alies explained what they were about to see, why, and where it had come from. The people listened, crowding closer and closer, making Rivière extremely nervous as he tried to protect the equipment—and his precious jeep—from the crunch of the curious. He was losing control, getting very upset, cursing, a little panicky. He would push the children back, his eyes wide and raging like a madman, the children almost falling over backwards with his shoving. All around were people of all ages in this clearing outside this village, a few huts off in the distance, a vagrant leaning against a tree, exhausted, his straw hat in shambles, and shoeless. Sometimes there would be as many as 1,000 spectators crushing in on the focal point, a standard-size film screen, the crowd barely visible in the blackness, the children pushing forward to see, any tree becoming a balcony seat, some heads inevitably silhouetted on the screen.

"It is your head!" Monsieur Alies would scream, pointing to the offender who did not understand he could not stand between the screen and the projector. "You can't stand there! Don't stand there!" Alies would rage.

It was always a big hit, but was it understood?

Little questionnaires were gathered after each screening, and soon it became obvious that the people were not getting all the messages. Even more explanation preceded the film; the film was projected a second time to reinforce the concepts. "She had another baby!" the people remarked incredulously. "Two babies so close together, and she was doing planning!" It became obvious the people had to be informed that it was a second screening.

Six months after the projections began, a study was conducted in twelve of the thirty localities with an open-ended nineteen-point questionnaire, again developed by Madame Hollant, reaching 312 people. Ninety-nine percent had seen at least one screening of the film; three of the four basic concepts the film had been designed to present had been understood by upwards of 73 percent of those questioned. The weak message? Preparation for childbirth. Only 24 percent got that one. On balance the data was very positive. The most vividly recalled image? Family planning, according to seven out of ten respondents. Over 12,000 people saw the film the first year alone; during the three "triangle" years it would be screened throughout the Cul-de-Sac Plain and in certain parts of Port-au-Prince, to the point of virtual saturation.

There is roving in Haiti. It gets pretty spectacular in the Haitian countryside during the Catholic season of Lenten penitence with wandering societies of costumed dancers, free and frenzied, merry-eyed and sweating bodies, making their way through the cane fields and countryside, after Carnival and before Christ's resurrection on Easter Sunday. The "RaRa" bands in particular generally feature the four-foot-long base-vaccine flutes, a veritable limb of bamboo, to keep the rhythm, smacking with its one-note cacophony, accompanied by baka drums and tymbals, flags, papier-maché figures, candelabra, and maybe an effigy of Judas, who was responsible for it all, dragging along in the dust.

Crow was in town on an evaluation visit, dining with the Bordeses at the gingerbready Grand Hotel Oloffson, just sitting there, sipping and enjoying the folk charm of the stage show, when Bordes began talking about Haitian traditions. He explained about the local dancers and musicians, the part they played in village life, the messages and stories they carried and spread as they wandered like medieval minstrels from place to place, earning their keep.

"The thought came to me and, perhaps, to Ary at the same time," Crow recalls—a folk troop with straw hats and colorful costumes, drums and instruments, lyrics with an educational intent and little skits enacting situations with a health message for the "triangle."

Enter Andre Dartiguenave, a tall, skinny man with a receding hairline and a scarecrow limberness about him, a remarkable hang-loose quality for a man in his sixties. He says song and dance have kept him young, and he's been at it since his school days. As he modestly explains, "From childhood I demonstrated a lot of talent for theater, song, preparation of speeches." Since 1932 Dartiguenave had been on the rural-education team of the Department of Agriculture, composing over one hundred skits for the education of schoolchildren, playing the harmonica, training teachers, holding a variety of positions around the country, and gathering a number of giant certificates with very impressive official-looking seals in the United States, where he spent some time taking little courses on writing for children and the development of educational materials at several universities and U.S. government agencies.

He is a real character and can burst into little songs at a moment's notice, lilting, gentle ditties, his eyes playful like a child enjoying his own birthday party; an iota of time later, his most expressive face, preoccupied, sincerely concerned about condoms. He has a condom story par excellence, biographical, alas, which dates from a certain traumatic Thursday, June 21—"I am not an archangel," as he says. He is a father. Most certainly Dartiguenave is most interested in everyone's "bf" (boyfriend) and "gf" (girlfriend) situation. He was a vigorous sixty-two-year-old man, perfect for the part of the leader of the folk troop charged with training seven young people in song and dance and drama on health. He would keep their performance level high with twice-weekly rehearsals; he would get into his part.

Announcements were made at the Croix-des-Bouquets clinic for likely candidates. Forty-one responded and were interviewed down to fifteen finalists. They sang. They danced. They spoke. They performed for four days of talent-testing on the porch of Dr. Narcisse's house, Madame Hollant, Narcisse, two nurses and a local schoolteacher having a marvelous time deciding who the final seven would be. They had to be local and rural so they could relate to the people; so they would be, with most coming from little villages outside of Croix-des-Bouquets. None had any formal musical training; they were just plain good. All were young and free, so they could perform evenings and weekends without any family constraints.

Dartiguenave had his assignment—develop a series of songs and skits on the subjects of maternal-child health and family planning. He selected from the rich folk tradition of Haiti he knew and loved, music forgotten by the younger generation in some cases, but which he well remembered and wanted to revive and restore to proper appreciation: the music of the great Haitian composer and political commentator Candio; the pianist Lamothe, who won the first Carnival competition for his work. Their music would get new lyrics like "Men Women O/Listen to the good news/Make a decision to do planning/Yes, yes do planning/ If you don't O/Child after child/It is a lot of problems/You better do planning."

While Dartiguenave was creating, the troop was learning about the objectives of the program, other educational methods, about sanitation and preventive medicine, family planning, breastfeeding, and immunization—six weeks of training by Narcisse and Madame Monpoint. Not only were they to entertain and educate the people, they must be able to answer their questions immediately on the scene, as well as twice weekly assist at the clinic.

Dartiguenave directed them for two months in preparation for their debut. "You don't have to be a great actor," he would say to the seven, "but you must PENETRATE into the subject . . . you must CAPTURE THE SPIRIT of the people." He would demonstrate the way to reach the public. A sad scene. A mother with six children and more pregnancies ahead in the future. His head would go down to one side, like a Picasso blue-period painting, his face a mask of tragedy, his voice changing pitch and tone, feminine now and morose, complaining, utterly believable. He cried out, "My God! What am I to do! I can no longer have children regularly like this!" The troop learned the method. By the time rehearsals were over, even the timid maniboula player had been dragged out of his shell.

Out in a cane field somewhere the jeep jumped around announcing their arrival with a "good evening" and the glad news to the sad rows of cane-cutter housing, like concrete-block motels, courtesy of the Haitian-American Sugar Company. Surrounded by nothing but the sugar railroad, as inevitable as original sin, were some pigs and goats feeding on the sparse blades of grass here and there in the bare dirt. The front yard of the luxury house of the HASCO manager, shaded by two mango trees, would be the "stage."

Slowly, the scrubbing stopped at the water pump and the people, in their best dresses and clean shirts, brought their chairs for comfort as the pink light began to hit the sky and the mountains took on the definite medium blue of Haitian evening. Even the migrant workers, some of Haiti's most desperate people, seemed to perk up a bit at the prospect of the performance ahead.

Dartiguenave put on his wide-brimmed straw hat in preparation, making his old face topping his polelike body look silly. Rivière had the electric generator going and a solitary lightbulb glowed in the evening, flung over a limb of one of the mango trees. Dartiguenave kicked away some animal excrement from the "stage." The performers took their places in their most bright red and patterned costumes, almost like Mexican Mariachis players, scarved and straw-hatted. Their leader took the mike.

"Good evening," he said to the audience. They replied gently in turn, the charm of Haiti. "We are going to do theater for you," he continued, "but it is not ordinary theater. It is not comedy to make you laugh. But it is a special theater which we call education—for your information. So you can put into practice different health advice and have a family in good health ... so pay close attention so you can understand what is being said."

Good point. There was a lot going on in the audience which crowded about the group, a little too close, almost overwhelming. Some of the tables and chairs brought for the occasion would be in pieces by the performance's end as the people climbed over one another to see— more than to hear. The music began, and quickly there was a lot of clapping and swinging to the songs, swaying of the hips to the music; the chief of section rolled with the rhythm, the rifle in his lap bouncing about dangerously in time with the drum beat; the children's heads bobbed up and down, tops thrusting forward from necks.

The troop enacted the importance of mother's milk and breastfeeding with the nurse in the skit called "Madame Monpoint," after the very one. More singing about breastfeeding: "I am happy my dream is coming true/I am going to have a baby/I will name the baby John/If it is a...." The troop's actress sang in her imaginary house, sewing a layette for her baby, the pillow of her "pregnancy" starting to slip a little under her dress as she threaded her fantasy needle and continued, "I will make a nice dress for the baby...." In the audience this one pushed that one; a child screamed because he was being squeezed; one woman pushed the woman who was squeezing her child; the young girls cursed the boys who had pinched their rears....

Dartiguenave joined in the next song, about immunization, dancing about waving a white handkerchief in the air, shaking hands with the crowd, getting roars of approval and laughter as he pulled one woman onto the "stage." More loud applause as he danced smoothly with her, she in turn following his direction impeccably. The troop carried on about the necessity for the complete series of three shots. Dartiguenave wiped his brow dramatically and kissed his partner's hand with a flourish, eliciting more roars of approval from the crowd. She went back to her spot, serious-faced, with arms-folded in defense of it all.

Another skit: Nurse: "I want to congratulate you on your husband's interest in your delivery."

Rora: "Ha! Thank you miss, he is a responsible man."

Nurse: "Now. Do you have all your vaccinations? Have you prepared the baby's clothes, the clean towel...."

The community agent moved among the crowd giving out coupons for family planning, for immunization....The children started to sing the group's recurring theme song. "Let us ... let us put ourselves together/Let us ... let us children and adults/Let us work for our community to be in good health/If we do we will be true citizens."

"Crick!" shouted out Dartiguenave.

"Crack!" responded the crowd, totally delighted at what was coming— a riddle!

"On the outside my body is rough; on the inside, sweet as sugar." He waited.

A pause, then a scream. "Pineapple!" yelled two members of the audience simultaneously, getting huge applause. The point? Proper nutrition. Explained. The next answer was eggs and nobody got it. But all eyes were aflame with pleasure and humor. More music ... more mothers dancing with their babies in arms ...

Dr. Narcissse now took "the stage," explaining in vivacious Creole about the clinic's purpose, its hours, about prenatal care, nutrition, vaccination, antitetanus treatment. "Do planning so you have the babies you want and time between babies and fewer troubles. Every three or four years is good enough," he continued, warming up and pointing out the community agent in the crowd, who acknowledged the introduction with a wave of his family planning coupon book. Narcisse was at his best now, full of energy and enthusiasm, good humor and good will. His explanation about condoms got a loud clap of approval from a man under one of the mango trees in the cleanest bluejeans. "Every man should have condoms," Narcisse stated firmly, getting loud laughter and applause, louder and louder applause, as he plunged into the merits of family planning. "Planning is like a soccer game," he concluded on a note of inspiration. "You can play the game, without scoring the goal!" Roars of laughter.

Now for the film, "Health Is Wealth", screened under the mango trees with all the mosquitoes in the neighborhood buzzing around the desk lamp set over the projector. Finally, that happy ending of Bernadette getting her pills. Just in time. The clouds that had visibly been gathering over the mountains, threatening, began to drip. Perfect timing. The people left, amused and informed.

[PART V]

14

THE HARVEST

"I felt we were the ones who should be determining the policies and in time I came to talk frankly with them [international organizations]. I had reached the time when I talked frankly with people—I agree with you or I am sorry, I disagree with you because.... You know we play games in every part of our lives and in public life you play games every day, and either you decide whether you want to be the winner, the loser, or have a draw.

"In the beginning when you start working with international organizations you have to learn about them and you have to play yourself down in order to learn. Until the time comes when you know them and you have your own base, then you can play to a draw. Then after a certain time you can try to play to win. Now I have reached a period in my life where I discuss with people and I tell them usually what I think....

"Now I don't think I can have much difficulty with internationals. ... I will not be angry with them and we will always keep good relationships because these are not personal questions, and if we disagree, we can disagree as gentlemen. We will stay friends and we will talk again. When we disagree, I will try usually to arrive at a consensus because I think it is very rare to have someone totally right or totally wrong. Usually people are partially right or partially wrong. And when you are in this field you must learn to negotiate also. I have read everything I could find on the art of negotiating. I remember reading something very useful once—that a good negotiation is one where everybody leaves feeling that he has won."

"Programs have to be adjusted to the situation in order to be continued and resist efforts to stop them. In a society in which things are highly personalized like in Haiti, a person who works here should know about that. And if he wants his program to be useful, should pay attention to that, to do his best to depersonalize it and concentrate on the principles and the ideas and not the person.... Otherwise the program has the full weight of the good and the bad side of the person who sticks to it and does not pull out when he should in order to have permanence of the program. That's the way I look at it and I do my best to decrease personalization. You have to find the proper moment to step out and have the program continue, always preparing for that transition, sharing knowledge and decision-making, opening things up for the time of replacement. I want to prepare others to head the division so I can step out any time without any trouble to the division because it would be very hard for me not to head the division and see it fall. It would be a great joy to step out and see it moving along, even getting better, that I had contributed to the division from that year to that year and now I look and see it flourishing and people continuing the work....

"My goal was reached at Croix-des-Bouquets so I stepped out. I wanted it to become a center for the training of medical students and that's happened and my job is finished and I should try to do something else. Now we have a national program and we have finished with the urban phase and now we are moving into the rural phase which will reach its momentum in the next two or three years. Then I should try to do something else ... to try and help another aspect of health in Haiti that is weak ... for instance, the drug issue ... strengthening of the administration of the health department in general ... the issue of use of the traditional folk network.... We have to integrate maternal-child health and family planning into the health department, and when it is done successfully, then I think it would be time for me to move on...." —Ary Bordes

In early 1977 staff from both the center and the division of family hygiene began the first of many trips to come taking them all over Haiti for the next few years as maternal-child health and family planning truly became "national." Both urban and rural methodologies were at last in the can ready for screening; cuts made—what did not work dropped; the highlights remembered—for premiere in the vast rural expanse of Haiti's mountainous countryside. Here lived four million people, their ills "cured" largely by a traditional folk system; only an estimated 20 to 30 percent with access to modern medical care.

The first trip in January was to Cap Haitien on the extreme northern coast; in February, to Cayes, on the extreme southern coast, and on it would continue through all the in-betweens of Haiti that year, and the next, and the next . . . national coverage, total extension, the original objective being realized.

It was an exciting trip, that first time out to Cap Haitien, almost symbolic to begin at the shrine of Haitian independence and evidence of this country's most remarkable revolution, history's only successful slave revolt after twelve years of fighting, overcoming the most powerful nations of the day. This had been a long struggle, too, and the opposition as formidable, in its way—scraping at home and hustling abroad for finances; the sheer adversity of the physical environment; the slow and laborious construction of an infrastructure to support the program; the all-pervasive human factor in all its fear and grumbling, resistant to innovation, distressed by more work to be done, demanding more salary. It was twelve years too since the center had started its work at the general hospital in a building off to the side of the main courtyard surrounded by hospital business-as-usual.

Despite the passing of the years, the program was still new, strange, and apart as well, thus the reason for the trip: to conduct an intensive day-long seminar for all medical personnel—physicians on through sanitary agents—on how to integrate maternal-child health and family planning into health delivery in northern Haiti; followed by an intensive two-day seminar to brief teachers in all of Haiti's northern schools about teaching health, human reproduction, population, and eventually, family planning, at the higher grade levels. In short, take the program and the materials into the provinces. There was an aura of adventure about the group, a holiday feeling. They were starting something, a new phase, which they had all been working toward for years.

It had been an enormous investment of time, energy, money, labor, and laryngitis to get here.

While Bordes had plunged into his job as chief of the new division of family hygiene back in December of 1971, reporting, "the work to be done . . . is infinite"—it was a little difficult to accomplish since the division existed on paper only. It had been the usual problem, a little bit of reliving of those days as director of school health services—no organization, office, staff, material, transportation, budget. Bordes waited for fourteen months; then, threatened to resign. "It is absolutely impossible to continue to direct a division that is legally constituted, but deprived of . . . every means needed to work."

He was heard. On April 7, 1973, the new offices of the division were formally inaugurated, found in a former rehabilitation center, moved out to the general hospital to make way for maternal-child health and family planning on the move. The inauguration was a white-suit occasion for Bordes with secretaries and subsecretaries of state everywhere, army officers, internationals, guests galore, and the U.S. Agency for International Development representatives roaming all over Port-au-Prince searching for Haut de Turgeau at the corner of Avenue Jean Claude Duvalier and Behanzin. They would send a letter of apology for their absence.

In his address Bordes outlined his three-phase plan, already begun with all existing public and private family-planning activities now coordinated through the division under defined conditions. Five clinics had reopened by that time—a little over a year since the shut-down communiqué. Bordes wanted, first, an urban family-planning project; then, its absorption by the division as part of a national family-planning program; next, expansion into the capital and surroundings and later to all the cities of the country; and finally, into the vast rural area, the greatest challenge.

This was the scientist speaking—a very large part of Ary Bordes, but there is much more to him and he exposed more, reaching deep within to speak some true feelings of what this moment meant to him, this inauguration ceremony of some office space devoted to maternal-child health and family planning. It had been twenty years since a just-returned Haitian physician with a master's degree in public health medicine had fired off those first furious letters, demanding action on these very issues from the ministry of health. There was a serenity now from many, many recognitions, a quiet radicalism that was really unadulterated hope.

"And we have the good hope," he told the audience, "that this will result in a program designed for our standards, responding to the needs of our people. Year after year, our women and mothers will enjoy better health, our children will be sound and blossom into robust and vigorous adults.... And one day, as we knew in our past glory, we will liberate ourselves, not this time from the irons of slavery, but from the intolerable pillory of underdevelopment, of suffering and of sickness." He so concluded his inauguration speech.

That was the plan and the philosophy to be implemented. It would never change. Bordes constantly insisted that everything done contribute to building this structure; the foundations, sound, consistent, relevant, planned and perpetuable, he would repeat over and over and over while he maintained a tight check rein. Anything that smacked of the playful, testful, experimental, the let-me-go-home-now-and-write-my-paper had little chance under Ary Bordes's leadership. A nationally-controlled family planning program within a strong health department was his priority at every step along the way.

It began to be articulated a matter of days after the creation of the division and his appointment as chief during discussions with the Pan

American Health Organization, in full swing at the center, since the division would not get its offices for many months to come. The setting was strategic because the battles would be territorial in nature. On the surface it seemed that the issue was simply how best to turn over activities at the general hospital, continue and extend them throughout the capital, and ultimately, the country—but a lot more was happening. It was to be another uphill fight in a long series of mountains. The base camp was supportive and health minister Theard would come through in the crunch . . . and the internationals know how to squeeze.

"You see," explains Wishik, "outside money was so important that any Haitian who fell out with the U.N. or PAHO, he would be the one to get axed, not the outsider." The United Nations Development Program Officer actually had the status of ambassador in Port-au-Prince, and any Haitian "could have been through if he developed any opposition with the U.N. representative. He would be just let go."

It was delicate, requiring a balancing act worthy of the circus with the resiliency of Tinkerbell, just in case. It was like a circus at times with all the simultaneous acts, three rings, a few clowns, and a ringmaster trying to direct attention appropriately.

Sue Klein observed some of the comings and goings of consultants at the time and developed some outspoken opinions. "This young shit coming in and from the day he arrived, he was telling people what to do . . . not exactly appropriate," she sums up her impression. "I remember being at a meeting and thinking, 'Boy, this guy is coming on pretty strong for someone who hasn't been around very much . . . without knowing the territory.' He seemed bright, but he was just coming on too strong! From my recollections, there were some very intense feelings . . ." she laughs. But it wasn't very funny at the time. A lot was at stake.

Bordes's position in the discussions was to work with compromise, to make progress toward the greatest need—money—while going as far as he could in the direction he believed best for a Haitian national program, yielding when it was the only way to continue the negotiation and get financial assistance. It was not an easy spot to be in, especially for a nationalist like Ary Bordes, who has angrily stood up in an audience at the Haitian-American Institute and told Selden Rodman, an American who has done the most to bring recognition to Haitian painting—". . . there was painting in Haiti before you came, you know!" No, it was not easy . . . all around.

Bordes remembers: "From the beginning of the discussion I started to fight against the attitude of the consultants who would not keep their proper place and give the proper place to the local technicians." In short, executive power versus advisory status, who had what and how much. Bordes continues: "I felt it was a government program and should be directed by the government and a Haitian, with the PAHO person as a consultant. I took this position right at the beginning of the discussions, but it was not easily accepted—not at all. . . ." It would be years before Ary Bordes was in a strong enough position to march down the hall of the division and tear the "Director" sign from the PAHO consultant's door and inform him in no uncertain terms that he was "the advisor." It was a question of proper timing in the "circus" of international assistance where a lot of conflicts are NEVER resolved. The next PAHO consultant got the message immediately, "I feel sorry for you because of your predecessor," Bordes said at their introduction.

It would always be a struggle, with Bordes maneuvering constantly to keep the Haitian government in control, from the signing of the agreement with the United Nations Population Fund Activities on April 13, 1972—for $194,577 the first year; $177,846 the second; and $373,310 the third. Haiti Project 4900, ratified by PAHO in May of that year, was to develop an institutional mechanism for a national maternal-child health and family planning program at two maternity centers in the capital and to study the acceptance of services by the people and the staff. The pilot phase included not only services, but training programs, education for the community, a corps of community agents, as well as the obvious administrative structure and materials. Services were to continue at the general hospital and expand to the Maternity Chancerelles and Isaie Jeanty—and be directed by a Haitian, Dr. Evariste Midy, trained in public-health medicine in Venezuela and assistant chief of the division of family hygiene. It was to be an experimental project, paving the way for the national program and based on the model developed by Bordes at the general hospital, dating back to 1965. The center had been recognized for its public utility by presidential decree, April 7, 1972, the week before the U.N. grant was announced.

Haiti Project 4900 was the finale of all the documents dating back to Sam Wishik's initial report in 1968, followed by years of talks, revisions, redrafts, pauses . . . why so l-o-n-g??????????

With his many years of experience as an international public health specialist, Wishik is in a good position to comment: "PAHO came in and dilly-dallied . . . just plain United Nations bureaucracy," he sums up simply. "The United Nations Fund for Population Activities has a slow, laborious procedure. They do not take over direct operations, but they select another part of the United Nations family of agencies to be the executing agency, and PAHO became the executing agency for the Haiti grant. So you have UNFPA, PAHO, the Government of Haiti, usually represented by Ary Bordes, in the discussions and a half dozen other parties all trying to cross the t's and get it done. Then, they dragged it out so they exhausted the funds for that fiscal year and so they would start again the next fiscal year. And it goes on and on and on. . . .

"An official is sitting in a certain position and he has to be important!" he continues. "And so he finds details and then the next time somebody else comes in and he finds new details, and so it goes on and on and on. . . ."

It is also true, as the saying goes, "Nature abhors a vacuum." The Haitian initiative in the beginning had been weak—not enough trained people in public health to hold up the Haitian banners of strong policy positions. So PAHO was filling in some of the emptiness, however badly; speed and efficiency are never the forte of large institutions, particularly when based thousands of miles away. Then, PAHO became acclimated to its role of determining and implementing Haitian programs—inappropriate and a habit difficult and painful to break—for everybody. Part of the Haitian vacuum clearly was its own bureaucratic reluctance to act, described well by Dr. Laraque, compounded by the pattern of Haitian politics of frequent ministerial changes to maintain a power balance. Since the founding of the Haitian health department in 1945, there had been thirty-one ministers of health, their average tenure, a year; one exception lasted five years—generating a great deal of speculation as to why. Political continuity rests in the presidency and technical continuity with the technicians of Haiti, and this makes things more difficult at times. But there had been gradual movement forward on the Haitian side during those years, helped along by the growing public recognition of the need for family planning, easing the bureaucrats out from under their security blankets, electric, and turned up to ten.

In April 1974, an interdisciplinary team of UNFPA-PAHO-World Health Organization officials from Washington, Mexico, and Haiti, as well as Haitian government officials, submitted a 120-page evaluation of Haiti Project 4900. Their conclusions were good. "Most of the objectives established for the pilot phase of the project have been achieved," the report concluded; successful enough to merit a five-year extension, beginning January 1975, with the objective of providing maternal-child health and family planning to 20 percent of the total Haitian population—the national program Ary Bordes always dreamed about.

As always the movement forward had been accomplished by a collaboration of the Haitian government, private foundations, and international assisting organizations. About $700,000 had been invested by the Government of Haiti, the United Nations Population Fund Activities, and the Pan American Health Organization in the first two years alone of the planning phase and the pilot study in the capital. In addition, the U.S. Agency for International Development had kicked in nearly $175,000, mostly for building and clinic maintenance in the "triangle" project, with the U.S. Pathfinder Fund adding another $110,000-plus for drugs and equipment.

As expressly stated in the two-year evaluation of the pilot phase of the national program, the "triangle" project "has been translated into the objectives and target for the expansion of the maternal-child health-family planning activities in other parts of the country . . . and will continue to provide a learning experience for health workers. . . ." The "triangle" had established what was possible: one health center with comprehensive services could cover a population of 25,000, including, at the existing birthrates, 1,000 pregnant women and 5,000 preschool children. So the national program coverage targets were 75 percent for prenatal care; 50 percent for postpartum/postnatal care; 80 percent for preschool children; 80 percent for immunization; 20 percent of the women at risk for family planning.

The first year of the national program nearly 18,500 women received prenatal care; over 37,000 consultations were given; a great deal of progress was made in occupancy of delivery beds, with 25,000 hospital births recorded; nearly 160,000 pediatric consultations; over 165,000 inoculations immunizing children against a variety of communicable diseases. The results in family planning were "excellent"—95 percent of objective with nearly 16,000 new users and almost 55,000 visits for family planning information and service. By the end of 1975, twenty-four health facilities in cities around the country had integrated maternal-child health and family planning into their services, all but four, government institutions.

The following year, 1976, seemed to be the time for consolidation, a qualitative rather than quantitative emphasis, and revving up for the plunge into the second phase of the national program—rural extension. By this point maternal-child health and family planning had been integrated into all of Haiti's eleven health districts with the necessary logistical supports as much as possible. There were nearly 500 people staffing the program, and results were up despite the attention to consolidation, including nearly 80,000 family-planning consultations, with almost 36,500 new users—more men than women—21,000-plus men and 15,000-plus women. It was a continuation of that extraordinary male breakthrough in the "triangle."

In addition, by the second year, 139 community agents had been trained by Norine Jewell and Dr. Eustache and others and had made nearly a quarter of a million home visits, the coupons flying for prenatal, pediatric care, family planning. Plus, 486 midwives had been certified in cities throughout the country, using the "triangle" methods developed by Madame Monpoint and others, another monumental achievement. The child health course now was available in every major city, a cooperative effort between the Red Cross and the health department. The health education section of the division of family hygiene had been busy with seminars for doctors about to take their rural residencies; the same for nurses; and many others, even drivers of public vehicles in the metropolitan area.

The radio-broadcast school "Health Class" was overflowing with listeners, indexed in response to the contest—over 25,000 participants from 191 different localities, compared with the forty-four respondents when the contest began. Beaming into virtually every nook and cranny of the country, "Radio Doctor" continued to be a huge success. When an administrator had a problem—women not coming for services, discontinuing the pill, whatever, Madame Souvenir was invited to visit and set things straight by sound-truck communication. The Jacmel administrator asked her to come for three days because the women no longer seemed to be seeking services—and he sent her home after two . . . too many women to accommodate.

The total program was go, the urban phase well on its way by 1976. Oh, there were gaps and weaknesses, but basically the major job had begun and the finishing touches would come with time. Extension had been achieved, rather than a Rolls-Royce style of medicine in a few locations available to very limited numbers of people. Now it was a question of refinement and the resources to do the job. Next, rural extension, the second and final phase, planned from July 1976, to June 30, 1979, when the United Nations grant was to expire and the Haitian government to take over responsibility for absorption and continuity—another major undertaking further down the pike, and something Ary Bordes already was planning for.

In short, Ary Bordes had succeeded in creating a model of maternal-child health and family planning; most importantly, he had institutionalized it into the Haitian government, Haitian urban life, and now was about to do the same for Haitian rural life. His pioneering work at the general hospital, his key position as chief of the division of family hygiene, his evolution of the "triangle" methodology, his leadership during all negotiations and ensuing developments had achieved the goal. For his part Bordes always pointed to a carefully built, competent, highly spirited staff at both the center and the division of family hygiene. And it had been a team effort, that was sure—but there had been a team leader. "He kept family planning on the map in Haiti," Wishik says flatly. "Without him family planning would either have just disappeared or just limped along. There would have been nobody to turn to. . . ."

"Nobody except Dr. Bordes with his tenacity could have done this," agrees researcher Dr. Laraque. "His is a very, very big contribution. For myself, there were so many obstacles I retreated to my private practice. ... The people who say they will help but never do, the self-interest, the money, it is all so discouraging. Dr. Bordes did what I knew should be done, needed to be done, but could not stand doing."

Even the new director of the Croix-des-Bouquets clinic, Dr. Jean Raymond Derosena, a young puppy of a public health physician reluctant to give credit where credit is due, acknowledges, "His contribution is enormous." Duvalierist Dr. Fourcand comments categorically, "If it were not for Dr. Bordes, family planning would have died in Haiti." He was in a position to know. And on the accolades go from all quarters, at home and abroad, to Bordes's utter embarrassment.

Dr. Berggren sums it all up well: "Just take the position of a Haitian mother living in a village within a reasonable walking distance of any of the health centers which now exist. Just compare her situation now since the division of family hygiene has been active under Dr. Bordes and her situation before that time. This mother now can bring her child to the clinic and have free immunizations. She can come for family planning education at any time. She has free prenatal care. There are community agents—people she knows and most often respects—who will come to her door to see how she is and encourage her to seek health care. If she's in an area where the local staff is able to go out with mobile-clinic equipment which Dr. Bordes has brought to the division, she won't have to walk all the way to the clinic to get her child's second or third immunization. Because she's getting prenatal care and immunization she need never lose another baby again to umbilical tetanus or whooping cough or any of these other diseases that most likely have killed her children in the past. If she doesn't want to deliver her baby in the dispensary there's a trained midwife in her area who will come to her with a box that contains sterilized packages to cut the umbilical cord of her baby in as clean a way as possible. The midwife is also trained to know what the dangers are of her delivering at home, and if she begins to bleed or has signs of convulsions. . . . Because she's made friends with the doctor or nurse at the clinic she might be willing when she is ill or needs medical help for different reasons to come to someone who is qualified to help her. She knows about family planning because someone has come to her door and told her about it, and if she's an acceptor, somebody will even come to her door and deliver it. In the past immunization has been inconsistently available . . . babies have needlessly died of dehydration. . . . Now, because of this program, many of these things are available to this mother.

"And I think this is a TREMENDOUS contribution in this country that there are centers that offer these services to the mothers in the most desperate need. This is a TREMENDOUS step forward, and Dr. Bordes deserves a great deal of credit."

Thus, the trip to Cap Haitien, passing the word and work on to medical and school personnel in Haiti's north, rural extension from the community level, reaching two million Haitians by the expiration of the United Nations grant. The rural phase was to proceed, first, by expanding the area of influence of each urban clinic with mobile teams going out to four different points, establishing "satellite clinics" serving 4,000 people. Second, certain rural points were to be picked out for special rural dispensaries offering family planning and visited once a month by a medical team from the district headquarters, forty-five of them by 1979, reaching 450,000 people. Third, the division planned to work with a large development organization in the Artibonite Valley, using specially trained agents chosen from each community. The coverage potential was enormous, half a million people living in Haiti's midriff. Fourth, each clinic had a quota of training fifty midwives each year, 1,000 midwives a year who would reach into the small huts of rural Haiti with maternal-child health and family planning information— 4,000 people. Second, certain rural points were to be picked out for 11,000 midwives in the country.

It was a beautiful trip north to Cap Haitien, full of the unique quality of fact and feeling that is so hauntingly Haitian, an intensity of experience, a richness of stimulus that makes this country so full of life. The center and division jeeps drove past the Telestar antenna in the middle of a cane field, sulfur baths for rheumatics, portals of old colonial plantation gates, a market lady burdened with a basket of breadfruit on her head with two big patches on the front of her dress where the material had been worn through by her bouncing breasts as she high-stepped along. They barely swerved past tap taps, tatooed with art and slogans. Bordes liked the one called, "All Is Only Vanity"—that's true, he laughed. It was his first trip to Cap Haitien in two-and-a-half years and he was enjoying it.

At St. Marc the jeeps turned inland over the arid, prickly growth of the lowlands of the Black Mountains, a sad-looking land with lots of cactus plants redeemed by an occasional tall yellow pompom jutting out incongruously like a foolish flower caught by mistake in a candelabra. "See the chocolate trees," he said, keeping up his running commentary. "The people of the North sing their Creole." "Limbe is known for its very sweet sugarcane." "What is St. Marc known for . . . what is Gonaïves known for?" he wondered aloud, getting no answer, because if he did not know, nobody else did, either. He later expressed the desire to spend a week in each of these provincial towns, hardly pulsing

THE HARVEST

with action. He wanted to know his country better and shook his head in silent disbelief when Madame Hollant fessed up never to having made the pony ride to Henri Christophe's citadel.

But the patchwork ricefields of the Artibonite Valley, their obvious fertility, inspired him most. Sunlight seared every blade, creating squares of neon chartreuse. Mixed in were the multicolored bandanas of bent-over peasant women and aristocratic, slender-necked white herron, and an occasional cow. "The rice season should be good this year," he started out with satisfaction, continuing on to the prospect for self-sufficiency, even export. They crossed the Artibonite River toward Gonaives, famous for historic monuments to General Dessalines. Gradually came the climb over the final bump of mountains before the coastal plain leading to the Atlantic northern coast of the country. It was turning dusky now, the air cool with an occasional hawk overhead, appropriately called "bad finish." Once a flock of heron broke through the mountain mist like a haiku come true. The Cahos Mountains looked like an expanse of undulating green velour speckled with lollipop mango trees and thatched huts.

"Flags," Bordes said, his head stuck out the jeep window. There they were by an obscure military outpost, three weary, tattered, faded flags, occasionally jerked by the breeze like a disturbed scarecrow. He was delighted. Past four historic cannons. More excitement. A change of mood. The jeep edged its way through a funeral procession in the small mountain town of Chatard, surrounded by Haitian screams of grief and rage at death, the coffin borne by uniformed soccer players.

Every so often Bordes would motion Ariste, the silent driver, to a stop and pull out a little notebook. It would be perfectly still with the engines cut. In the pause would pass the panorama of Haitian rural life, but Bordes's mind was elsewhere. He had been thinking about a pregnant woman puffing up one of those terraced hillsides off in the distance, so steep it looked like a struggle up a ladder. "That pregnant woman cannot find medical help," he mumbled, making notes, "unless medical care comes to her. She would have to walk all the way back to Plaisance or Ennery for antitetanus injections . . . she'll never do it. We need a combination of small medical outposts and mobile clinics," he summed up, slapping his notebook shut, having recorded a likely mobile-clinic site. He was thinking about rural outreach . . . almost an obsession. Madame Hollant leaned forward politely to listen to Bordes's continuing commentary, then leaned back to stare, glazed in silent saturation. Later at the hotel, she would collapse full-bodied into her hotel-room bed, exclaiming—"He sustained his interest FOR THE ENTIRE TRIP!"

He would be much the same at the Cap Haitien meeting where seventeen doctors and nurses gathered around a large conference table, arguing and interrupting—the doctors, that is. The nurses sat there very silent as always in the presence of physicians. Bordes constantly reached for a piece of chalk, drawing arrows on the blackboard and explaining what extension meant—reaching people. Going to THEM! Dr. Mark Angrand, the district health administrator with a master's degree in public health from the University of California at Berkeley, would be in there pitching, too. A big man by Haitian standards, with short salt-and-pepper hair, his face embossed with smile wrinkles, he had prepared the list of three mobile clinics and four rural points for the division chief's visit.

It was an interesting meeting and typical of what would be happening all over the country. There had to be persuasion. Many protested the idea of using the four existing dispensaries, unstaffed by doctors, but according to the plan, to have qualified auxiliaries just like Fond Parisien. Presentation of the three possible mobile clinic sites aroused another outburst. "The wrong places!" "How are the people going to know about them!?" Fear . . . reservations . . . almost a can't-do attitude. Bordes tried to soothe the frayed sensibilities at the thought of all those paraprofessionals carrying out health delivery. He spoke of the need to inform people of the facts of nutrition, to conduct simple but vital procedures such as vaccination, to assist pregnant women. . . . "We are not always going to have the maximum of materials. We know very well," he said flatly. "There will be a lack of things, but we can still offer help."

"No, it will never work," said one doctor vehemently, insisting that at least all the care be done at the dispensaries. "Too little organization . . . people all over . . . some healthy . . . some sick . . . some waiting for something . . . some just wanting to watch . . . it will never work!" He was upset. But it had worked in the "triangle," and Bordes had that argument ready.

The midwife training aroused the greatest flak, virtually all the doctors talking together; the district administrator trying hard to maintain order; Bordes shouting above the din. He was finally able to make his point. "The objective of the training of the midwives is to upgrade their skill level and with time, the traditionally untrained will give way to a new breed," he assured his colleagues, "but we have to go from one step to another . . . progressively." The midwives are part of the community and supported by the people, he emphasized, and in the future the people will ask for an improved level. "The traditional midwife as we know her now will disappear," a comment generating some peaceful silence. It was short-lived.

Next came family planning under fire . . . all the reasons it wouldn't work. But it had, again, in the "triangle." Resistance comes from the very young and those with a lot of children, Bordes told the group. The best ages are twenty-five to thirty-five, he said. Work there.

This is the way it would be in the beginning, just as at the general hospital more than a decade earlier, and in the urban integration of services in the capital during the pilot phase of the national program. In time, opposition turned to indifference, and later to acceptance, and even some enthusiasm. It would take more time . . . this was just the beginning. But now it was all part of Haiti's health plan and this really made a big difference. The word had been spoken from high above; Bordes was just the unwelcome—to some—messenger.

In 1976 Haiti officially presented its eleven health administrators with the first national health plan for the country, an extraordinary development, the result of three drafts and five years of intermittent discussion. It was a unique approach for Haiti for a variety of reasons, not the least of these being a commitment to carry health coverage to the masses; an emphasis on preventive over curative medicine; the execution of programs according to precise priorities; and development of an infrastructure employing a system of decentralized organization. Among many other points it reflected across-the-board the basic policy positions of the division of family hygiene. The second top objective of the entire plan, after eradication of communicable diseases—provide maternal-child health and family planning.

The moment the plan was adopted as national policy and practice, the division's task then became to supervise and organize those activities countrywide, according to the norms and rules of the health department, guided by the plan. At least on paper family planning was to be carried out by directive of the government as a routine activity in all health institutions in Haiti, not something piggybacked upon existing services, demanding extra salary or foreign funding—but right in there with setting broken bones and pulling teeth.

While Ary Bordes did not participate in the final discussions of the plan, his thinking and work profoundly influenced the direction of Haiti's maternal-child health and family planning policy, according to many Haitians involved, and particularly rigorously stated by Sam Wishik. He calls the Haitian policy "a direct outgrowth of Ary's program in a number of respects": local services using local people as primary-care units; decentralization into the country's health districts; a variety of family planning choices offered every Haitian woman; family-planning always accompanied with education. Wishik says Bordes's contribution to the plan was enormous, not his doing alone, but he deserved a lot of credit for the accomplishment, a recognition received at home as well as abroad. While Bordes very purposefully maintained a low profile in Haiti, where notice was not so helpful, he got his due. The monthly reports that had been requested widely from the first years of the center's operations in Port-au-Prince had grown into a variety of invitations to present his experience to other public health specialists internationally, struggling with some of the same problems. Bordes was an expert on how to use limited resources to organize a maternal-child health and family planning program, what the day-to-day problems were and the priorities. He knew the personnel, training, salary, material, etc. hassles all too well at this point.

In 1970 Bordes attended a nutrition seminar in Lima; in 1971, a seminar on family planning in Quebec and Montreal; in 1972, meetings in Barbados, Guatemala, and Guadeloupe, on family planning and child health. They became even more frequent and prestigious. In 1973 Bordes participated in a seminar on sterilization in Geneva; a few months later, he was in Costa Rica for discussions on sexual education; that November, in Washington, D.C., for a conference on the integration of nutrition and family planning; back to Geneva again for a World Health Organization meeting of experts on research techniques for the integration of family planning into health services; then off to Rennes, France, to teach a course on maternal-child health and family planning, reaching many French-speaking African medical professionals as well as French nationals, a yearly trip and seminar originated by Wishik. As the years passed and his reputation grew he would represent Haiti at the second international conference on voluntary sterilization in Tunis . . . be a member of the Haitian delegation to the executive council of the World Health Organization meeting in Mexico City . . . invitations constantly arriving . . . Honduras . . . Brazil . . . Israel. . . . In addition there had been two United Nations requests to share his Haitian know-how with two African nations, with Mali in 1974 and the Central African Republic in 1976, missions to help them better organize their maternal-child health efforts, geared to their respective national realities. Also in 1976 the Unitarian Universalist Service Committee had sponsored a seminar bringing thirteen public health specialists from eight Caribbean countries to Port-au-Prince for more exchanges of opinions and approaches. They had discovered common strengths and a need to nurture growing Caribbean partnership and possibilities for mutually beneficial collaboration in the future. The largest country in the Caribbean, Haiti was French-speaking and did not always interface with its predominantly English-speaking neighbors.

While the division of family hygiene had been very occupied "passing on" the methodology to the cities of Haiti, the past few years had been a time of reflection at the private center of family hygiene, maybe even of recuperation. The frenetic activity stage was past. Next had come some sitting down and just plain thinking, a continuing examination of what had been done. Were they on the right track? What corrections could be made? Data on effectiveness had been collected; now to further study.

Madame Hollant almost despaired as she looked at the stacks of folktroop questionnaires in the files, waiting for the time to get tabulated and evaluated by computer. It was a good approach, but she had to have the facts to prove it to the division. Three months earlier the Nursing Association had written the center, telling them of their troop. They had gotten the idea from the student nurses who had trained at Croix-des-Bouquets and seen the original troop in action. Soon she would be off to Curaçao to give a paper on "Utilization of Folk Media in Education Programs on Maternal-Child Health and Family Planning" at a conference of Caribbean family-planning educators sponsored every two years by the International Planned Parenthood Federation. The organization also expressed a strong interest in duplicating many of the center's educational materials. For her part, Madame Hollant was thinking of leaving Haiti, maybe joining a large international organization, maybe in Brazil.

Driver Rivière had a new son and, almost as good, was about to get a new jeep.

Community agent Dieumaitre Jacques had done very well. He lived in Pingano now, the "wealthiest" neighborhood in Fond Parisien, in a solid rural Haitian middle-class house with four rooms. His house was full of glasses and cooking implements, a radio, and a lantern—a great many other acquisitions. His wife ran the only store in the neighborhood. He had farm animals, a horse, and a bicycle; two hectares of land in four parcels, which he rented out to four tenant farmers. He had the same enthusiasm for the program.

The same nurse and auxiliaries were still in the Fond Parisien clinic wrestling with the same problems with good humor and good human relations and a respite on weekends in Port-au-Prince. They were ready for a change. Whereas before they spoke of how much they had gained and learned by working with the people, now the people were taking from them. The balance had tipped; they wanted advancement. Bordes was considering using some of them as trainers, they were so experienced.

Madame Monpoint was conducting an unofficial "Kola-sip" on her Croix-des-Bouquets front porch for a crowd of third-year nursing students who had been coming to the center for training since 1974. Generally she was appalled to discover it was their very first field experience, as was the case with this group, watching her draw out a diagram of extending medical services with mobile clinics on the blackboard she had set up. She was supposed to be on vacation. "After you graduate, you have to get a big straw hat because if you are going to do community medicine, you have to do the work in the sun . . . in the field. You must always be in the field," she told them.

Agronomist Depestre was now director general of the department of agriculture, the third-top post, continuing to spread the word about the integrated approach that had proved so successful in the "triangle," talking it up in the highest levels of government, channeling it into the government machinery. Actually the idea of an interdisciplinary coordination of development had been talked about by a subcommittee, including Bordes, under the national planning agency for almost four years. But it never seemed to really move until Depestre had joined in. Six months earlier the meetings had begun to take place on a regular monthly basis and in January 1977, the directors general convened a seminar of all technicians in their respective disciplines to improve cooperation.

Dr. Eustache was at the University of Puerto Rico getting a master's degree in public health medicine, annoying his brother even more, apprehensive himself about what he would be doing come two or three years, worried about a structure to fit into. "There is nothing to work with, no facilities, no materials," he spoke of his concern during a vacation period home. "There is no real public health field, really, except for Dr. Bordes," he said. While he was in his country some of his patients from Thomazeau came to call, seeking medical care, since he was no longer with them.

Dr. Dessources was in a small hospital in Petit-Goave, despondent, basically. "My idealism is not yet dead," he said, sounding dead, his face full of unsmiling fatigue. There was an aura of defeat about him from his many battles and adversities which appeared to have overwhelmed his spirit, exhausted him, making him old before his time, his movements slow. He was thirty-two—"that is a great privilege to have made it this far in this country with this mortality rate," he said. He was a peasant in a white doctor's coat—passive, accepting, not fighting anymore; ready to move if an opportunity presented itself, but not very hopeful. He wanted a scholarship to study abroad and come back and serve the people, "but, sadly, this program is not available to everyone," he said.

Dr. Narcisse was assistant director of a spanking-new fully equipped Croix-des-Bouquets Center of Health and Training, courtesy of the U.S. Agency for International Development. Dedicated November 22, 1977, the one-story sprawl of clinics, administration offices, a pharmacy, laboratory, and conference room, also featured classrooms. Just the previous

THE HARVEST

month another difficult dream had come true, unrealized throughout the "triangle" years. In October the medical school for the first time had formally scheduled classes in community medicine as part of the official curriculum for all third-year medical students—two weeks, thirty hours at the general hospital, and now at the modern Croix-des-Bouquets center. The culmination of many years of persuasion by Bordes and a few others, now every doctor before he got his degree would be exposed to public-health medicine—of incalculable value to the future of Haitian health.

Radio star Madame Souvenir was busy with a ten-year study on the impact of the broadcasting program and had just finished up her survey work in Petionville with ten neighborhood workers. Plus, she was producing still another radio broadcast, twice weekly, called "Family Radio." In the same spirit as "Radio Doctor," it had begun in 1975, with tapes made in Port-au-Prince and sent to all the radio stations in the provinces.

Consultant Norine Jewell had her farewell party at the center in December of 1976. Bordes spoke his good-bye in Creole, symbolic of her tie to Haiti. If she had any flaw, it was what was good carried too far, he commented, looking down on the floor, off to the left, as he does when he is feeling shy or embarrassed. Informed earlier of her great wish, he kissed her lightly on both cheeks, what she had really wanted from Bordes all along—a little caring. Her stateroom would be crowded with well-wishers and Bordes uncorking champagne bottles as she made the boat trip home, rather than the abruptness of a flight; separating gradually from a people who had absorbed her for three years.

Gerry Murray was a full-fledged Ph.D.; Sue Klein a successful consultant; the Berggrens had gone back to Harvard; Sam Wishik had retired from Columbia: Hal Crow . . . Dick Steckle had moved on and up; Alice Sheridan was grieving the loss of her husband; Laraque still researching; Laroche still pushing for preventive medicine; Titus still practicing pediatrics; Fourcand still in the know. . . .

It was the same in "the village," with Tante and Antoinisse, although their tubercular baby had died, and Tante herself had been very close to death, the near victim of an itinerant "charlatan" who had administered an injection causing her to fall over unconscious and remain rigid for some time afterwards. Papa Joie was not feeling too well, either. He sat in his "office," where a human skull stuffed with rags was the clear focal point. His face muscles sagged with the twinkle nearly gone from his eyes. "Gaz . . . tension," he complained.

In Fond Parisien, where once there had been no modern medical care; once only thirty latrines; once no organized sanitation or drinking water; once only a third of all children in school; once one of the highest rates of malnutrition in the country; once a high birth rate; once no cooperative spirit; once 10 percent of all babies dying of umbilical tetanus. . . . Now there was the crowded clinic and paraprofessional staff and trained midwives and no umbilical tetanus. Child mortality had been reduced by half. Two-thirds of all children were in school. Communicable diseases were under control through immunization. There were 122 latrines. Malnutrition came from poverty from persistent drought, not lack of information on proper food habits. More than 800 families, over a third of the families of Fond Parisien, were active in the family planning program with knowledge of contraception 100 percent. Forty percent of the men in the agricultural cooperatives were involved in the family planning program. All the children knew the family planning song. And—the villagers of Fond Parisien, 560 volunteers, were on the march each day "to bring the water down" from the Lastic River with financial help to complete the project to come from the CARE foundation. As biblical-looking as ever, Lemé Jacques was a prime mover, befitting the founder of the original cooperative, now occupying a kind of elder-statesman status. The community organization built up since 1972 was self-sustaining, engaged in its most ambitious undertaking.

As Dieumaitre said: "Before the people had to go all the way around the village because of the gulley and right now there is a little bridge that the people built themselves. In 1965 the gulley under the bridge needed cleaning and now the people themselves do it. But then nobody would do the work. Before when the irrigation pumps ran out of gasoline, they would sit there and not be used and now there is never a time there is no gasoline. As soon as it runs out, they are there. Before there were five or six fights a week and now they are rare. In the old days if a hurricane came the people would probably lie back and die. Now they would run around and try to find whatever means they can to try and pull themselves together."

He concluded: "I think the people are beginning and will eventually understand that they can do just about anything if they are willing to do it themselves. But that it is all in their hands."

For his part, Bordes for the very first time was beginning to feel the understandable fatigue of holding down two full-time jobs plus "interests." He wanted more time for planning at the center and less day-to-day executive responsibility and was thinking of proposing assistants in the next funding request. In short, more and more time for organizing—his first love; less and less time for managing—the least acceptable part of the job. His wife, Lillian, would be pleased. While he did not bring his work home much, save for a particularly difficult problem or decision, his 8-to-7 workdays did not bring him home enough. In short, too much time for the work and not enough time for the wife. "I receive that critique, oooohhhh!"—he shook his lowered head—"that is my permanent critique. . . . I must say I have the desire to change, but it has not been implemented yet," he continued methodically, always the planner. He wanted to try for tighter organization, more delegation, more time for a more balanced life. He was fifty-three, and while his energy level was enough to wear out almost anybody alive, he had started to understand the fatigue he had caused others in the past with his many demands.

But there were all these things he wanted to do—Haiti needed a more defined population policy, he believed, particularly after his United Nations missions to Africa . . . there was his book on the history of Haitian medicine, now in its fifteenth year of preparation . . . more attention had to be paid to the potential of the traditional folk system for rural extension . . . maybe to people's pharmacies, where the government could purchase drugs in bulk and provide greater availability . . . then perhaps vending machines to provide contraceptives rather than rely on the medical establishment solely . . . all these ideas . . . dreams. . . .

A few weeks after his Cap Haitien trip Bordes sat at the desk of his private center, behind the nearly foot-high confusion of a mess of reports, correspondence from all over the world, books and medical journals in piles, all cleared away once a year, he claims. The walls were upholstered with Haitian art constantly squeezed by new additions. Bordes looked contentedly at home, relaxed and well, even better after he got a very excited telephone call from Dr. Laroche. A second floor was to be added to Bordes's original center at the general hospital, according to a decision that day by the health department and the medical school. It was to house a department of preventive and social medicine, finally, after seventeen years, and the downstairs to be used for on-the-job training. Bordes laughed with pleasure at the news, and as he replaced the telephone receiver in its cradle, he spoke with a softness of tone, a certain mellowness, reserved generally for the wise:

"These things take time and that's why I believe in the future all the time. Because I know that if you work hard, four, or five years, you can have it. . . . There are very few things in life you can have quickly. Of that I am certain. But once you know what you are doing is worthwhile and that you are moving in the right direction, you just have to try and make your efforts. Try and do all you can. And give it time. . . . I have learned respect for time. If you plan your action for instant success—then you had better quit."

APPENDIX

Fond Parisien Demographic Profile

	1966	1975
Population	4.220	4.700
Birth Rate	36.9 per thousand	24.9 per thousand
Death Rate	12.5 per thousand	11.2 per thousand
Population Growth Rate	2.4	1.4

Mortality Rates 1966-1975

	1966	1975
General Death Rate	12.5 per thousand	11.2 per thousand
Infant Mortality Rate IMR 1966-1970 = 95.3 per thou. IMR 1971-1975 = 81.9 per thou.	108.8 per thousand	86.2 per thousand

	1966-70	1970-75
Maternal Mortality Rate	3.1 per thousand	3.2 per thousand

Child Mortality as a Percentage of General Mortality	1966	1975
0-5 Years	54.6 per hundred	30.1 per hundred
0-11 Months	32. per hundred	18.8 per hundred
1-5 Years	22.6 per hundred	11.3 per hundred

Neo-Natal Mortality

1966 to 1970 (640 Live Births)	5% (32 infant deaths)
1971 to 1975 (610 Live Births)	1.97% (12 infant deaths)

Fond Parisien Total Number of Births Per Year

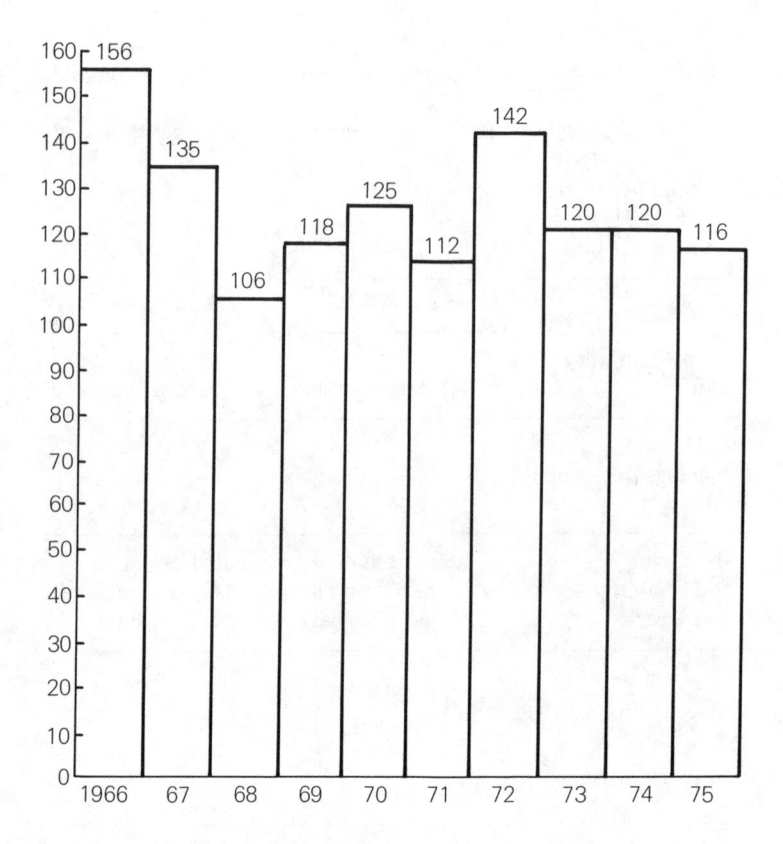

Year	Births
1966	156
67	135
68	106
69	118
70	125
71	112
72	142
73	120
74	120
75	116

Fond Parisien Cumulative Family Planning Acceptance by Year

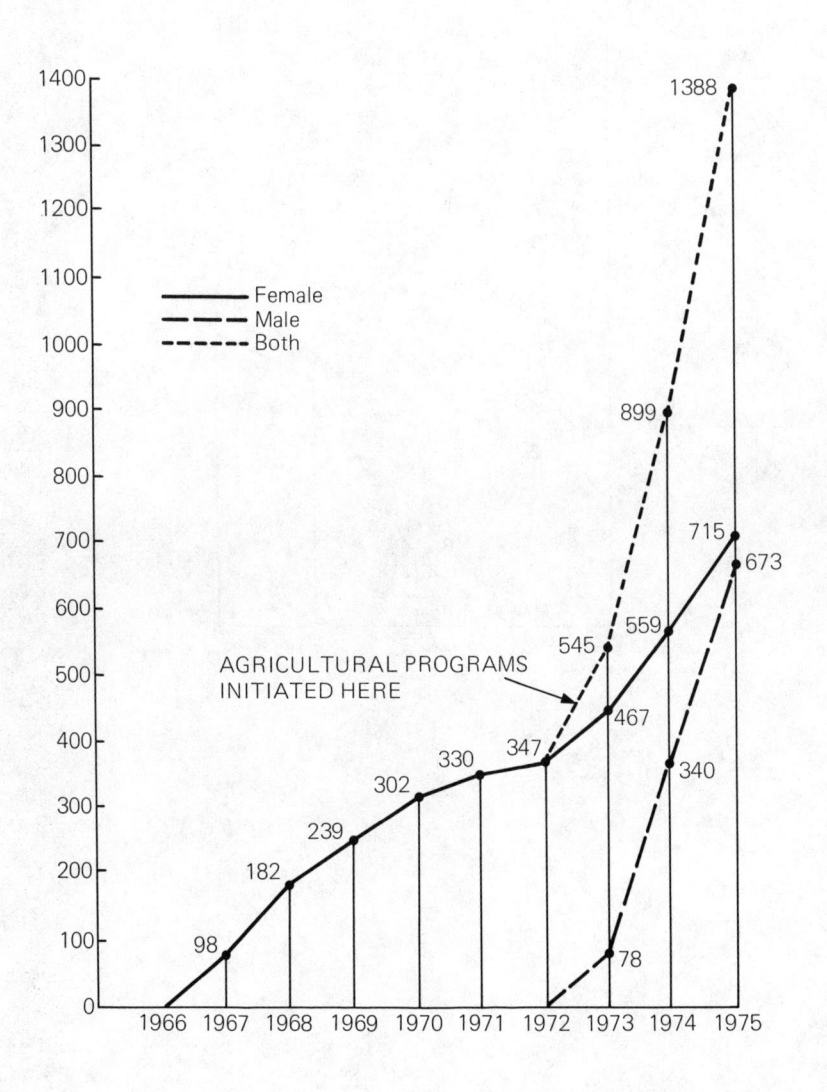

Family Planning in Cooperatives in Fond Parisien
(Percentage of Members Practicing Family Planning)

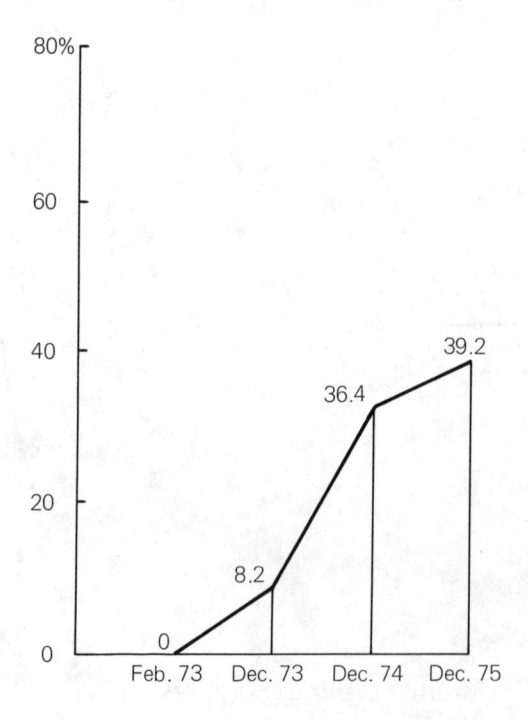

Economic Cooperative Loan Program (1972–75)

Names of Group	No. of Members	No. of Loans	Total Loans	Deposits	Total Profits	Individual Gains
Bois-de-Mieux	48	8	$6,490	$324.50	$1,298	$27.04
Pengano	39	5	2,700	135	540	13.84
Gaillard	28	5	1,650	82.50	330	11.78
Ganthier	24	6	2,800	140	427	17.79
Dagout	64	5	13,300	665	3,325	51.95
Riguad	39	4	7,700	380	1,900	48.71
Dieudon	35	4	5,100	255	1,275	36.42
Cabronet Cassé	32	4	2,500	125	1,000	31.25
Nan Plaisir	64	1	135	6.75	—	—
Association of Women of Bois-de-Mieux and Pengano	34	2	436	21.80	218	6.41
Total	407	44	$42,811	$2,136.55	$10,313	—

INDEX

Abortion: 118, 120
Absenteeism: 181-182
Absolutist rule: 25, 28
Adolphe, Max A.: 152, 162
Adventists: 222
Advertising, of health: 196, 250-251
Agriculture: 19-21, 26, 40, 184, 226-227, 238; crops, 2, 35, 91-92, 94-96, 179, 277
Albert Schweitzer Hospital: 114, 118, 121, 133-134, 162, 203
Alies, Philippe: 246-247, 248, 259, 260
Alvarez, Maria D.: 201
Ambroise, Ulrick A.: 72, 86
American Friends Service Committee (AFS): 123
American Revolution: 27
American Sanitary Mission: 115
Angrand, Mark: 278
Animals: 10-11, 32, 94
Architecture: 46
Ariste: 277
Armand, Maurice: 118, 123, 161
Art, Haitian: xiii-xiv, 86-87, 90, 251, 252
Artibonite River: 35
Artibonite Valley: 118, 184, 203, 276, 277
Association of Medical Students: 51
Audouin, Fritz: 128
Authoritarianism: 34

Auxiliary School of Nursing: 183
Azuey, Lake: 93, 151, 186

Bas Boen: 143-144
Batraville, Benoit: 29
Bauxite: 35
Bellanton, Théoma: 228, 231, 237
Berggren, Gretchen: 121-122, 125, 161, 203, 275-276, 284
Biassou, Jean-François: 24
Birth control pills: 80, 88; dropout rate, 145; preference of, 82, 109, 146, 149, 208; side effects, 81, 116, 118
Birth rate: 100-101
Bizoton: 28
Black Mountains: 276
Blaise, Marie Carmelle: 257
Bois-Caiman: 24
Bois-de-Mieux: 220-221, 224, 226-230, 233, 234
Bolívar, Simón: 27
Boncy, Paul: 161
Booklets: 136-141, 146-147, 247-249
Bordes, Ary: administrator, 74, 133-135, 146, 195; boyhood, 45-52; education, 52-55; nationalism, 22, 90-91, 167; objectives, 64, 241-242, 267; philosophy, 1-2, 31-32, 41, 67, 159, 192-194, 217; political practicality, 52, 67-68, 75-76, 113, 266

Borno, Raymond P.: 116
Boukman: 24
Boulos, Carlos: 123, 124, 162
Boyer, Jean Pierre: 26, 27
Brandt family: 184
Bureaucracy: 126, 208
"By the Year 2,000": 140-141, 247, 249

Cabello, Octavio: 149
Cacos War: 29
Cahos Mountains: 277
Calabash booklets: 136-137
Camus, Albert: v
Cancer: 116, 118
Candio: 262
Cap Haitien: 45, 89, 255, 267, 268, 276, 277-278
CARE: 123, 284
Catholic Church: see Roman Catholic Church
Cayes: 255, 267
Center for Maternal-Child Health: 59, 62
Central School of Agriculture: 29
Cham, Revalin: 242-243, 250
Charcoal production: 92, 184
Charles V, King: 23
Charles X, King: 27
Chatard: 277
"Childbearing, Sickness and Healing in a Haitian Village": 201
Children: 4, 9, 11
Children's Bureau: 149, 150, 165
China: 119
Christophe, Henri: 25, 26, 27, 30
Church World Service: 123, 127, 232
City Rurale: 98, 186
Clothing: 5, 7, 8
Coffee: 45, 46
Collectivism: 30
Colombia: 27
Columbus, Christopher: 23, 34
Comacho, Ruth: 127, 128
Communications: 40
Condom: 145, 240
Congress of Panama: 27
Continuity of care, concept: 106-107, 213
Contraception: 70, 80, 114, 161; see also Birth control pills; Condom; Family planning; IUD

Cooperatives: 219-234, 239-240; in Bois-de-Mieux, 219-221, 233
Creole: see Language
Croix-des-Bouquets: 172, 185; clinic, 151, 172-176, 180-182, 187, 190, 200, 204, 212, 215, 267, 275, 281-282; diseases, 181, 187, 190; family planning, 197-198, 242-243; location, 89, 151, 178-179; midwives, 253-255; pharmacy, 215-216; propaganda, 250-251; radio education, 89, 184, 187; sanitation, 183; sales project, 236-238; school, 247; social structure, 179-180; water, 214, 247
Crops: see Agriculture
Crow, Harold: 174-176, 212-213, 243, 251, 252, 255, 260-261, 283
Cuba: 30
Cul-de-Sac Plain: 2, 144, 151, 168, 169, 171, 236, 244, 249

Damballah: 19
Damien: 223
Dartiguenave, André: 261-264
Data, importance of: 100, 106, 124, 196-197
Daumac, Lucien: 59
Death: 12, 100; see also Infant mortality
Death rate: 101, 107
Deforestation: 92-93, 96
Dehydration: 18
Department of Agriculture and Natural Resources and Rural Development: 188
Department of Public Health and Population: 165, 188
Depestre, Marcel: 221-239, 246, 282
Derosena, Raymond: 275
Dessalines, Jean-Jacques: 25, 27, 277
Dessources, Phyat: 200, 208-211, 282
Development: 176, 213
Diarrhea: 37-38, 63, 69, 101, 181, 195
Dieudonne, Mme E. Antoine: 253

Index

Dieumaitre: see Jacques, Dieumaitre
Diphtheria: 190
Discipline: 4
Division of Family Hygiene: 165
Dominican Republic: 29, 92, 95-96, 100, 104, 169
Dresse, Francois: 128
Drexler, Anthony: 171, 187
Drought: 95, 184, 232
Duffaut, Préfète: 251, 252
Duvalier, Francois: 30, 43, 57, 114, 117, 118, 128, 160, 163, 174, 180
Duvalier, Jean Claude: 30, 39, 161, 163, 164, 177

Education: flexibility in, 34; level of, 30, 31, 70; of midwives, 103, 107-108, 133, 142, 253-255, 278; nutritional, 44, 78-80
"The Effectiveness of an Oral Contraceptive": 115
Elites: 26, 28, 33, 36, 46, 50, 208
Equipment: 193, 206-207, 209, 211
Estimé, Dumarsais: 30, 51, 93
Eustache, André: 205-208, 211, 216, 273, 282
Evangelicalism: 87-88, 206, 222
Exorcism: 13, 37

Family Hygiene Center: 135
Family life: 3, 9
Family Planning International Assistance (FPIA): 171, 173-174, 176-177, 213-214
Family planning program: 65, 69; approach, 72, 73, 82-83, 113-114, 145, 242, 248; Croix-des-Bouquets, 197-198; Fond Parisien, 108-109, 137-140, 199, 239-240; national, 124-129, 141-150, 160-165, 189; negativism, 137; radio broadcasts, 120, 122; religion and, 84, 118, 120-121; success, 76, 80, 118, 175, 278-279; Thomazeau, 208
"Family Radio": 283
Farming techniques: 226-227
Faucher, Lauvinski: 152
Faustin: xiii, xiv

Films: 85, 255-261, 264
Fishing: 110, 150-151, 184
Folk medicine: see Voodoo
Fond Parisien: 135, 151, 175; climate, 92-96, 107, 284; commerce, 92-94; cooperatives, 219-225, 232-239; development efforts, 92-112, 209-211, 221-222, 238-239; disease, 99, 100, 107-108, 187; Dominican border, 95-96, 104; family planning, 108-109, 145-146, 148, 188, 199, 249, 284; fishing, 110; irrigation, 92-96, 232-233, 238; language, 137; literacy, 111-112, 137, 140, 251; midwives, 103, 107-108, 187; nutrition, 97, 109-111, 284; pharmacy, 215-216; road to, 44, 175, 186, 199; schools, 140; village elite, 208-209; voodoo, 99-103, 202, 209-210, 243; water, 214, 236
Food: 8, 36, 69
Ford Foundation: 123, 170, 172, 173
Fort Dimanche: 164
Fougère, William: 96-97
Foundation for International Child Health of New York: 43, 65-66
Fourcand, Jacques P.: 117-119, 275, 283
France: 23-24, 26, 28
Funari, John: 172

Gaillart: 224, 233, 237
Galette Chambons: 210
Ganthier: 111, 143-144, 145, 186
General Services Foundation of St. Paul: 188
Germany: 28
Gold: 23
Gonaïves: 45, 276-277
Gran Colombia: 27
Grand Bois: 207
Grand Rivière du Nord: 52-53
Guadeloupe: 25, 46
Guiana: 30

Haiti: absenteeism, 181-182; agriculture, 19-21, 40; boundaries, 33; climate, 5, 91; com-

munications, 40; economy, 26–29, 39–40, 42, 207; education, 18, 30, 34; government, 25, 27, 28, 30, 57, 116–117, 126–129, 152, 159–165, 177, 188, 207; health, 36–38, 44; historical background, 22–30, 34, independence, 27, 90, 268; international relations, 22, 26–27, 29; imports, 35; mores, 2–17; natural resources, 35; population, 35–36, 119; social structure, 33; topography, 2, 34–35, 45, 91, 207, 277; trade, 23; underdevelopment, 31–32, 167; U.S. aid to, 28, 30, 65; U.S. occupation of, 27, 28–29, 50–51
Haitian American Community Help Organization (HACHO): 123, 124
Haitian-American Sugar Company (HASCO): 93, 184, 262
Haitian Dark Ages: 27
Haitian Institute for Social Welfare and Research: 117
Haiti Project 4900: 272, 273
Hall, Lee: 175
Haut de Turgeau: 269
"Health Class": 147, 190, 246, 247, 248, 274
Health, Culture and Community (Paul): 60–61
"Health Is Wealth": 258–259, 264
Hepatitis: 13–14
Hollant, Edith: 86–87, 136–141, 147, 151, 160, 163, 190–191, 201, 215, 243, 247–251, 255–261, 277, 281
Homer: 2
Home visits: 243
"Houngan macoute": 18–19, 99, 101, 103, 201, 209–210, 243
Housing: 8, 9, 36, 46, 49, 180
Human resources: 31, 90
"The Human Tide": 251–252
Hurricanes: 96, 284; Flora, 94; Hazel, 57, 94; Inez, 87, 94, 107
Hygiene: 12, 37
Hysterical paralysis: 17

Illiteracy: 5, 34, 85, 111–112, 187, 249; visual, 137, 250

Immunization program: 65, 77, 108, 135, 186, 198, 201, 212
India: 119
"Infant Malnutrition: Cultural Factors": 44–45
Infant mortality: 17, 37, 60, 99, 101, 108
Infants: 9, 12
Institute for the Study of Human Reproduction: 171
Insurance system: 58
Interamerican Institute of Children: 42
"An Interdisciplinary Laboratory for Community Medecine and Family Planning": 204–205
International Planned Parenthood Federation (IPPF): 117–118, 123, 125, 173, 281
Intestinal parasites: 38, 62, 207
Irrigation: 92–97, 150, 218
IUD: 114–115, 118; complaints, 82, 144; demystifying, 73; extractions, 144–145, 199; insertion abuses, 161–162; preference for, 109, 119, 146, 149, 175, 208

Jacmel: 45–46, 87, 221, 251, 274
Jacques, Dieumaitre: 95–99; 101–105, 108–109, 112, 138–140, 144–145, 148, 186, 204, 210, 215, 223, 238, 242–243, 244, 246, 281, 284
Jacques, Lemé: 219–221, 224–225, 228–232, 237, 240, 284
Jacques, Louis: 62
Jamaica: 30
Jérémie: 45
Jewell, Norine C.: 245, 273, 283
John, Sister: 57, 97, 104
Johnson, Lyndon: 105, 188
Joseph, Aurele: 126, 128
Julien, Marie José Moreau: 211
Juste, Louis: 242, 244
Justin, Vierginie: 211

Kennedy, John F.: 30, 44
Klein, Sue: 121, 123, 145–146, 163, 169, 171, 187, 270, 283
"Kola-Sips": 142, 281
Kwashiorkor: 12, 69, 194, 196

La Gonave, Gulf of: 33

Index

Lamothe: 262
La Navidad: 23
Language: 11, 26, 33-34, 87, 137, 139
Laraque, Felix H.: 115-120, 125-126, 149, 159, 162, 163, 165, 275, 283
Laroche, Victor: 61, 209, 283, 285
Lastic River: 92, 93, 232, 234-235, 238, 284
Leandre, Michael: 216
Legros, Gerard: 68, 73
Le Nouvelliste: 122
Leonidas, Jean-Robert: 195-196, 202
Leopard Corps: 30
Lescot, Elie: 29, 30
Levine, Samuel: 43, 44, 45, 63-66, 91, 130
Loans: 226-227, 232, 236
Louisaux, Rosemarie Pierre: 211

Magloire, Paul: 30
Malaria: 38, 43
Malnutrition: 43, 44, 181; causes, 36, 69, 108, 111, 284; folk theory, 195; statistics, 36, 60, 97, 101; symptoms, 4, 5, 7, 12, 73
Marasmus: 12, 17, 69, 73, 196
Martinique: 25
"Maternal and Child Health in Haiti": 62
Maternal death: 60
Maternity Chancerelles: 149, 271
Maternity Isaie Jeanty clinic: 118, 123, 271
May, Cordelia Scaife: 130, 168, 173
Mellon, Andrew William: 130
Mellon family: 130-132, 152, 187, 188
Men: attitude towards family planning, 82, 84, 89, 145; daily life, 16, 18, 195
Mennonites: 218, 222
Mental health: 17, 91, 94-95, 187, 195
Midwives: certification, 273-274; training, 103, 107-108, 133, 142, 253-255, 278; voodoo ritual, 15-16

Midy, Evariste: 271
Miranda, Francisco de: 27
Mirebalais: 184
"Modern Time Is Different from the Old Time": 255, 259
Monpoint, Carmen: 81-82, 84-85, 139-142, 145, 160, 163, 216, 245-246, 252-253, 254-255, 262, 274, 281
Murray, Gerald F.: 200-204, 283

Napoleon: 24
Narcisse, Antonio: 180-181, 198, 211-212, 245-246, 251, 255, 261, 262, 264, 282
National Bank, 28, 29-30
National Council of Family Planning: 118
National Council on Development and Planning (CONADEP): 148
National Railway Company: 28
National Seminar on Haitian Nutrition: 42, 62, 65
News of Fond Parisien: 138, 150-151, 235
Nursing Association: 281
Nutrition program: 65, 69, 73, 77-78, 110

Oral contraception: *see* Birth control pills
Organization of American States (OAS): 42

Pan American Health Organization (PAHO): 71, 123, 127, 128-129, 150, 160, 162-163, 190, 270, 271, 272
Paratyphoid: 38
Parents: 4, 7
Pathfinder Fund: 119, 123, 136, 273
Paul, Benjamin: 60-61
Paul, Eugene: 247
Pediatrics: 76, 189
Pengano: 224
Peniciliin: 53
Péralte, Charlemagne: 29
Personal approach: 71-72
Peters, Father: 92
Pétion, Alexander: 25, 26
Petit Goave: 45
Pharmaceuticals: 206, 215-216

Physicians: ratio of, 38-39; rural residency, 178, 180, 192-194
"Pictorial Illiteracy in Rural Haiti": 136
Pierre-Noel, Lucien: 116
Pincus, Gregory: 116, 118
Pingano: 281
Polio: 169, 190
Polynice, Bonard: 215-216
Population Council: 119, 123, 173
Population Reference Bureau: 123
Portail de Leogane: 62
Portail St. Joseph: 17
Port-au-Prince: 33, 51, 179; family planning programs, 114-115, 141, 150; hospitals, 38, 39, 59, 62; population, 36; sanitation, 37; slums, 36, 70
Port-de-Paix: 45
Practical approach: 195
Pregnancy: 14, 62, 136
Prenatal care: 108
Preventive medecine: 58, 68, 96, 120, 198, 279
Price-Mars, Jean: 52
Prindle, Richard: 150
Privacy: 9
Private practice: 58

Race: 24, 26-29
Radio broadcasts: 87-89, 112, 120, 122, 246, 283
"Radio Doctor": 89, 112, 138, 147, 184, 190, 246, 274, 283
Records: see Data, importance of
Red Cross of Haiti: 77, 85, 148, 187, 274
Reflections of a Doctor (Bordes): 122
Religion: 7, 33, 84, 197-198; see also Roman Catholic Church; Voodoo
Research Corporation: 65
Respiratory diseases: 60, 69, 73, 181
Rivière: 134-135, 140, 148, 259, 281
Roads: 40, 44, 178
Robert Sterling Clark Foundation: 188
Rockefeller Foundation: 170
Rodman, Selden: 270

Rolland, Gerard: 150
Roman Catholic Church: 33, 84, 102, 116, 118, 120-121, 208
Rural Code of 1826: 26
Rural extension program: 165, 268-269, 276-277; see also "Triangle" project

Saint Marc: 45, 276
St. Vincent's School for the Handicapped: 57, 97
Saldun de Rodriguez, Maria Luisa: 42, 65
Sam, Vilburn Guillaume: 28
San Domingo: 1, 23-24
Sangor, Margaret: 198
Sanitation: 37, 44, 181, 183, 185, 187, 214
School(s): 4, 11, 18, 179, 248
Service Committee: see Unitarian Universalist Service Committee
Sévère, Lovinsky: 88
Sewage system: 37
Sexual mores: 7, 9, 90, 203
Sheridan, Alice: 42-45, 62-65, 74-75, 91, 98, 111, 113-115, 128, 130, 214, 283
Shirer, William Lloyd: 127
Slaves: 1, 23-25, 27, 46, 91, 268
Slum life: 36, 70
Smith, John Palmer: 174-175
Smith, Sam: 65-66
Social structure: 26, 33-34, 46, 50
Souvenir, Monique: 71-75, 83, 88, 160, 246, 274, 283
Steckel, Richard A.: 130-132, 152, 168-173, 176, 283
Stine, Raphael: 256, 258
"Syllabus of the Haitain Family": 249

Tenant farming: 220
Tetanus: 16, 18, 60, 99, 107-108, 133, 138, 189, 190
Theard, Alix: 164-165, 270
Thomazeau: 151, 184, 204, 211, 214, 255; cooperatives, 236, 238; progress in, 207-208; provincialism, 185, 202, 248; statistics, 185-186, 194-197
Titus, Henec: 57, 59, 91, 161, 283
"Tonton macoutes": 30

Toussaint: 24, 25
Treaty of Ryswick: 23
"Triangle" project: economics, 219-234, 236, 239; family planning 212, 279; funding, 168, 172-180, 188, 214, 236, 237; goals, 151-152, 203; methodology, 204-205, 208, 215-216, 273, 274; planning, 163, 169-170, 175-178, 182, 186, 188-189; records, 196-197; staff, 198, 200, 206; statistics, 204; vaccination campaign, 190-191, 212
Trowbridge, John: 170, 172
Trujillo, Raphael Leonidas: 29
Tuberculosis: 18, 37, 38, 76-77, 190
Typhoid: 38, 77, 93

Umbilical tetanus: 37-38, 133, 135, 142, 181, 187
Underdevelopment: 31-32, 167-168
Unitarian Universalist Service Committee: 42, 64, 65-66, 68, 79, 111, 119, 130-131, 172, 188, 235, 237, 280
United Nations: 171, 172, 270
United Nations Children's Emergency Fund: 43
United Nations Development Program Officer: 270
United Nations Food and Agricultural Organization: 42-43
United Nations Population Fund Activities (UNFPA): 271, 272
U.S. Agency for International Development (AID): 123, 161, 171, 172-174, 176, 273, 282
U.S. State Department: 164
United States: aid to Haiti, 28, 30, 65, 173; materialism in, 90; occupation of Haiti, 27-29, 50-51; prejudice in, 54

Vaccination programs: 62, 77, 93, 96-97, 169, 183, 190-191
Veatch Committee of the North Shore Unitarian Society: 188
Vincent, Stenio: 29, 51
Violence: 10
Volunteers: 142
Voodoo: 6, 13, 18-19; medicine vs., 101-103; pregnancy and, 14, 70; preventive medecine with, 96, 201-203; and underdevelopment, 33-34, 37

Walker, Edwin S.: 87-88, 112, 120
Washington, George: 27
Water: 36-37, 181, 183, 185, 195, 214, 235-236, 247
West Indies Mission: 87
"When We Grow Up": 139-141, 247, 249
Whooping-cough: 190
Williams, Charles: 127, 128
Williams-Waterman Fund of New York: 43, 44, 65-66, 97, 122
Willison, Robert E.: 130-132, 168-170, 172, 173
Wishik, Samuel M.: 79-80, 89, 91, 106-107, 109, 111, 121, 126-132, 148, 149, 150, 152, 168-169, 171, 182, 201, 270, 271, 274, 279-280
Women: attitude towards program, 80, 83, 104-105; in cooperatives, 237; daily life, 6, 17; status, 75
Worcester Foundation: 119
World Church Service: 119, 149
World Health Organization (WHO): 43, 121-122, 127, 129, 148, 149, 151, 160, 272
World Population/Planned Parenthood: 123, 172

Yaque del Norte: 23
Yaws: 43
Yellow fever: 25